Traumatic Brain Injury

A Clinical Approach to Diagnosis and Treatment

A Clinical Workbook (Edition 2.0)

Published in the United States of America by Millennium Health Centers, Inc.
Traumatic Brain Injury: A Clinical Approach to Diagnosis and Treatment (Edition 2.0)

ISBN: 978-0-9904630-1-6

Mark L. Gordon M.D., FAAFP — Author

Jim Huth — Editor

Alisa Vidor — Editing Assistant

Jayne DeVries — Cover Design

Other Books by the Author

The Clinical Application of Interventional Endocrinology (2007)

The Clinical Application of Interventional Endocrinology: The Handbook (2013)

The Laboratory of Interventional Endocrinology (2016)

Hormones and the Brain (2016)

Special Thanks

It is greatly appreciated that Access Medical Laboratories provided Millennium Health Centers with a grant for the laboratory evaluation of 100 military veterans with mTBI (PTSD) sustained while on active duty. We salute Ryan El-Hosseiny, CEO of Access Medical Laboratories, and his family, for their kindness to our veterans.

Recently, University Compounding Pharmacy of San Diego California sponsored a $100,000.00 grant for our veteran patients to cover any prescriptions for compounded medications. Joe Grasela and John Grasela have been strong supporters of our Support-A-Veteran program and continue to provide the best in compounding medicines.

The Warrior Angels Foundation, a 501(C)(3), founded by SFC Andrew Marr (retired) is a beacon of hope for many veterans who have found that their handful of prescription medications failed to protect and promote a quality of life. Along with the Millennium-TBI Network hope is being restored.

The Final Inspection

The soldier stood and faced God,
Which must always come to pass.
He hoped his shoes were shining,
Just as brightly as his brass.

"Step forward now, you soldier.
How shall I deal with you?
Have you always turned the other cheek?
To My church, have you been true?"

The soldier squared his shoulders and said,
"No, Lord, I guess I ain't,
Because those of us who carry guns,
Can't always be a saint.

I've had to work most Sundays,
And at times my talk was tough.
And sometimes I've been violent,
Because the world is awfully rough.

But, I never took a penny,
That wasn't mine to keep,
Though I worked a lot of overtime,
When the bills just got too steep.

And I never passed a cry for help,
Though at times I shook with fear.
And sometimes, God forgive me,
I've wept unmanly tears.

I know I don't deserve a place,
Among the people here.
They never wanted me around,
Except to calm their fears.

If you've a place for me here, Lord,
It needn't be so grand.
I never expected or had too much,
But if you don't, I'll understand."

There was a silence all around the throne,
Where the saints had often trod.
As the soldier waited quietly,
For the judgment of his God.

"Step forward now, you soldier,
You've borne your burdens well.
Walk peacefully on Heaven's streets,
You've done your time in hell."

- Anonymous

Dedication

To Pvt. Charles H. Kuhl, of L Company, U.S. 26th Infantry Regiment, who reported to an aid station of C Company, 1st Medical Battalion, on August 2, 1943. At the time, Kuhl had been in the U.S. Army for eight months, and attached to the 1st Infantry Division since the 2nd of June 1943. He was diagnosed with "exhaustion," a diagnosis he had been given three times since the start of the campaign. Arriving at an aid station he was subsequently transported to the 15th Evacuation Hospital near Nicosia for further evaluation, being started on treatment with sodium amytal. Notes in his medical chart indicate that he was suffering from "psychoneurosis anxiety state, moderately severe — this soldier has been twice before in hospital within ten days. He can't take it at the front, evidently. He is repeatedly returned."

Patton arrived at that hospital on the same day, accompanied by a number of medical officers, as part of his tour of the U.S. II Corps troops. He spoke to some patients in the hospital, commending the wounded. He then approached Kuhl, who did not appear to be injured. Kuhl was sitting slouched on a stool midway through a tent ward filled with injured soldiers. When Patton asked Kuhl where he was hurt, Kuhl reportedly shrugged and replied that he was "nervous" rather than wounded, adding "I guess I can't take it." Patton "immediately flared up," slapped Kuhl across the chin with his gloves, then grabbed him by the collar and dragged him to the tent entrance. He shoved him out of the tent with a kick to his backside. Yelling "Don't admit this son-of-a-bitch," Patton demanded that Kuhl immediately be sent back to the front, adding, "You hear me, you gutless bastard? You're going back to the front."

Corpsmen picked up Kuhl and brought him to a ward tent, where it was discovered he had a temperature of 102.2 °F (39.0 °C). He was later diagnosed with malarial parasites. Speaking later of the incident, Kuhl said, "At the time it happened, [Patton] was pretty well worn out. I think he was suffering a little battle fatigue (1) himself." Kuhl wrote his parents about the incident, but asked them to "just forget about it." That night, Patton recorded the incident in his diary: "[I met] the only errant coward I have ever seen in this Army. Companies should deal with such men, and if they shirk their duty, they should be tried for cowardice and shot."

I also dedicate this book to all the patients of the Millennium Health Centers.

I am who I am because of all of you who have challenged me to find an alternative approach to wellness in light of your suffering and loss of hope. And all of you who trusted the literature that I read finding answers that had already been discovered and ignored for years before dusting off layers of cobwebs. Not always an issue of selecting the right pill, but more so, in listening to what you had to say. Not about treating laboratory numbers, but accepting that we are not all made equally.

Pushing the envelope on interpretation of standard labs in a non-standard manner and treating to replenish the chemicals, hormones, and minerals that are found to be less than optimal, and redefining the use of the terms — deficiency and insufficiency — with possibly more apropos terms of healthy and non-healthy. For all these reasons and more, I dedicate this book to you.

— Mark L. Gordon M.D., FAAFP

About Dr. Mark L. Gordon

Upon completing his residency training (after graduating first in his class and receiving highest honors) and then receiving his board certification in Family Medicine in 1984, Dr. Mark L. Gordon advanced his medical education through Clinical Orthopedics (1990), Cosmetic Dermatology (1993), Sports Medicine (1995) and, in 1997, Interventional Endocrinology (a term he coined to best describe his approach to age-management medicine). In 2005, Dr. Gordon also obtained his exempt pharmacist license from the State of California.

Always a strong advocate for Integrative Medicine, and the promotion of preventive medicine through the correction of underlying hormonal deficiencies, he was instrumental in promoting the recognition of traumatic brain injury as a cause of hormonal deficiency in the hallmarked presentation on ESPN's Outside the Lines (January 2007). Dr. Gordon's book, The Clinical Application of Interventional Medicine (2008), continues to be recognized by his peers as the definitive primer for the standards of care and assessment in Interventional Endocrinology (age-management medicine). His academic standards and medical knowledge have been recognized by UCLA and USC, where he holds the position as Voluntary Associate Clinical Professor at the Keck School of Medicine (1998-date). As Medical Director of CBS Studios (2001-date), he has participated on projects with HBO, ESPN, CNN, FOX, Good Morning America, and a number of international programs.

In January 2014, Dr. Gordon was on the Joe Rogan Experience **(#438)** where the discussion on traumatic brain injury and hormonal dysfunction generated national and international interest. A second Joe Rogan program in November 2014 **(#574)** with Dr. Gordon also included Jason Hall, the screenwriter for American Sniper, and ex-petty officer and Navy Seal Corpsman Matthew Gosney, who spoke at length about his blast trauma, gunshot wounds, surgery, depression and 16 different medications that did nothing to prevent his attempted suicide in January 2014. Gosney shared his experience of being evaluated by Dr. Gordon, and of starting a hormonal replenishment protocol that led to him being able to discontinue 14 of his medications within six weeks, as well as the resolution of his deep depression. In February 2015, Dr. Gordon appeared on the Dr. Drew program, along with ex-Navy Corpsman Jordan Cordova, to discuss their experiences with military traumas, hormonal deficiencies, and recovery from anxiety and depression on a hormonal protocol. Dr. Gordon continues to work with veterans groups, providing full and partial funding for those with injuries received while in the theater of war.

In February of 2015, Dr. Gordon and SFC James Andrew Marr (retired), founder and CEO of Warrior Angels Foundation (WAF), joined together to provide funding, comprehensive biochemical evaluation and treatment for Veterans suffering from the signs and symptoms of trauma, either brain or stress related. In September 2015 (**#700**) another presence on the Joe Rogan Experienced allowed for Andrew Marr to share his experience before and after starting his Millennium Protocol. Additionally, Andrew Marr explained the goal of his federally accepted non-profit organization and what it means to veteran suffering from TBI or PTSD.

Table of Contents

Disclaimer

This book is a compilation of over 5000 published peer-reviewed articles that were used to develop clinical parameters for patients electing to have a neuroendocrinological work-up and hormonal treatment. Results of over 1000 patients have been cited in a number of anecdotal cases (according to medical dogma). We see it a little differently in that the results do speak for themselves. Nonetheless, this book is for educational purposes only and does not profess to provide diagnoses or treatment for your patients. These are the findings and results from our patients at the Millennium Health Group under the auspices of the Millennium-TBI Network.

Additionally, in the transformation of the originally produced digital version of this book, which had over 1600 embedded hyperlinks to abstracts, full articles, and educational institutes, they were removed. It is our intention, in the future, to have a document with these references provided to you.

Foreword

Muhammad Ali defeated more champions and top contenders than any heavyweight boxing champion in history. Although his prime was a little before my time, I always enjoy watching the old footage of him "float like a butterfly, sting like a bee." The black and white films of Ali being interviewed in his 20s showed him speaking gracefully and eloquently. He was never at a loss for words, often referring to himself as "the greatest." Unfortunately, he is also the most notable and greatest athlete that comes to my mind when I think of traumatic brain injury.

After 22 years of professional boxing, at 42 years of age, Ali was diagnosed with Parkinson's disease. It saddens me to know that one of the most extraordinary athletes of all time was transformed into a very old man as a direct result of receiving multiple head blows. Yet, outside of sports stars, traumatic brain injury (TBI) is more common than we tend to think. Apparently, a brain injury occurs every seven minutes and results in death every five minutes.

Being a triathlete, I have had my share of accidents. One of the several cycling accidents I have been involved with occurred when I was riding with a group of cyclists. We were going down a road very fast when the lead cyclist hit a pothole, and suddenly there was a major crash with ten of the cyclists. I was fortunate enough that I flew into the ditch on the other side of the road, and even more fortunate there was not a car coming down the road. In another close call, I was snowboarding when the edge of my snowboard hit a patch of ice. Immediately, my snowboard and I went out of control, up in the air, and then I slammed my head hard on that sheet of ice. I can still remember thinking, as I was flying through the air, that I was going to lose consciousness and suffer from head trauma. Luckily, that helmet saved me from certain head injury. Lying there, I was thanking God that I wore my helmet that day.

Being an Endocrinologist and having done a fellowship in critical medicine at one of the country's top medical centers, University of Pittsburgh, I was involved with resuscitating the many unfortunate trauma victims — usually from motor vehicle accidents. Most of the outcomes were poor in terms of regaining their state of independence, as brain damage with neurological deficits usually resulted. During my fellowship in critical care medicine, I was exposed to NIH clinical trials in that I made the rounds on TBI patients who were on trial drugs, and so I would read the numerous NIH studies to see if a special anti-cytokine or some medication could reduce inflammation of the brain after TBI. Sadly, none of those studies showed any significant improvements.

Those memories of TBI have stayed with me. Now, years later, my latest children's book, *Your Awesome Brain*, addresses the dangers of head injuries, while demonstrating to children and adults what happens to their fragile brain over time, and guiding children on the "secrets" to always having a healthy brain. Based on the belief that it's easier to build up a child than repair an adult, my passion is to educate our youth so that there may come a time when TBI is rare, or at least not causing a death every five minutes.

Until that day, we have the exciting, emerging science that Dr. Mark Gordon brings to us in this, his newest book. For example, the importance of balancing hormones as being critical for helping the brain to recover from TBI. Progesterone is a simple and inexpensive hormone that has been used in many clinical trials on TBI, and has been shown to be very promising — especially when compared to the very expensive new drugs. Progesterone receptors, which are in the brain, are no longer thought of primarily in terms to help women become pregnant. I prescribe bioidentical progesterone in my patients to help prevent Alzheimer's disease. It has also been shown that estrogen, progesterone and testosterone can be neuroprotective.

The current test of recalling three previously stated words is of little use — unless someone has experienced severe brain injury. TBI does not have to be from an explosive injury, from playing professional football, or from years of boxing. I have seen many cases of subtle TBI from playing high school football, falling from ladders, falling from a horse (without wearing a helmet), crashing in motocross or being involved in motor vehicle accidents. This is why the correct testing needs to done for TBI, and Dr. Gordon addresses this topic exceedingly well — far better than anyone else has even attempted.

Additionally, another of Dr. Gordon's areas of expertise has to do with growth hormone, and the science of secretagogues to release growth hormone. In fact, he knows the literature on the hypothalamic pituitary liver pathway of growth hormone better than most clinical endocrinologists. His passion and expertise in traumatic brain injury are unprecedented. When I first met Dr. Gordon in 2010, he was reciting to me the latest research articles about TBI. And since then, at every national meeting where I meet with him, he is tirelessly lecturing about the latest on TBI. He is a true leader in this field and I am excited that his book will be shaping the future of care for TBI.

Together, we can make a difference in treating, and hopefully preventing, traumatic brain injury.

— **Edwin Lee, M.D., FACE**
Founder of the Institute for Hormonal Balance
Best-selling author
Assistant Professor of Internal Medicine at the University of Central Florida College of Medicine

Chapter 1: An Overview and Introduction

"Adapt or perish, now as ever, is nature's inexorable imperative."

— H.G. Wells

Let's Begin

Traumatic brain injury (TBI) is nothing new, having been developed in the rising of man and the socialization of war. In the time of Australopithecus, as depicted by Stanley Kubrick's 2001: A Space Odyssey, an early hominid learned how to use a bone as a tool, and then as a weapon to kill another hominid. Archeological records represented by skulls, and not friable papyrus, tell us the stories of traumatic brain injury before there were stories to tell.

It is unlikely that those unearthed skulls found with depression fractures of the frontal, temporal, or occipital bones were the result of a motor vehicle accident, an improvised explosive device, or a slip-and-fall — and all of which have now become the hallmark of our socio-economic evolution in the here and now.

In survey of countries that have weathered their own unique social growth over the past two hundred years, we have seen a significant rise in the occurrence of traumatic brain injury from a diversity of causes. In those individuals less than 20 years of age, motor vehicle accidents (mainly DUI related) make up the majority of cases, while those over 65 succumb to overmedication, Frailty Syndrome, and vitamin D deficiency — which all cause gait instability and falls, the second most common cause for TBI.

The landscape between 20 and 65 years of age is filled with assaults, slip-and-falls, sports injuries, motor vehicle accidents, blast trauma, occupational, and recreational injuries as causative factors.

Although not perceived literally as a trauma, strokes (hemorrhagic and ischemic), hypoxia, severe hypoglycemia, ionizing radiation, and prolonged surgical procedures can lead to the same pathophysiological pathways and changes in cognition and personality as those produced by direct force trauma to the skull.

Alzheimer's disease (AD) is now being linked to the occurrence of traumatic brain injury. The hallmark of AD has been the accumulation of Amyloid-β and the disruption of microtubules with tau protein disruption which is also being found in TBI. (1) The same critical processes that lead to the loss of executive function and cognitive abilities are the same chemical pathways in both conditions. (2) A 1999, report by the American Journal of Epidemiology acknowledged that those with TBI developed Alzheimer's at the same rate as those with a history of TBI, but developed it much sooner than statistically anticipated and at an earlier age. (3) Adding to this was a study commissioned by the NFL reported that Alzheimer's disease or similar memory related diseases(dementia) appear to have been diagnosed in the league's former players infinitely more often than in the national population — and at 19 times the normal rate for men ages 30 through 49. (4)

The core of this book, chapter by chapter, is about the overwhelming number of individuals who have sustained a mild traumatic brain injury (mTBI) and don't even know that it has occurred. They are the ones who develop progressive cognitive, neurobehavioral, and psychosocial changes that appear as behavioral issues that can manifest even after a delay of 30 years. (5) These are the individuals that have forgotten the injury, and therefore instead of looking beyond the superficial presentation of their apparent "illness", are placed on psychotropic medications to mask the underlying cause referred to as the "Stealth Syndrome." (6)

This book and the associated three-day TBI Symposium will provide the fundamental knowledge to assist healthcare workers in how to recognize the parameters associated with TBI-related hormonal dysfunction and how to diagnose and treat the individual. Chapter by chapter, you will find an abundant amount of information that cross-relates and was difficult to avoid redundancy at times. Therefore, I will apologize in advance for these redundancies which, if they were not present, would otherwise lead to a list of once stated facts whose salient points would be lost.

Epidemiology of Non-Combatant Traumatic Brain Injury

TBI is a major cause of traumatic death and disability. In individuals younger than 45 years of age, injury is the primary cause of death in the

United States and other developing nations. (7) The general incidence of TBI in developed countries is approximately 200 per 100,000 population at risk. This estimate is skewed since the statistics are based upon those patients with TBI that are hospitalized while the majority of those sustaining a TBI never seek medical attention. (8)

Based upon a 2010 report looking at only the United States, a brain injury occurs every seven seconds and results in death every five minutes, representing about 4.5 million brain injuries and 53,000 deaths a year. (9) A prior CDC evaluation of TBI cases between 2002 and 2006 reported 1.7 million cases per year with 80.7 percent emergency room visits, 16.3 percent hospitalizations, and 3.0 percent deaths. (10) But again, this only took into account those individuals who ended up in the medical system immediately after sustaining their TBI while the majority were lost or delayed from inclusion.

Contrary to general belief, the majority of TBI cases are mild in nature and therefore, the bulk of the injured never seek medical attention, that is, until the subtle neuropsychological changes start occurring, forcing medical assessment. By that time, the association between the mild TBI (mTBI) and symptomatology is lost. Unfortunately, this creates erroneous data by underestimating the frequency of mild forms of TBI and overestimating the proportion of moderate to severe TBIs.

Approximately 50 percent of TBIs are the result of motor vehicle, bicycle or pedestrian–vehicle accidents. Falls are the second-commonest cause of TBI (20 to 30 percent of all TBI), being more frequent among the elderly and the very young population. Violence-related incidents account for approximately 20 percent of TBI, almost equally divided into firearm and non-firearm assaults. (11)

Several classification scales are used to rate TBI severity with the post-resuscitation Glasgow Coma Scale (GCS) being the most widely used. The GCS is based on the patient's response (eye opening, verbal and motor function) to various stimuli. Fifteen is normal with a score of 13–15 considered mild, nine to twelve moderate and ≤8 severe TBI. (12) Clinical severity of TBI is also defined by duration of loss of consciousness (LOC), loss of memory for events immediately before or after the accident (post-traumatic amnesia) and identified intracranial lesion. (13, 14) Radiological findings by computed tomography (CT) may be helpful in TBI severity evaluation, and the most used radiological scale is the Marshall's CT classification of TBI. (15) Functional outcome after TBI is usually evaluated by the Glasgow Outcome Scale (GOS), a descriptive and easy to use scale, describing five outcome categories (death, vegetative, severely disabled, moderately disabled, and good recovery). (16)

Given all these excellent resources to assess those with TBI, it still does not equate out to effective care when you consider that almost 66 percent of those who need help fail to make it into the medical system. Those that do, the system fails them in limiting diagnoses and treatment to antiquated superficial markers of injury instead of looking deeper into the new science of traumatic brain injury. But, it's here now.

Epidemiology of Combatant Traumatic Brain Injury

Traumatic brain injury (TBI) has been described as the "signature wound" of the conflicts in Iraq and Afghanistan. Improvised explosive devises (IED), mortars, tank cannons, hand grenades, and even repetitive fire from an M-16 or M-4 Carbine, can produce the mechanical factors predisposing a soldier to mTBI. This micro-impact trauma of repetitive gun fire is a frequently omitted cause of TBI.

Of the total 178,876 TBI cases since 2000, 137,328 have been mild, 30,893 have been moderate, 1,891 have been severe, 3,175 have been penetrating, and 5,589 have not been classifiable, but all are suffering the sequela of brain trauma with psychological, physiological, and physical impairment. (17) The majority of these soldiers are without loss of consciousness or overt physical trauma and are now classified as Post-Traumatic Stress Disorder (18) experiencing symptomatology that parallels that of mild TBI.

On March 4, 2009, a USA TODAY headline was *360,000 Veterans May Have Traumatic Brain Injury*. The story followed with, "Washington — Pentagon officials estimated for the first time Wednesday that up to 360,000 Iraq and Afghanistan veterans may have suffered brain injuries. Among them are 45,000 to 90,000 veterans whose symptoms persist and warrant specialized care." (19)

Chart 1.1: Annual PTSD diagnosed in all branches of the service from 2000 – 2013.

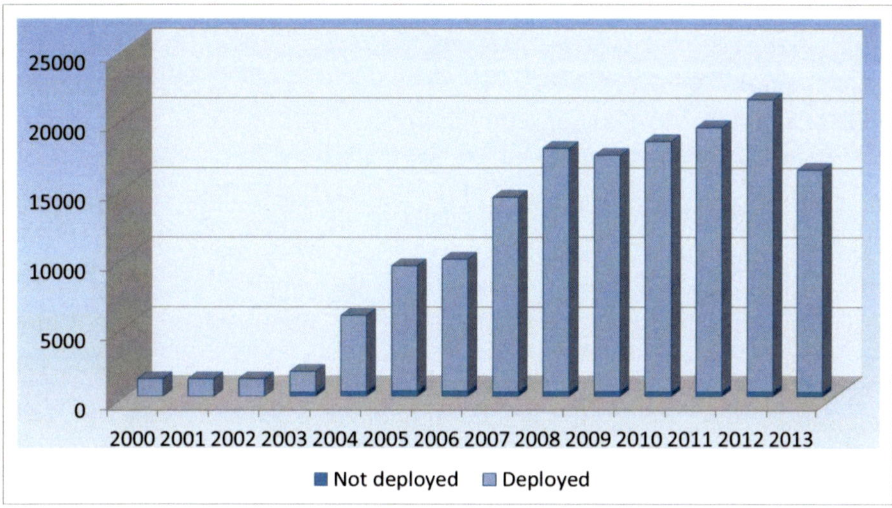

Blast injuries can cause brain damage with significant long-term and often delayed neurological consequences. Blast injury can be a complex clinical syndrome or "poly-trauma" caused by the primary blast wave where air filled structures such as the sinuses, ears, lungs, and intestines are most vulnerable leading to bleeding, alteration of ventilatory mechanisms with hypoxia, and tissue damage. The blast wave can cause a sudden rotation of the brain leading to shearing forces that can sever cerebral capillary and long axons responsible for intra-lobular communication (diffuse axonal injury).

Individuals exposed to a blast frequently manifest loss of memory for events before and after the explosion; confusion, headache, impaired sense of reality, and reduced decision-making ability. Patients with brain injuries acquired in explosions often develop sudden, unexpected brain swelling and cerebral vasospasm despite continuous monitoring. However, the first symptoms of blast-induced neurotrauma (BINT) may occur months or even years after the initial event, and are therefore categorized as secondary brain injuries. (20) The broad variety of symptoms includes weight loss, hormone imbalance, chronic fatigue, headache, and problems in memory, speech and balance. These changes are often debilitating, interfering with daily activities. Because BINT in blast victims is underestimated, valuable time is often lost for preventive therapy and/or timely rehabilitation. (21)

Consistent with the civilian population, laboratory assessment for hormonal disruption is infrequently performed over the course of the individual's rehabilitation for their physical trauma. An initial or baseline level is rarely obtained, thereby missing the 56 percent of those injured with TBI that do have one or more hormonal deficiencies by three months. (22) Failure to recognize and correct the underlying hormonal deficiencies (insufficiencies) may compound the physical and psychological complications of TBI and interfere with rehabilitation. (23)

The Military's available programs are comprehensive but limited. They might be seeing the literature and acknowledge that there is an association between mTBI and hormonal dysfunction, but they rarely pursue testing as recommended by the American Association of Clinical Endocrinologist and others. (24) Since 2009, the Millennium Health Centers, Inc. has offered a free laboratory assessment for military personnel that have sustained a mTBI with a Glasgow Coma Score of 13 to 15. (25) The free laboratory testing has been made possible through a privately funded grant from Access Medical Laboratories of Jupiter, Florida and the El-Hosseiny family.

Epidemiology of Sports-related Traumatic Brain Injury

Andre Waters was not the first, Dave Duerson was not the second, and nor will Junior Seau be the last to succumb to the secondary psychological consequences of hormonal deficiencies precipitated by traumatic brain injury that led to their depression and ultimate suicides. (26)

Their suffering and ultimate sacrifice has shaken the very fiber of the sports world, not only in football but in all contact sports, awakening us to the need for better protection, assessment, restrictions, and treatment for those who have sustained a TBI on and off the field. Presently, a player can be taken out of a game if their bench-side evaluation (after a suspected TBI) shows any sign of impaired brain functioning. Injured players will no longer have their jerseys just brushed off and be sent back into the game, they will be restricted from playing until their neurological evaluation has normalized.

Nonetheless, there will be many players, even decades after their last head injury, who will seek medical attention due to altered personality, bouts of anger and rage, and both cognitive and functional impairments. Hopefully, at that time, their medical care will include an initial history of trauma and a TBI hormonal assessment as opposed to being placed on a psychotropic medication first and ask questions later. Furthermore, if the athlete is found to be hormonally insufficient, and not necessarily deficient, they will be allowed to have replenishment to raise the levels to a more physiologic one as opposed to being denied a potentially life-saving treatment protocol. (27, 28, 29)

Both the physical and social impacts of sports related TBI have become a political bailiwick with congressional hearings and threats of banning football and all contact sports. Head injuries suffered by the likes of Patrice Bergeron, Pierre-Marc Bouchard and Marc Savard have raised awareness to new heights, so much so that the NHL instituted in the 2010 season, Rule 48, banning blindside hits to the head. This was seen as a way to reduce the public health risks and the consequential financial burden on insurance companies, families and the team leagues. (30)

Consequently, there are many NFL veterans who are still struggling post-career. A 1994 survey from the players' association found a significant numbers of retirees were depressed, fat and managing chronic pain. A 2006 Scripps Howard report found that of 3,850 deceased players, NFL players were more than twice as likely as Major League Baseball players to have died before their 50th birthday. Frequently, their much heavier bodies failed in retirement. (31)

What about our children? Football accounts for nearly two-thirds of the estimated 62,816 TBIs incurred in high school sports each year, according to a 1999 survey published in the Journal of American Medical Association. (32)

Traumatic brain injury (TBI) has been associated with hypopituitarism in general and GH deficiency (GHD) in particular; the consequences of this on growth and development are likely to be critical in children and adolescents in the so-called "transition phase". At three months, hypopituitarism was present in 34.6 percent, and at twelve months, hypopituitarism was present in 30.3 percent. Growth hormone deficiency (GHD) and secondary hypogonadism were the most common acquired pituitary deficits in this age group. These results show the high risk of TBI-induced hypopituitarism also in the transition age. Thus it is recommended that pediatric endocrinologists follow-up pituitary function of children and adolescents after brain injuries. (33) I think there is little else to say here, but more later.

Neuroendocrinology of TBI (Chapter 3)

Post-traumatic hypopituitarism (PTHP) was first recognized and described in 1918 by Cyran, but at that time it was thought to be a rare occurrence. (34) More recently, TBI has been recognized as a frequent cause of hypothalamic–pituitary dysfunction and impairment, contributing to a delayed or diminished capacity for recovery. (35, 36, 37, 38, 39)

PTHP following a traumatic event can be divided into an acute phase, during which there are transient alterations in the production of pituitary hormones such that they are either increased or diminished, and a delayed phase, when those alterations in hormones fail to return to normal regulatory production as a result of permanent damage at the pituitary and/or hypothalamic levels. (40)

The pituitary gland responds to acute trauma with two secretory patterns: adrenocorticotropin (ACTH), prolactin (PRL) and growth hormone (GH) levels increase, while luteinizing hormone (LH), follicle-stimulating hormone (FSH) and thyrotropin (TSH) levels may either decrease or remain unchanged, associated with an independent decrease in activity of their target organs. Changes in circulating hormone levels become apparent during the first hours or days following trauma, and may persist for the duration of the acute critical phase of injury. These alterations represent part of the acute adaptive response to the injury, and may be influenced by the type of injury and pharmacological therapy used in treatment during this early phase (glucocorticoids, narcotic analgesics or dopaminergic agents). (41)

Accepting the premise that trauma to the brain leads to a progressive disruption of hypothalamic control of hormonal production by both the anterior and posterior pituitary glands, would make it reasonable to test for the adequacy of production of those central hormones directly regulated by the hypothalamus. This would include anterior pituitary hormone markers such as thyroid stimulating hormone (TSH), growth hormone (GH), and adrenocorticotropic hormone (ACTH), and posterior pituitary markers such as anti-diuretic hormone (ADH) and vasopressin. (42)

In addition to those hormones, we need to look at IGF-1, IGFBP-3, fT3, fT4, rT3, free testosterone, total testosterone, dihydrotestosterone (DHT), DHEA-s, estradiol (E2), estrone (E1), progesterone, pregnenolone, and cortisol. These are used to establish the presence of a primary hormonal deficiency (peripheral failure) that could pre-date the impact of TBI. Additionally, all these hormones have beneficial effects on the central nervous system as either neurosteroids (NS) or neuroactive steroids (NAS). Therefore, identifying those that are deficient early in the course of injury allows for development of comprehensive treatment protocols. (43)

Our recent understanding of neurosteroids (NS) is mind boggling. These steroid hormones were once thought to pass into the brain through the blood-brain-barrier(BBB) having been produced in the periphery. Today, science shows us that these hormones are regionally manufactured de novo in the brain starting with cholesterol. Pregnenolone, progesterone, allopregnanolone, and DHEA, and their sulfonated active metabolites, are a few of the prominent neurosteroids. Each has important functions to protect nerves from oxidative stress (ROS), reduce inflammatory cytokines, reduce interleukins, promote neuroregeneration, and to regenerate myelin. (44, 45, 46) An interesting finding in the frontal lobes of patients with Alzheimer's disease is a significant deficiency of allopregnanolone (47, 48, 49, 50) which is also found in traumatic brain injury. (51)

So, the issue becomes when is the best time to assess the potential of neurotrauma related hormone dysfunction? The answer comes as no surprise in being as soon as possible after the head trauma. Unfortunately, as indicated above, most individuals with head trauma fail to seek medical attention until subtle or overt symptoms start to creep into their life, years later. The initial testing, if early, will represent the baseline hormonal levels with follow-up hormone panels at three months, six months, and twelve months from the date of the initial testing (injury). In a 2006 study by Schneider and Schneider, after followed new TBI cases for a period of one year, one or multiple hormone deficiencies were found at 56 percent and 36 percent, at six and twelve months, respectively. (52)

A more recent article in the Journal of Neurotrauma (2012) addressed the persistency of *Pituitary Hormone Deficiency after Traumatic Brain Injury*, acknowledging that 69 percent of the patients had at least one pituitary hormone deficiency, where GH deficiency was more prevalent (severe: 40.0 percent; partial: 23.6 percent) than corticotropin (27.3 percent) or thyrotropin (21.8 percent) deficiencies. (53)

Diagnosing the TBI Hormone Dysfunction Syndrome (THDS) can be challenging for the majority of clinicians, as well as for the trained endocrinologists. This is because of the new paradigm in what constitutes a laboratory result as being insufficient or low-normal as well as the controversial of whether-or-not to treat the insufficiency? Many of the hormone tests have reference ranges that are very broad, representing two standard deviations so that the numerical distance from the low-end to the high-end can be immense as in the case of Total Testosterone; 270 ng/ml to 1730 ng/ml. So, if a patient has a result of 280 ng/ml is that deficient, insufficient, or normal?

The majority, if not all, of traditional physicians would call that "within the normal range" and not address the myriad of associated complaints and elect not to treat. Fortunately, this is slowly changing and physicians are treating patients with appropriate physiological doses of replenishment hormones to achieve a level that is from the median of the range (50th percentile for age) to the 75th percentile.

Neuropathophysiology of TBI (Chapter 4)

The majority of mild traumatic brain injury (mTBI) cases, if not all, are of the non-penetrating type where the force of the trauma is conveyed to and through the skull (blunt force, blast waves, or ionizing radiation). Nonetheless, there are two phases of injury that occur to the brain: an initial mechanical injury (primary injury) associated with contusion, hemorrhage, edema, ischemia, and axonal shearing, and this is followed with a biochemical-inflammatory assault (secondary injury) associated with expanded neuronal loss resulting from the activation of one or more of the injury cascades — Necrosis, Apoptosis, Autophagy, and Parthanatos. (54, 55)

These events, mechanical and biochemical, can co-exist depending upon the magnitude of damage, but frequently in mTBI, the primary injury is short-lived while the subtle and insidious secondary injury can linger on for years taking its toll cell by cell. It is the impact of these biochemical processes that are most important for understanding the cause-and-effect relationship between TBI and hypothalamic-pituitary dysfunction (HPD) and the disruption of hormonal homeostasis.

The primary impact is frequently followed by the development of vasogenic and cytotoxic edema and impairment of energy metabolism (ATP and mitochondrial loss). This sets in motion a cascade of biochemical events both extra- and intracellular causing an indolent progression to cellular death. That is, indolent until there is impact upon a region of brain that regulates right and wrong and self-preservation.

Neurons that escaped the initial mechanical trauma (shearing) are exposed to a secondary mechanism that few cells can escape. At the immediate area of contusion and also remotely, neurons that succumbed to the initial trauma release an array of physiological cellular components into the intracellular space that accumulates to toxic levels; nitric oxide (NO), reactive oxygen species (ROS), glutamate, excitotoxicity, cytokines, and interleukins create an environment of collateral cellular damage as the oxidative stress (OS) increases. This is the non-neuropermissive environment (NPE) that like a pebble dropped in water leads to concentric rings of expanding cell death. Over time, the accruement of dead and dying brain cells leads to the signature changes that have come to represent not only mild traumatic brain injuries but all degrees of neurotrauma. (56)

Compounding the condition, capillaries that are torn leak red blood cells and plasma into the environment only to be degraded to a more reactive hemoglobin/iron (OS). As damage includes blood vessels there is the loss of the autoregulatory function of the cerebral vasculature with intravascular fluids leaking into the white and gray matter spaces causing edema. Owing to the edema, the intracranial pressure (ICP) increases and the brain is crushed against the unyielding cranium increasing the risk for uncal herniation, as well as further diminution of vascular blood flow, cerebral spinal fluid circulation, and death. The ensuing ischemia, hypoxia, hypoglycemia and further neuronal damage all cause acceleration of oxidative stress and expansion of the involved area. (57)

Although these processes have an overt appearance of a negative net affect upon the brain, in fact, we are learning that the ultimate goal of these neurochemical cascades is to help preserve and limit damage to the brain and its neurons. Think of it as a back fire in a blazing forest which is set to control the path and extent of the initial fire, but with a complexity that has been orchestrated into the following four types.

Necrosis may be the only process that does not stand out as a bad-good mechanism to help cells survive like Apoptosis and Autophagy. In necrosis, which has classically been regarded as uncontrolled cell death, recent research is now suggesting that its occurrence and progression might be tightly controlled. This is based upon finding signs of organized processes like mitochondrial dysfunction, ATP depletion, increased ROS, cytoskeletal proteolysis by Calpain, and disruption of the cell membrane. It is this loss of cell membrane integrity that precipitates irreversible cell death. (58, 59)

Apoptosis, or programmed cell death, has always implied that the cell dies in an organized and programmed manner, which is heralded by condensation of nuclear chromatin with DNA fragmentation, cell shrinkage, and the formation of apoptosomes that are subsequently cleared by phagocytosis. In this process, an organized removal of an irreversible damaged cell ensues in a surgical manner. The process of apoptosis is focused on the containment of intracellular components that can trigger inflammatory responses that if allowed to float freely into contiguous cell spaces will precipitate collateral damage. Contrary to necrosis, in apoptosis there is little collateral inflammation and no significant release of chemotactic agents that would bring the immune defense system into play. This is more of a quiet process that saves the surrounding cells and their morphology from a potential logarithmic process of destruction. (60)

Autophagy also called the type 2, non-apoptotic cell death mechanism, differs from apoptosis in that it doesn't necessarily terminate in cell death. On the contrary, autophagy is probably the most cell protective mechanism against cell execution. (61, 62, 63) In the event that damage occurs to a cytoplasmic organelle, which brings with it the risk of leakage of its content into the cytoplasm, autophagy would encapsulate it in an autophagosome. Once engulfed, the organelle would be processed with lysozymes digesting it into its principle components for reutilization for other cell structures, a form of cannibalization that can also occur during cell starvation where the cell is forced to ingest its own parts (organelles) for survival. (64)

Finally, and the most recent addition to the cell death mechanisms is Parthanatos which is initiated by release of mitochondrial apoptosis-inducing factor (AIF) and its translocation to the nucleus. (65) Apoptosis-inducing factor is a mitochondrial flavoprotein contributing to both cell life and death. Under physiological conditions, AIF maintains mitochondrial structure and plays an essential role in oxidative phosphorylation. Conversely, under pathological conditions, AIF enters the nucleus and facilitates poly (ADP-ribose) polymerase-1 (PARP-1)-dependent cell death. (66) In the process, mitochondrial transmembrane potential dissipates, chromatin condenses and large DNA fragmentations are formed. Unlike apoptosis, it does not cause apoptotic body formation or small scale DNA fragmentation. It is worth noting that PARP-1-mediated cell death involves loss of membrane integrity similar to necrosis, yet it does not induce cell swelling. Parthanatos is distinct also from autophagy as it does not involve autophagic vacuoles formation or lysosomal degradation. (67)

Traumatic brain injury in humans results in a pattern of neuronal loss that seems to preference the cortex, hippocampus, cerebellum, and thalamus (hypothalamus). (68) In the acute post-traumatic period, injured neurons appear swollen then become shrunken and eosinophilic with condensation of chromatin. This pattern suggests the presence of both necrotic and apoptotic processes. Under the electron microscope, these degenerating neurons appear swollen, with swollen mitochondria, vacuolated cytoplasm and Pyknotic nuclei, indicative of necrosis. (69) In the delayed or chronic post-traumatic period, there is a progressive but indolent process of neuronal degeneration that differs in the pattern seen in the acute phase, reflecting the apoptotic component of post-traumatic brain injury. (70)

Knowledge of the different biochemical cascades associated with each of the above processes has led researchers to develop compounds that can interrupt the progression of neuronal destruction and cognitive impairment. (71) Though, it might take three to five years or longer before we see any of them in our local pharmacies. Until that time, we can use prescriptive and alternative products that are available, but are not being utilized due to the lack of awareness and skills in how to use them. (72)

Neuroradiology of TBI (Chapter 5)

It was November 2006; I had just given my classical lecture, Traumatic Brain Injury – The Hormone Dysfunction Syndrome, to about 400 attendees of the ACAM symposium focusing on neurological illnesses. As I walked off the stage and down the side aisle, a voice from behind called out "I got it, I got it". I turned around and asked in a demanding manner "What do you got?" The doctor repeated herself and said, "I got it. I got it." Again, "What do you have?"

She introduced herself as a Neuroradiologist who reviews the CTs and MRIs of patients who have sustained anywhere from a mild to severe TBI. She explained that she rarely sees any structural abnormalities in those patients with mTBI even months or years post-trauma even though the patients are being studied for progressive functional impairment. She added that almost all of the moderate to severe TBI cases have recognizable contusions of the brain, large areas of diffuse axonal injury, and if not frank intracerebral bleeding (subdural hematomas), punctuate areas of intracerebral bleeds.

This is the paradigm that is finally changing due to advancements in radiologic technology and the unraveling of the biochemical mechanisms that activate both apoptosis and autophagy creating the telltale micro-calcified scars. In the past, these microscopic remnants of injury were missed due to the smaller Tesla coils (magnetic strength) but now with a 3.0 Tesla coil the resolution can identify these micro-calcifications which are found within neuronal tissue representing scarring precipitated by axonal damage (DAI), microhemorrhages, and necrosis. (73)

The importance of this technology was clearly defined in the paper by Orson and Handson in 2009 when they showed that 76 percent of non-combatant individuals who sustained a TBI had positive findings with only 14 percent involvement of their pituitary gland. (74) This, in my mind, opened the door to looking beyond the pituitary gland as the poor recipient of all things bad and turn attention to other areas of the brain. In fact, in this same paper, over 59 percent of findings involved the Hippocampus (memory and the ability to learn new information) and 29 percent diffuse axonal injury (DIA). Together, these describe the foundation for the majority of symptoms experienced by patients with mTBI and above.

Using newer software enhancements to this MRI technology (DTI-MRI) allows for images to be formed that look at the directional flow of water within neurons from the bodies down the microtubules into the axons. Diffusion Tension Imaging (DTI) or Tractography can delineate the course and continuity of long axonal connections between one or more cerebral hemispheres. Traumatic or neurochemical (necrosis, apoptosis or autophagy) damage to these neuronal conduits can be seen as though they were cut wires. It is in these areas where there is loss of continuity and connectivity that produces the alterations in brain functioning that we see as change in the personality and cognitive abilities of the individual. (75)

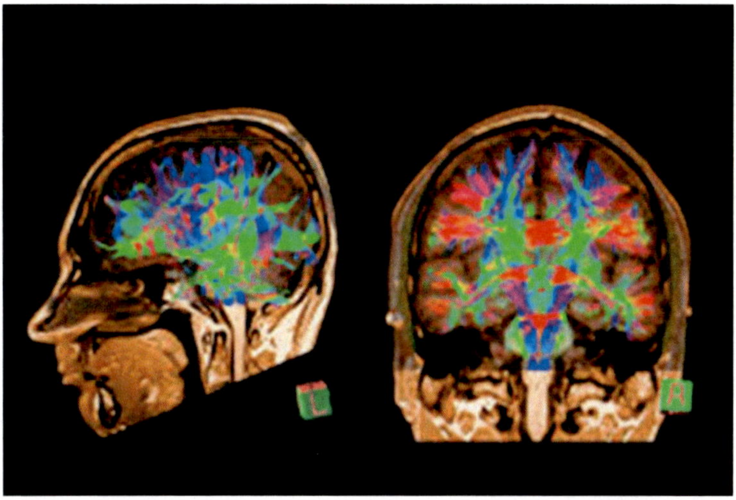

Image 1.1: Diffusion tension imaging MRI or tractography follows the flow of H_2O within the axons of neurons.

The functional MRI (fMRI) is another neuroimaging technique that can display patterns of brain activity based upon increases and decreases in regional blood flow (hemodynamic). After sustaining a TBI, there can be a significant redistribution of the hemodynamics reflecting the changes in blood flow with alterations in both glucose and oxygen utilization. (76)

There are a number of other technologies like SPECT, PET, and Fusion scans that will be discussed in Chapter 5.

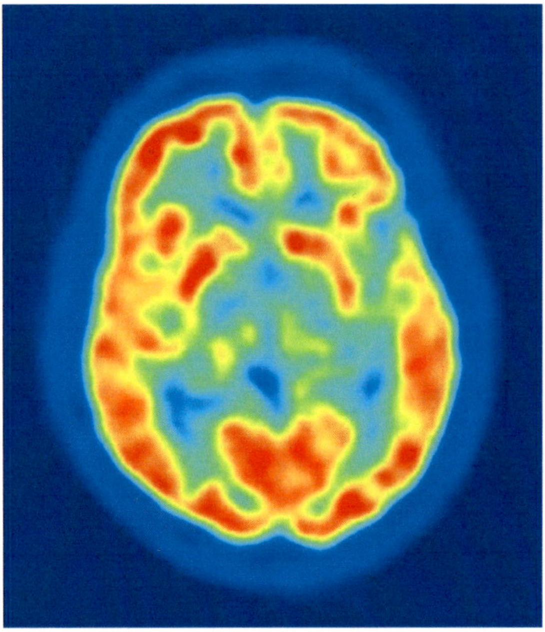

Image 1.2: Functional MRI showing preferential regional blood flow into areas of the brain that are actively being used.

The Laboratory of TBI (Chapter 6)

In Ireland Dr. Amar Agha, in Italy Drs. Ambrosio and Amaretti, in Serbia Dr. Popovic, and here in the United States Drs. Ronald Swerdloff and Daniel Kelly, have published, as a group, thousands of articles discussing the relationship between TBI and hormonal dysfunction. In 2007, on ESPN Outside the Lines, Dr. Dan Kelly and I were on the January 21st program discussing the relationship between hormone deficiencies and sports related TBI. So, it would make sense by now, almost ten years after the fact, that everyone would have an idea as to the ideal hormonal panel to use in the evaluation of anyone with TBI. Right? NOT YET!

The Millennium-TBI panel (3624) consists of 26 specific tests that allows for both direct and indirect assessment of the neurosteroid and neuroactive steroid pools. In the initial assessment of the patient it is important to determine if any of the hormonal deficiencies are of a primary nature with failure of the peripheral glands or of a central origin due to damage to the

HP axis. The findings of low tetraiodothyronine (T4) and elevated thyroid stimulating hormone (TSH) is a classical pattern of Primary Hypothyroidism while a finding of low TSH and a low T4 would be more suggestive of a central or Tertiary Hypothyroidism. Furthermore, having a normal TSH, low-normal T4, normal T3 and a high level of rT3 would indicate a Low T3 Syndrome with impact on mood with predilection for depression, poor sense of well-being, fatigue, diminished cognition, dry skin and brittle hair.

Without the full complement of testing you will be left with insufficient data points to make an accurate assessment of deficiency to formulate an optimal treatment protocol. The end result might be some improvement, but not optimal.

Biomarkers of TBI

The search for a viable biomarker for traumatic brain injury, which can identify the presence and progression of neurotrauma and be predictive of outcome, is under intense scrutiny. The goal here is to identify a reliable marker that is only present after TBI, is detectable in a peripheral blood sample, and can reflect the intensity of damage based upon the magnitude of the results. Additionally, this ideal marker would also reflect improvement or resolution in the bio-chemical processes that precipitate the indolent damage to the brain.

Creatine Kinase	**CK**	Special energy requirements of different neuronal and glial cell types.
Glial Fibrillary Acidic Protein	**AFAP**	Intermediate filaments form networks that provide support and strength to cells.
Lactate Dehydrogenase	**LDH**	Marker for brain aging/damage
Myelin Basic Protein	**MBP**	Comprises about 20% of the myelin sheath in neuronal axons.
Neuron-Specific Enolase	**NSE**	Rapidly detected in serum after TBI. Elevated in brain tumors.
* S-100 Proteins (19 types)	**S-100 β**	S 100β is detected in TBI patients.
Spinal Fluid IL-6	**SPIL-6**	Inflammatory cytokine.
Serum Cleaved Tau Protein	**CLT**	Microtubule protein.
Caspase -3	**Cap3**	Messenger of Death.
α II-Spectrin	**AIIS**	In CSF 24-72 hrs post-TBI.
* Neurofilament 68 Protein	**NF-68**	Information on the pathophysiology of dendritic and axonal damage after TBI.

Table 1.1: These are bio-markers of proteolytic damage to brain that are found in the cerebral spinal fluid within hours to days of neurotrauma.

Table 1.1 is a short listing of the most prominent biomarkers of TBI that are actively under evaluation. Unfortunately, many are only obtainable from the cerebral spinal fluid and not present in the peripheral circulation to any usable extent.

Neuropsychiatry in TBI (Chapter 7)

In this 2002 study, patients who had suffered traumatic brain injury were evaluated to determine the occurrence of psychiatric disorders during a 30-year follow-up period. Of the 60 patients, 29 (48.3 percent) had had an Axis I disorder that began after traumatic brain injury, and 37 (61.7 percent) had an Axis I disorder during their lifetimes. In this study, the most common disorders associated with post-traumatic brain injury were major depression (26.7 percent), alcohol abuse or dependence (11.7 percent), panic disorder (8.3 percent), specific phobia (8.3 percent), and psychotic disorders (6.7 percent). Fourteen patients (23.3 percent) had at least one personality disorder. The most prevalent individual disorders were avoidant (15.0 percent), paranoid (8.3 percent), and schizoid (6.7 percent) personality disorders. Nine patients (15.0 percent) had DSM-III-R organic personality syndrome. (77)

A 2009 Australian study commented on 100 post TBI patients, "Post-injury, 65 percent received a diagnosis, of which major depression became the most common (45 percent), followed by anxiety (38 percent) and substance use disorder (21 percent). Frequency of depression, generalized anxiety disorder, post-traumatic stress disorder, panic disorder, and phobias rose from pre-injury to post-injury. More than two-thirds of post-injury depression and anxiety cases were novel and showed poor resolution rates." They concluded: "A high frequency of post-injury psychiatric disorders was evident up to 5.5 years post-injury, with many novel cases of depression and anxiety. Individuals with TBI should be screened for psychiatric disorders at various time points post-injury without reliance on history of psychiatric problems to predict who is at risk, so that appropriate intervention can be offered." (78) The high rate of psychiatric disorders found in this study emphasizes the importance of psychiatric follow-up after traumatic brain injury.

This brings us to the recent office case of Bill who played rugby between the ages of 18 and 22, during which time he sustained five significant head traumas with loss of consciousness on three separate occasions and one which precipitated a hospitalization. At 36 years of age, and after nearly ten years of self-medication with alcohol Bill was interred for evaluation and treatment for severe depression. Once he was detoxified from the alcohol addiction, he was treated with a number of SSRIs that did not fully resolve his depression (treatment resistant depression). Ultimately, Bill's psychiatrist placed him on three medications and acknowledged and accepted the persistence of mild depression.

Five years later, at age 41, and after being on psychotropic medication for five years, Bill became aware of traumatic brain injury causing hormonal deficiencies that can be causative of depression and substance abuse. Bill came to our offices in Los Angeles from Boston, at which time he had our TBI-panel performed. In review of his TBI intake forms, there was a suggestion of testosterone deficiency.

Bill was given a 60mg injection of our blended testosterone and sent home with instruction to call in one week to review any response to this "Provocative testing". At the time Bill informed me of an appointment he had scheduled with an Orthopedist to discuss his chronic right shoulder pain and "turf toe" (frozen left 1st toe). His appointment was two days after our initial appointment.

On that Thursday, Bill called the office and when we spoke he asked me to remind him why he went to the Orthopedist. When I jokingly reminded him that it was for his shoulder pain and frozen toe, he said that he awoke that morning and the shoulder pain was gone and the toe was moving. He also stated that he slept the night of his injection better than he had in years. He also noted a rise in his libido and a calming of his depression.

Making this long story short, after two months on hormone replenishment treatment (self-administering a shot of testosterone once a week), Bill started working with his psychiatrist to taper him off of the anti-depressants. At six months, not only did Bill's depression abate but he was off his SSRIs, had mental clarity, slept very well, was emotionally stable, had a new girlfriend, had a return of his libido, and was working out harder in the gym with improved recovery.

A recently published book by Springer (2011), entitled Acquired Brain Injury — an Integrative Neuro-Rehabilitation Approach, provides a comprehensive dissertation on neuropsychiatry and traumatic brain injury. The chapter brilliantly written by Dr. Angela Scicutella discusses the clinical manifestations, assessment, and treatment for an array of psychological complexes (depression, mania, anxiety, psychosis, agitation, arousal and attention, dementia, and sexual dysfunction) that are acknowledged as being associated with traumatic brain injury. (79) Unfortunately, each section contains a clinical case where every single patient is ultimately placed on one or more psychotropic medications foregoing any laboratory assessment for hormonal homeostasis. This is in light of the thousands of articles showing the correlation between changes in neuropsychobehavior and hormone dysfunctioning. (80[L])

Women with anorexia and low testosterone levels were found to be the most resistant to traditional treatment with antidepressants. After low-dose replacement testosterone therapy the Anorexic patients' cerebral metabolism increased in the posterior cingulate, subgenual anterior cingulate, premotor cortex, right caudate and right parietal lobes as compared to the control group of Anorectic patients with improvement in their depression. (81)

For whatever reason, we seem to be focusing in on only the superficial aspects of psychological conditions without going after the cause (neurochemical); a patient presents with depression put them on an antidepressant and increase the dosing until the symptoms resolve. I was unaware that humans can have an antidepressant deficiency and therefore, replacement is all that is needed. Medicine has become shortsighted in the quest for health and wellness vying for a quick fix rather than a potential cure.

PTSD versus mTBI

I believe that the use of the term PTSD is a misnomer and should be replaced with the more accurate term; mTBI. The use of PTSD implies that there is a psychological or emotional propensity that is precipitated by a non-physical trauma or a trauma that does not create an overt or enduring physical injury. (82)

Looking at the work by Kessler and Gelea; approximately 7.7 million Americans suffer from PTSD, with the most common causes of PTSD in the civilian sector being motor vehicle crashes and assaults. (83, 84) These are both conditions that involve acceleration-deceleration type injuries and the possibility of blunt trauma. The underlying biomechanical forces that are involved are commonly seen in all levels of TBI. The fact that there is a delay in the onset of neuropsychological symptomatology should not dispel the presence of TBI, as causative, over PTSD since delays in the onset of symptoms have been recorded up to 17 years post TBI and frequently appear as Alzheimer's Disease. (85)

A 2009 article looking at the use of functional neuroimaging techniques to distinguish between TBI and PTSD did not convince me that these differences were exclusively associated with PTSD or TBI. It may be that a particular pattern of neurotrauma generates the patterns that they are promoting or that these patterns were pre-morbid to the event that caused the PTSD. Either way, the symptomatology is the same and the beneficial results that the Millennium has achieved in both PTSD and mTBI are the same. (86)

Supplementation for TBI (Chapter 8)

The use of supplementation concurrent to hormonal replenishment is necessary in order to reverse the non-neuropermissive environment (inflammatory) that was precipitated by the secondary phase of neurotrauma. (87) Additionally, supplementation must be used to counter any side effects associated with treatment, such as diminution of pregnenolone and DHEA from down-regulation caused by testosterone.

An increase in generation of reactive oxygen species (ROS) occurs as a by-product of damage to the cellular energy management system involving mitochondria. The loss of a competent cell surface ion exchange mechanism (ion-gated flux) allows for the random influx of calcium, chloride, and potassium leading to the precipitation of apoptosis or parthanatos. In an attempt to compensate for the loss of energy to regulate the ion-gate, mitochondria increase their production of ATP with an increase in oxidative stress. Free radicals foster inflammation creating a non-neuropermissive environment that does not foster the ability of cells to repair. Therefore, supplements with the ability to scavenge free radicals as well as to decrease inflammation can yield a more neuropermissive environment for cellular recovery. (88)

As a consequence of TBI initiated cellular depletion of ATP reserves, there is a reduced in ubiquitous mitochondrial creatine kinase (uMtCK), an enzyme implicated in the energetic regulation of Ca2+-pumps and in the maintenance of Ca2+-homeostasis. It is when Ca2+ levels increase in the cytosol that irreversible cell death mechanisms are initiated (Caspase-3, the messenger of death). The use of Omega-3 fatty acids supplements normalized the levels of uMtCK after traumatic brain lesions and helps the cell to maintain calcium balance. (89)

Oxidative stress due to the production of ROS, NO, peroxyl, and nitryls along with blood by-products such as *heme*, damages the cell membrane's composition of lipids generating an increased concentration of harmful the end products. Peroxidation appears to be important in atherosclerosis and in worsening the initial tissue injury caused by ischemic or traumatic brain injury. Oxidative stress can damage many biological molecules such as proteins and DNA, and are often more significant targets of injury than are lipids, as well as the finding that lipid peroxidation often occurs late in the injury process. (90)

N-acetyl cysteine (NAC) has been available for about 40 years as Mucomyst being used for pulmonary issues and also as the antidote for acute acetaminophen toxicity, in the emergency room. An impressive group of recent articles (17,500) found that NAC has both antioxidant and anti-inflammatory benefits in traumatic brain injury. Michael Hoffer, et al 2013, used NAC in an active theater of war (Iraq and Afghanistan) study on mild and moderate TBI cases produced by blast trauma. The studies clearly showed that initiation of treatment with NAC within 24 hours of injury led to better outcome in terms of headache, confusion, memory loss, and sleep issues. (91, 92)

Remember nothing is free. When we replenish levels of testosterone we do at the risk of precipitating a negative feedback loop that causes a decrease in the migration of cholesterol into the inner membrane of mitochondria where it is converted to pregnenolone. This appears to be set in motion by the level of luteinizing hormone (LH) which is down-regulated by supplementation with testosterone. Therefore, it is imperative to supplement with all the neurosteroids diminished by treatment with testosterone or estrogens for that matter. Otherwise, you diminish the magnitude and speed of a healthy response by the patient; testosterone decreases endogenous pregnenolone and DHEA pathways causing a transient increase in cholesterol.

Treatment for TBI (Chapter 9)

I wish there was something cryptic I could say about this section, which deals with treatment of mTBI based upon laboratory confirmed hormonal disruption, but there isn't. Insufficiencies are generally looked at as being within the "normal" reference ranges, and therefore, they are never considered to be causative or participating in the clinical presentation of the patient. We need to reassess our thinking about what represents healthy hormonal levels based upon individual responses and not what an acceptable numbers looks like on paper. Treatment must be tailored to the patient with the goal of optimizing all hormones based upon functional outcome. What? You think this is unprofessional and not the way medicine should be practiced? Let's see. What are the objective laboratory tests that a psychiatrist performs prior to loading the patient up with medication? There are none! The psychiatrist starts the patient on treatment empirically and monitors their response (subjective at best).

As far as objective results for the treatment of TBI, a 2002 review article entitled "**Outcome Measures for Clinical Trials in Neuro-Trauma**" clearly indicated that dozens of medication trials were stopped prematurely due to their failure to improve the condition of patients with mild to severe TBI. The medications and procedures that were being evaluated did not work at best and many worsened the patients' condition. (93) Not a single article addressed the associated hormonal deficiencies or insufficiencies.

Another prominent treatment modality is hypothermia or cooling during which an unconscious patient with severe TBI has their body temperature decreased to 32–35°C (89.6-95°F) in order to protect neurons from ischemia and hypoxia caused by cerebral edema. Unfortunately, the attached 2009 review, published their assessment of the benefits of "cooling" in TBI stating "...our present knowledge on the use of active cooling in TBI patients has not been shown to be effective for outcome after TBI...." (94)

In light of these and hundreds of other articles addressing the lack of beneficial effects, hypothermic treatments continue to be used while the literature promoting the positive outcomes from the use of Growth Hormone, IGF-1, Testosterone, DHEA-s and DHT on neuropsychiatric, cognitive, and physical sequelae are ignored. (95, 96, 97, 98, 99, 100, 101, 102)

It is my opinion that the major reason why hormone treatment protocols are being ignored is because the literature has been weak in supporting the benefits from their use. This arises from the flawed perception that monotherapy for TBI is all you need. A greater understanding of the importance of neurosteroids in neuroendocrinology and the impact of TBI on their production will lead to more complete treatment with greater beneficial outcomes for the patients. The growing science on neurosteroids is clearly showing that they are responsible for the integration, modulation, and maintenance of neuronal functioning, protection and repair. Failure to address the need for optimal neurosteroids in treatment can only mean failure to the patient's abilities for recovery. (103, 104, 105, 106)

Nonetheless, when treating cases of mTBI we must replenish all hormones to at least the median physiologic levels. Then, add secondary hormones that can be lost, such as Pregnenolone and DHEA, when using testosterone. This will maintain optimal levels of NAS and NS and provide for added protection against oxidative stress and promote remyelination of damaged neurons. The addition of specific antioxidant regimens by oral or IV routes is encouraged along with a number of potential Nootropic products (L-Deprenyl, amantadine, and neurotransmitter precursor amino acids). (107)

Knowing the mechanisms behind the subtle progression of nerve damage can only help us to provide a means of diminishing their long-term effect on brain functioning so that we may maintain who we are for a longer period of uninterrupted quality of life.

Summary

Traumatic brain injury is rapidly become the number one cause of functional disability worldwide. Anywhere from 100 – 250 persons per 100,000 population are succumbing to the progressive development of symptoms that can create hordes of socially dependent individuals.

Mild traumatic brain injury (mTBI) and not post-traumatic stress disorder (PTSD) is associated with a physical component that leads to the interruption of both cellular connectivity and functional neurochemistry. The disruption of cellular membranes precipitated by blunt trauma, penetrating projectiles, motor vehicle accidents, any given Sunday, radiation, chemotherapy, ischemic strokes, hypoxia, blast trauma, repetitive gun fire, and starvation leads to the loss of cell integrity. As the gradient of cellular damage unfolds anyone of the neurochemical processes of the secondary phase of neurotrauma; necrosis, apoptosis, autophagy, and parthanatos, will regulate the ultimate outcome in both cognitive and emotional functioning.

Movement of the brain against the various ridges and bony protuberances of the anterior (frontal) and middle (temporal) fossae is particularly injurious to the temporal and frontal poles and the ventral anterior, medial, and lateral temporal cortices, and the frontal cortices. Acceleration or deceleration injuries are maximal on axonal projections and small blood vessels within and from the brain stem, the parasagittal white matter of the cerebrum, the corpus callosum, the gray-white junctions of the cerebral cortex, and especially at gray-white junctions in the ventral and anterior frontal and temporal lobes. This pattern of injury is associated with an almost predictable group of neurobehavioral conditions that can include depression, anxiety, altered executive functions, rage, aggression, mood disorders and suicide.

Lateral and rotational forces add further injury to the central areas of the brain that includes the pituitary gland, hypothalamus, thalamus, hippocampus, amygdala, optic chiasma, and olfactory bulbs. This accounts for the development of hyposmia or anosmia, hypogeusia or ageusia, hypothalamic-pituitary dysfunction with loss of hormonal homeostasis, faltering memory, and fatigue.

The acute use of neuroradiologic studies is to detect skull fracture, subdural hematoma, intracerebral bleeding, and cerebral edema. In the post-acute phase the use of MRI, DTI-MRI, PET or SPECT scans can help determine the impact on structural and functional integrity. Scarring, cavitation, diffuse axonal injury, altered cerebral blood flow can all be identified and followed for improvement based upon treatment.

Ideally, treatment will be based upon the performance of a comprehensive laboratory assessment that will look at the continuation of hormonal homeostasis predicated by a normal HP axis. In the event that damage impaired the brain's ability to maintain optimal hormonal production, replenishment of those hormones would be mandated to avoid the consequences of neurobehavioral and physiologic dysfunctioning. Furthermore, to avoid missing a patient that has a relative hormonal deficiency or insufficiency, we will need to apply the new interpretive paradigm in which the median of the range is used instead of the ineffective "reference range."

Neurobehavioral conditions have been found in association with the presence of neurosteroid and neuroactive steroid alterations. Both groups of steroids have been found to modulate communication between neurons in all centers of the brain maintaining optimal functioning. Disruption of healthy neuronal communication involving shearing of neurons and loss of hormonal modulation can account for the many psychobehavioral changes witnessed in the post-TBI period. The traditional approach using SSRI's has obviously failed to provide recovery since the majority of individuals are on combination therapies due to treatment resistant depression (TRD); a telltale sign of an underlying hormonal deficiency.

Supporting the neurosteroids' ability to promote recovery is an array of supplements that function to reduce the presence of oxidative stressors (OS). Only with a return to a more neuropermissive environment (NPE) can the process of reconnection of neurocommunication and modulation of neurotransmitters be accomplished. Until the state of a healthier NPE is met, the individual will continue to struggle and delay a return to their pre-injury status.

Finally, treatment will be primarily based upon the use and interpretation of the Millennium-TBI panel 3426 with the objective being to raise all the hormones to the median (50 percent) of the range and above, if needed. Once treatment is started the patient is assessed by a monthly treatment questionnaire (MTQ) and a small laboratory follow-up test. Based upon the results of an objective blood test and a subjective self-assessment, their treatment protocol can be adjusted up or down. Many times, we add additional supplements to improve mitochondrial functioning along with free radical scavengers, like PQQ.

At the time of writing this segment of the book, we have started using progesterone oral drops (at bed time) to increase the presence in the blood of its metabolite allopregnanolone, which has been found, along with estradiol and DHEA-s, to provide significant neuroprotection, neuroregeneration, and recovery over the long-term, and lessening of “brain fog” in the short-term.

Chapter 2: Neurology in TBI

"Once lost it cannot be regained, twice lost you're not the same, thrice lost and improvement is sought."

— Mark L. Gordon

As we begin our strategic buildup toward chapter nine and the treatment of TBI, it is important to appreciate that this collection of information entitled, "Traumatic Brain Injury: A Clinical Approach to Diagnosis and Treatment," is my clinical workbook more than a traditional textbook. It represents more than ten years of effort to understand what happens immediately after the primary phase of insult, and then the conditions that arise during the secondary phase causing chronic inflammatory that creates the non-permissive environment (NPE) leading to both cognitive and neurobehavioral alterations.

Also, just as this chapter is not a textbook on neurology, this book is not the final word on neurotrauma and neurorehabilitation. Rather, it contains a significant amount of relevant and accurate information; which, like pieces in a puzzle, are waiting to be put together — thereby providing you with ample material for your own epiphany... your own "aha moment" of recognition.

Introduction

Trauma, head trauma, neurotrauma, and traumatic brain injury are all synonymous with processes that can cause a loss of physical, electrical, and biochemical connectivity within the brain. (1) Superficially, this can present as alteration in personality with mood and cognitive changes. Depending upon the type and intensity of the trauma, it may help us to predict some or all of the expected sequelae that can develop either immediately after the injury, or those issues that can take years to fully unfold. (2r)

Thus, the recognition that there are two major injury phases: the primary, where the acute injury can cause physical loss of brain cells and tissue volume (penetrating injury), compression of tissue (hematoma and edema); and the secondary, which is precipitated by the primary injury initiating a dynamic interlude between ischemia, hypoxia, inflammation, and cytotoxic processes (oxidative stress, excitotoxicity, BCL2, and Caspase), thereby causing indolent processes that can take years to present as progressive dysfunctioning. (3r)

It has been the general consensus that once neurotrauma has occurred, there is little hope of a full recovery. Nonetheless, medical research has suggested alternate potential outcomes based upon treatments that address Caspases (messengers of cell death), damage from oxidative stress (reactive oxygen species- ROS), axonal demyelination (diffuse axonal injury, also known as DAI), microtubule disruption (Tau protein), and stimulation of neuron regeneration (IGF-I & II), which all carry the potential of improvement through neurorehabilitation. (4r)

Over the years, a significant number of articles have promoted an associated decline in cognitive functioning with low levels of testosterone, estrogens, progesterone, thyroid hormones, growth hormone, and DHEA-S. (5[L]) These same hormones have also been reported in association with depression, psychoses, schizophrenia, anxiety, panic, paranoia, and an addictive personality when deficient.

Therefore, when TBI (A) causes a disruption in hormonal homeostasis (B), and the resulting insufficiencies of these hormones are associated with the onset of neurobehavioral and cognitive changes (C) it makes sense by the most basic transitive relationship (A=B and B=C and therefore, A=C) that TBI is at the root of mood disorders that develop, over time, due to the loss of hormonal homeostasis. (6)

Again, this is not a textbook on neurology, let alone a textbook at all, but a compilation of my readings, thoughts, and clinical observations on the science that was extracted and applied to individuals that were suffering both with the neurotrauma and the deleterious effects from ineffective treatment. Our journey begins by looking at the cells of the central nervous system, their function, and the different lobes of the brain (frontal, parietal, temporal, occipital) as it all pertains to traumatic brain injury and loss of functioning. This will help you to understand why, possibly, the majority of individuals on behavioral medications fail to improve.

Cells of the Central Nervous System

Scientists have organized the cells that make up the nervous system into two groups: neurons, which are the primary signaling cells; and glia, which support neurons. Recent research has in fact found that these glia have more than just a supportive role — they also interact with the propagation of signaling down neurons. (7a) Considering that the human brain contains around 100 billion neurons and somewhere between ten to 50 times as many glial cells, all the help we can get is appreciated.

Neurons and macroglia were once thought to derive from different embryonic stem cells, but we now know that both can be derived from the same stem cell precursors. Their fate is determined in part by exposure to growth factors and by developmental programs that ultimately restrict the precursors to either glial or neuronal fates. Neural stem cells persisting in the adult nervous system participate in plasticity and regeneration, but they have the immunocytochemical markers of glia. (7b)

A neuron is an electrically excitable cell that processes and transmits information by means of electrical (action potentials) and chemical signals (neurotransmitters). Neurons are the core components of the nervous system (8), which includes the brain (9), spinal cord (10), and peripheral ganglia. (11) Neurons connect to each other to form neural networks. (12) A number of specialized types of neurons exist: sensory neurons (13) respond to touch, sound, light and numerous other stimuli affecting cells of the sensory organs (14) that then send signals to the spinal cord and brain.

The typical neuron possesses a cell body, dendrites (15), and an axon. (16) Dendrites are thin structures that arise from the cell body, often extending for hundreds of micrometers and branching multiple times, giving rise to a complex "dendritic tree." An axon is a special cellular extension that arises from the cell body at a site called the axon hillock (17) and travels for a distance, as far as one meter in humans. The cell body of a neuron frequently gives rise to multiple dendrites, but never to more than one axon, although the axon may branch hundreds of times before it terminates. At the majority of synapses, signals are sent from the axon of one neuron to a dendrite of another.

All neurons are electrically excitable, maintaining voltage gradients across their membranes by means of metabolically driven ion pumps (18), which combine with ion channels (19) embedded in the membrane to generate intracellular versus extracellular concentration differences of ions such as sodium, potassium, chloride, and calcium. Changes in the cross-membrane voltage can alter the function of voltage-dependent ion channels. These ion gradients are maintained by the production of ATP by the mitochondria which pumps the specific ion across cell membranes and synapses. (20) If the voltage changes by a large enough amount, an all-or-none electrochemical pulse called an action potential (21[1]) is generated, which travels rapidly along the cell's axon, and activates synaptic connections with other cells.

Neurons do not undergo cell division. In most cases, neurons are generated by special types of stem cells. (22) Astrocytes (23), a type of glial cell, have also been observed to turn into neurons by virtue of the stem cell characteristic pluripotency. (24) In humans, neurogenesis terminates during adulthood except in two brain areas, the hippocampus and olfactory bulb, where there is strong evidence for generation of substantial numbers of new neurons.

In traumatic brain injury, a combination of physical damage to the neuronal axon (shearing) and the subsequent loss of membrane integrity lead to the interruption of the action potential and loss of neuron-to-neuron signaling. The number of neurons that are damaged is not always proportional to the degree of functional impairment and neither is the intensity of the initial injury. It appears that there are a number of factors that influence the gradation of damage to neurons. Some of those factors identified are the neurosteroids produced de nova from brain cholesterol by the Purkinje neurons. (25[1])

Purkinje Neurons

These cells are some of the largest neurons in the human brain (Betz cells being the largest), with an intricately elaborate dendritic arbor, characterized by a large number of dendritic spines. Purkinje cells are found within the Purkinje layer in the cerebellum. Purkinje cells are aligned like dominos stacked one in front of the other. Their large dendritic arbors form nearly two-dimensional layers through which parallel fibers from the deeper layers pass. These parallel fibers make relatively weaker excitatory (glutamatergic) synapses to spines in the Purkinje cell dendrite, whereas climbing fibers originating from the inferior olivary nucleus (26) in the medulla provide very powerful excitatory input to the proximal dendrites and cell soma. Parallel fibers pass orthogonally (27) through the Purkinje neuron's dendritic arbor, with up to 200,000 parallel fibers forming a Granule-cell-Purkinje-cell synapse (28) with a single Purkinje cell.

Each Purkinje cell receives 500 climbing fiber synapses, all originating from a single climbing fiber. Both basket and stellate cells (found in the cerebellar molecular layer) provide inhibitory (GABAergic) input to the Purkinje cell, with basket cells synapsing on the Purkinje cell axon initial segment and stellate cells onto the dendrites. Purkinje cells send inhibitory projections to the deep cerebellar nuclei, and constitute the sole output of all motor coordination in the cerebellar cortex. Purkinje neurons are also responsible for the production of a number of neurosteroids from cholesterol, especially pregnenolone, progesterone and allopregnanolone. (29)

Glial Cells

These are non-neuronal cells providing support to neurons in both the central and peripheral nervous systems through their ability to surrounding and hold them in place, supply nutrients and oxygen, producing myelin to insulate one neuron from another, and acting as part of the immune system (microglia) to destroy pathogens and remove dead neurons. (30)

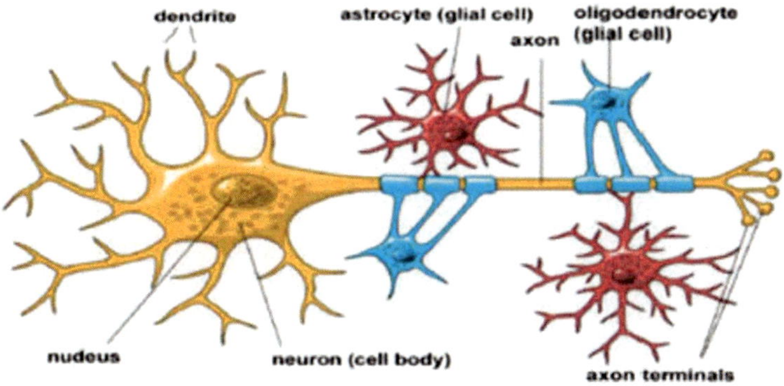

Astrocytes

Astrocytes, or astrocytic glial cells, are a sub-type of glial cells in the central nervous system. They are involved in the physical structuring and support of the brain, ensheathing synaptic junctions, associating with nodes of Ranvier (31*), and mount a respond to disease and injury by clearing cellular debris, secreting trophic factors and forming scars. The name refers to their stellate or star shape but they are not limited since some astrocytes span the entire width of the brain radially from the hollow ventricles to the pial surface, providing scaffolding along which neurons migrate during fetal development. Others stretch from blood capillaries to neurons, transporting ions and other substances to sustain neurons and to regulate the extracellular environment. The prevailing view, based on histology, has been that the stellate processes of astrocytes form a tightly intermingled web throughout the brain, but now it seems that these cells are much larger than previously thought, and the processes of adjacent astrocytes do not overlap extensively. Thus, parts of the brain (such as the hippocampus where memories are formed) are divided by astrocytes into separate compartments, each one the sole domain of an individual astrocyte. (32)

It is by this configuration that they regulate both the transmission of electrical impulses down the neuronal axon and provide for the crucial clearance of neurotransmitters from within the synaptic cleft, and also prevent the toxic buildup of neurotransmitters such as glutamate (excitotoxicity). (33)

Several forms of astrocytes exist in the CNS including fibrous, protoplasmic, and radial glial cells. The fibrous glial cells are located within white matter and exhibit long unbranched cellular processes with "vascular feet" that physically connect the cells to the outside of capillary walls. The most prevalent protoplasmic glia are found in grey matter and exhibit short and highly branched tertiary processes. (34) Being among the earliest cells to differentiate in the early CNS, they provide support for neuronal migration during embryonic brain development; provide instructive and neurotrophic signals required for the survival, proliferation, and differentiation of neurons; and may be multi-potential progenitor cells that give rise to various cell types, including neurons. (35)

Astrocytes are the most abundant cells of the human brain performing functions that include biochemical support of endothelial cells that form: (1) the blood-brain barrier; (2) provision of nutrients to nervous tissue; (3)

maintenance of extracellular ion balance; and (4) a role in the repair and scarring process of the cells of the brain and spinal cord following traumatic brain injuries.

Oligodendrocytes

Oligodendrocytes are another type of neuroglia with main functions to provide support and to insulate the axons in the central nervous system. By virtue of the electrical activity in neurons, ATP is released which serves as an important stimulus for myelin formation. This ATP does not act directly on oligodendrocytes; but, it instead causes astrocytes to secrete cytokine leukemia inhibitory factor (36), a regulatory protein that promotes the myelinating activity of oligodendrocytes. This suggests that astrocytes have an executive-coordinating role in the brain to regulate the oligodendrocytes that create the myelin sheath (37), which is 80 percent lipid and 20 percent protein. A single oligodendrocyte can extend its processes to 50 axons, wrapping approximately one μm of myelin sheath around each axon. Each oligodendrocyte forms one segment of myelin for several adjacent axons.

Oligodendroglia arise during development from oligodendrocyte precursor cells (38), which can be identified by their expression of a number of antigens, including the ganglioside GD3 (39), the NG2 chondroitin sulfate proteoglycan (40), and the platelet-derived growth factor-alpha receptor subunit PDGF-αR. (41) Most oligodendrocytes develop during embryogenesis and early postnatal life from restricted periventricular germinal regions. They are the last cell type to be generated in the CNS. Myelination is only prevalent in a few brain regions at birth and continues into adulthood. The entire process is not complete until about 25 to 30 years of age. Oligodendrocyte formation in the adult brain is associated with glial-restricted progenitor's cells, known as oligodendrocyte progenitor cells. (42*) These cells migrate away from germinal zones to populate both developing white and gray matter, where they differentiate and mature into myelin-forming oligodendroglia. It has been suggested that some undergo apoptosis and others fail to differentiate into mature oligodendroglia but persist as adult oligodendroglial progenitors. Myelination is an important component which has been found to directly correlation with white matter and intelligence. People with greater white matter had higher IQs. (43*)

Microglia

The third major glial population, microglial cells are ubiquitously distributed in central nervous system (CNS), being the first elements that react to the pathophysiological stimuli; thus, they participate in all brain pathologies, either chronic or acute. In response to these different triggers, microglia change shape, motility, expression of innate and adaptive immune molecules and function; they release various cytokines, chemokines, reactive oxygen species, prostaglandin metabolites, bringing a major and direct contribution to neuroinflammation, the basis for all neurodegenerative disorders. (44)

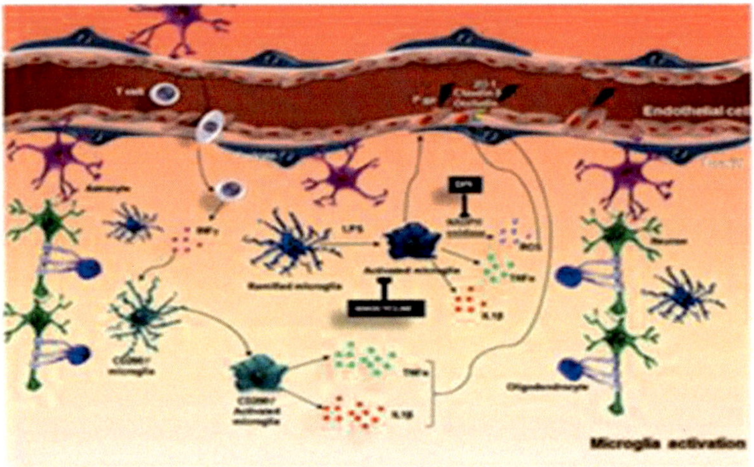

These microglia are homologous to peripheral macrophages having the capacity to phagocytosis and protect neurons of the central nervous system from infectious agents. (45) Microglia constitute 15 to 20 percent of the total glial cell population within the brain and are mobile and can multiply when the brain is damaged or set upon by infectious agents. They act as the first and main form of active immune defense in the central nervous system. In the healthy central nervous system, microglia are constantly scavenging the CNS for plaques, damaged neurons, and infectious agents. Microglia (and astrocytes) are distributed in large non-overlapping regions throughout the brain and spinal cord. (46*)

The brain and spinal cord are considered "immune privileged" organs in that they are separated from the rest of the body by a series of endothelial cells known as the blood-brain barrier (BBB), which prevents most infections from reaching the vulnerable nervous tissue. In the case where infectious agents are directly introduced to the brain or cross the blood-brain barrier, microglial cells must react quickly to decrease inflammation and destroy the infectious agents before they damage the sensitive neural tissue. Due to the size limitation of the BBB, most antibodies are unable to cross into the brain, microglia must be able to recognize foreign bodies, engulf them, and act as antigen-presenting cells activating T-cells. Since this process must be done quickly to prevent potentially fatal damage, microglia are extremely sensitive to even small pathological changes in the CNS. They achieve this sensitivity in part by having unique potassium channels that respond to even small changes in extracellular potassium. (47)

Blood-brain Barrier

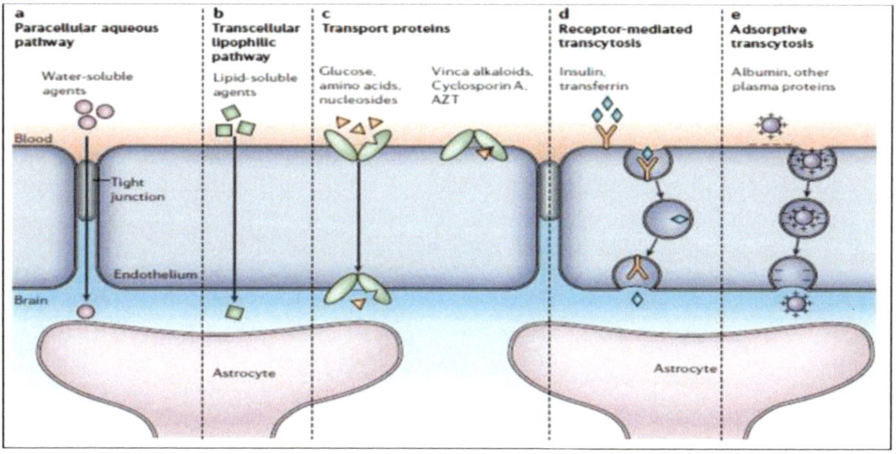

Astrocytic end-feet encircling endothelial cells were thought to aid in the maintenance of the blood-brain barrier, but recent research indicates that they do not play a substantial role; instead, it is the tight junctions and basal lamina of the cerebral endothelial cells that play the most significant role in maintaining the barrier. However, it has been shown that astrocyte activity is linked to blood flow in the brain, and that this is what is actually being measured in fMRI scans. (48)

In addition, astrocytes contain glycogen and are capable of glycogenesis. Astrocytes located in the frontal cortex and hippocampus store and release glycogen to their adjoining neurons. Thus, astrocytes can fuel neurons with glycogen during periods of high rate of glycogen consumption thereby protecting them for a short period of time during ischemia (49) secondary to stroke or cerebral edema arising from a traumatic brain injury. Once the glycogen stores are exhausted, a state of hypoglycemia occurs which is recognized as a trigger for apoptosis.

Electrophysiology of Neurons

Years of analytical research on cellular electrophysiology has elucidated the sensitive nature of timing of neural activity associated with covert abnormalities in brain function associated with overt behavioral deficits commonly seen post-TBI. These are brought about by alterations in electrophysiology that regulates neuron-neuron, glial-glial, and neuron-glial interactions that modulate all that is held holly (and wholly) in our brain. The disruption of these important communication relationships allows for the loss of regulatory mechanisms that are manifested in personality disorders and cognitive decline. (50[1])

The Action Potential

Propagation of an action potential down the axon of a neuron requires a complex series of chemical events. Action potentials are generated by special types of voltage-gated ion channels (ATP dependent) embedded in a cell's plasma membrane. When a neuron is not sending signals, the inside of the neuron has a negative charge relative to the positive charge outside the cell. Electrically charged chemicals known as ions maintain the balance of positive and negative charges. (51)

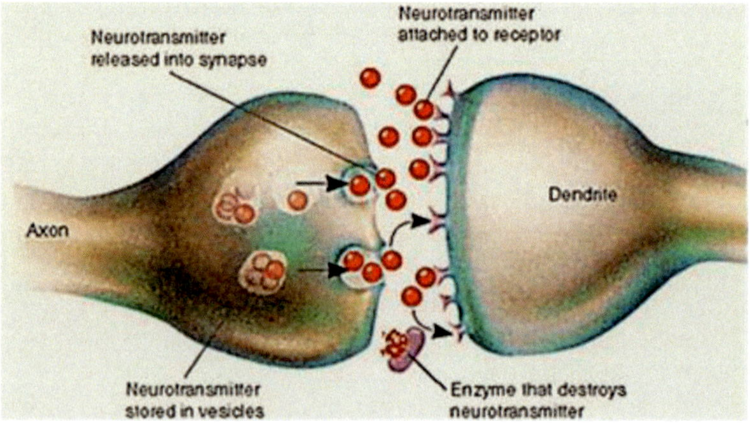

The movement of positively charged ions (Na^+,K^+,CA^{+2}) from outside the neuron to inside, and negatively charged ions (Cl^-,) from inside to outside the cell causing a rapid increase in the positive charge of the nerve fiber.

When the charge reaches +40 mv, an impulse is propagated down the nerve fiber; an all-or-none event.

As the current travels down the axon, support from astrocytes, oligodendrocytes, and other glial cells, modify the rate and propagation of the impulse (action potential) so that it reaches the end of the axon at the synaptic bulb thereby, causing the release of neurotransmitters into the synaptic gap. On the other side, the post-synaptic receptors respond to the neurotransmitter by initiating an action potential that continues the propagation of the originating signal.

When at rest, the cell membrane of the neuron allows certain ions to pass through while preventing or restricting the movement of other ions. In this state, sodium and potassium ions cannot easily pass through the membrane. Potassium ions, however, are able to freely cross the membrane. The negatively charged ions inside of the cell are unable to cross to the outside of the barrier (Cl-). The cell must activity transport ions in order to maintain its polarized state. This mechanism is known as the sodium-ion pump. For every two potassium ions that pass through the membrane, three sodium ions are pumped out. These processes are heavily ATP dependent. (52)

Compositional changes in the intra-neuronal ionic pool, can lead to death of neurons and glia as is the case with leakage of potassium from neurons, which is rapidly picked up by astrocytes causing them to swell and die. Additionally, secondary inflammation is associated with elevation in an array of oxidative stressors (ROS: e.g., superoxide radical, peroxynitryl, hydroxyl radical and hydrogen peroxide), each causing neuronal death. (53)

In terms of electrical activity of the brain, the neurons are the only cell type that generates an action potential. Astrocytes, in terms of brain electrical activity were thought to be inactive as they do not generate any electrical activity on their own being considered non-excitable and, therefore, unable to communicate. This concept or perception has changed. The finding that astrocytes can be excited non-electrically has expanded our knowledge of the complexity of brain communication to an integrated network of both synaptic and non-synaptic routes. (54)

As technical abilities evolved, astrocytes are now recognized as expressing voltage-gated channels (potassium ion), neurotransmitter receptors, control of synapse formation and function, adult neurogenesis, and brain vascular tone. Astrocytes have been found to express plasma membrane transporters such as glutamate transporters for several neurotransmitters, including glutamate, ATP, and GABA. More recently, astrocytes were shown to release glutamate or ATP in a vesicular, Ca^{2+}-dependent manner. When neurons are active, they release potassium, increasing the local extracellular concentration. Because astrocytes are highly permeable to potassium with a high density of potassium channels, they rapidly clear the excess accumulation in the extracellular space. If this function is interfered with, the extracellular concentration of potassium will rise, leading to neuronal depolarization resulting in epileptic neuronal activity with the potential of cell death. (55)

Brain tissue has a relatively high consumption of oxygen and glucose, and depends almost exclusively on oxidative phosphorylation for energy production. Focal impairment of cerebral blood flow restricts the delivery of substrates, particularly oxygen and glucose, and impairs the energetics required to maintain ionic gradients. With energy depletion, membrane potential is lost and neurons and glia depolarize allowing for the leakage of Ca2+, Na+, K+, and Cl^- into the cell. (56)

Diffuse Axonal Injury (Shearing/Ionic gradient)

One of the most significant factors causing secondary brain injury is the excessive release of excitotoxins (such as glutamate and aspartate) that occurs at the time of the primary injury. These excitotoxins act on the N-methyl-D-aspartate channel (NMDA), altering the cell wall permeability causing an increase in intracellular calcium and sodium. As the ionic balance regulated by both calcium and sodium fails, the neuronal axons are destroyed. Concurrently, potassium is also released from traumatized cells and is absorbed by astrocytes trying to maintain the extracellular ionic balance. Unfortunately, the battle to preserve this ionic balance is lost with swelling and subsequent death of the cells thereby, losing focal regions of functioning showing up as diffuse axonal injury. (57*, 58*)

Neurotransmitters

A dissertation on the intricacies of each of the neurotransmitters is beyond the scope of this book; however, an understanding of their function and disruption of function is pertinent to the individual's ultimate treatment. Therefore, weaved throughout this chapter, and the rest of this book, will be expounding information that is context sensitive to your knowledge-base.

The amino acid L-glutamate is recognized as the major excitatory neurotransmitter in the central nervous system while γ-aminobutyric acid (GABA) is the major inhibitory neurotransmitter. It is the continuum of interactions between these neurotransmitters and their receptor that eventually leads to who we are and how we think, and also how we emote. Both cognition and affect are regulated by a complex array of interrelations that can easily be disrupted when the neurochemistry of the brain is impaired. (59)

Neuroexcitatory

Glutamate is used at the great majority of fast excitatory synapses in the brain and spinal cord. It is also used at most synapses that are "modifiable," i.e., capable of increasing or decreasing in strength. Modifiable synapses are thought to be the main memory-storage elements in the brain. Excessive glutamate release can overstimulate the brain and lead to excitotoxicity causing cell death resulting in seizures or strokes. Excitotoxicity has been implicated in certain chronic diseases and conditions including ischemic stroke, epilepsy, Amyotrophic lateral sclerosis, Alzheimer's disease, Huntington disease, Parkinson's disease, and traumatic brain injury. (60)

Neuroinhibitory

GABA, a major inhibitory neurotransmitter, mediates fast synaptic inhibition by activating ligand-gated chloride channels. Binding of 3α-reduced neurosteroids (Allopregnenolone (3α, 5α-THPreg), Progesterone, 3α, 5α-THDOC) to $GABA_A$ receptors results in either inhibition or potentiation of the inhibitory effects of GABA. Therefore, anticonvulsive, anesthetic and anxiolytic effects of neurosteroids are mediated by their capacity to positively modulate $GABA_A$ receptor function; via stimulation. Neurosteroids achieve this effect by increasing the frequency and duration of chloride channel openings. Under the right scenario, inhibition of the $GABA_A$ receptor function by neurosteroids such as Pregnenolone-sulfate and DHEA-sulfate can increase the susceptibility to excitability, anxiety, and seizures. Many sedative/tranquilizing drugs act by enhancing the effects of GABA. Additionally, GABA is in itself a neurotransmitter that specifically inhibits dopamine and norepinephrine. (61)

The Neuro-regulatory Receptors

Modulation of electrical and chemical influences on neuronal transmissions can affect the expression of many personality and disease states. The flow of communication from one neuron to another is generally perceived as being a synaptic event with little else influencing it. What has developed over decades is an understanding that mood (affective) disorders, memory and learning abilities are influenced by an almost synchronous interaction of an array of receptors exemplified by GABA, NMDA, AMPA, and Sigma-1. Furthermore, these receptors and their subsets are found to be modulated by the presence of endogenously produced neurosteroids. (62*)

Neurosteroids exert their effects on the central nervous system either by regulating the expression of specific hormone-sensitive genes or by modulating the activity of neurotransmitter receptors, such as the type A γ-aminobutyric acid (GABA), the N-methyl-D-aspartate (NMDA), the nicotinic, the dopamine D1, and the sigma-1 (σ1) receptors and the α1 adrenoreceptor. (63)

GABA Receptors

Gamma-Aminobutyric acid (GABA) is a major inhibitory neurotransmitter in the vertebrate central nervous system. It is estimated that close to 40 percent of the synapses in the human brain work with GABA and therefore have GABA receptors.

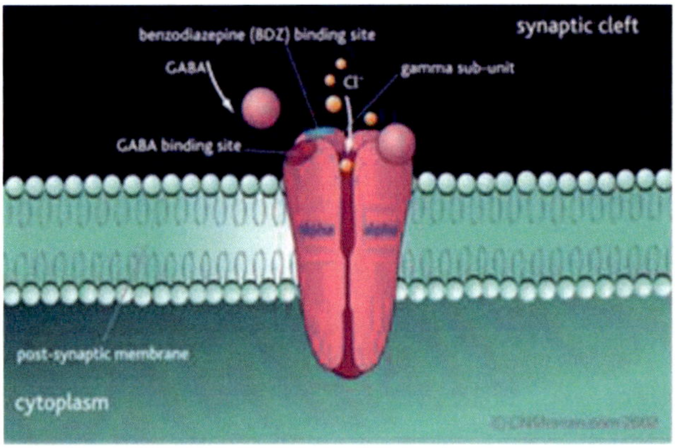

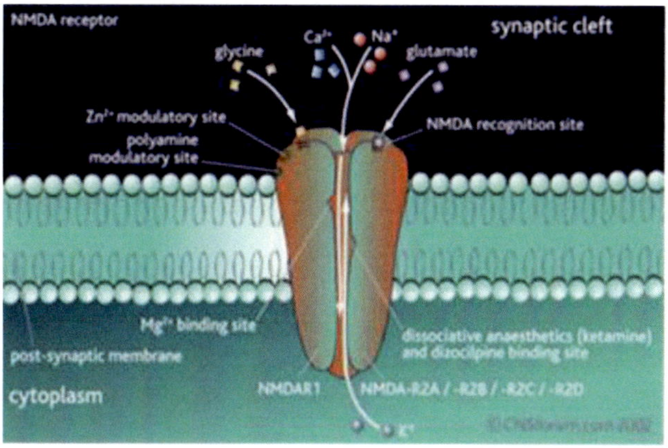

The $GABA_A$ receptor is composed of five sub-units — two alpha, two beta and one gamma sub-unit. Two molecules of GABA activate the receptor by binding to the alpha sub-units. Once activated the receptor allows the passage of negatively charged ions through a channel and into the cytoplasm, which results in hyperpolarization and the inhibition of neurotransmission. The $GABA_A$ receptor directly gates a Chloride ionophore and has modulatory binding sites for benzodiazepines, barbiturates, neurosteroids and ethanol. (64)

NMDA Receptors

The NMDA receptor belongs to a family of ionotropic receptors for the excitatory amino acid glutamate and is characterized by high affinity for glutamate, a high unitary conductance, high calcium permeability, and a voltage-dependent block by magnesium ions. (65*)

During excitatory neurotransmission, presynaptic release of glutamate activates glutamate receptors in the postsynaptic membrane, resulting in the generation of an excitatory postsynaptic potential. (66)

Activation of the receptor and concurrent depolarization results in the development of a relatively slow-rising, long-lasting current mediated primarily by the influx of Ca2+. Calcium entering the cell can also mediate longer-lasting cellular responses. NMDA receptors appear to have a pivotal role in long-term potentiation (67), long-term depression (68), and developmental plasticity. Over activation of NMDA receptors, however, appears to cause damage via excitotoxicity, which commonly happens in TBI. (69)

At a single CNS synapse, NMDA receptors usually coexist with either AMPA or KA receptors and are thought to be involved in amplification of the glutamate signal, although examples of primarily NMDA- mediated synaptic responses have been reported. At resting potentials, NMDA channels are normally blocked by Mg^{2+} and there must be sufficient concurrent depolarization of the postsynaptic neuronal membrane before the Mg^{2+} block is relieved and the NMDA channel can contribute to the electrical response of the cell. The level of concurrent depolarization depends on AMPA/KA activation and/or other modulatory postsynaptic signals controlling depolarization. (70)

Precise modulation of NMDA channel activity is required for normal neuronal function, and, as expected, there are several regulatory sites on the NMDA receptor/channel complex which control NMDA- mediated activity further. The binding of glycine to the receptor/channel complex increases the frequency of agonist-induced channel opening. Glycine binding appears to be an absolute requirement for NMDA channel activation. Studies of the NMDA receptor/channel complex at the molecular level indicate that binding of two glycine and two glutamate molecules is required for channel activation. The receptor/channel complex also includes a polyamine binding site which, when activated, potentiates the NMDA current by increasing channel open probability. This is due, in part, to an increase in glycine binding. (71)

The NMDA receptor/channel complex can also be inhibited via a Zn^{2+} binding site. Thus, there is capacity for several different mechanisms for both positive and negative control of NMDA channel function. (72)

Sigma-1

Sigma-1 receptors are associated with Alzheimer's disease, major depressive disorders, and schizophrenia. These receptors show pro-growth/anti-apoptotic properties via their chaperoning functions to counteract ER (endoplasmic reticulum) stress, to block neurodegeneration, and to regulate neuritogenesis. (73)

Activation of sigma-1 receptors (Sig-1R) reportedly has antidepressant-like action. Limited data suggest that Sig-1Rs also modulate anxiety-related behaviors. Sigma receptors (SigRs) are non-opioid, non-phencyclidine, intracellular receptors that modulate multiple signal transduction and neurotransmitter systems. The Sig-1Rs are widely expressed within the limbic systems and brainstem motor structures. The highest levels of Sig-1R were observed in the olfactory bulb, hypothalamus and hippocampus, with the caudate-putamen, septum, nucleus accumbens and amygdala. (74[1])

In animal models, blockade of Sig-1Rs is known to attenuate the rewarding and toxic properties of drugs of abuse, including psychostimulants and ethanol. Conversely, activation of Sig-1R exerts neuroprotective effects and improves upon learning and memory impairments .(75)

Neuroactive neurosteroids, including progesterone, allopregnanolone, pregnenolone, and DHEA have been shown to act as Sigma-1 ligands exerting a potent neuromodulation on excitatory neurotransmitter systems, including the glutamate and cholinergic systems. (76)

Lobes of the Brain and Functioning

An understanding of the functional aspects of the different lobes of the brain can allow for a greater clinical assessment of the patient. As you will learn in the chapter on neuroradiology, not all types of injury affecting the functioning of the brain can be illuminated by CT or MRI scans. Therefore, the ability to recognized specific functional weaknesses in clinical assessment can help to arrive at a preliminary diagnosis involving one or more areas of the brain. The Millennium has developed a clinical assessment tool called the Clinical Brain Injury Locator (CBIL)® which can assist in qualifying where brain injury has impacted neurological functioning. A copy of this document is included in this book's supplement, which is entitled, *Office Documentation for TBI.*

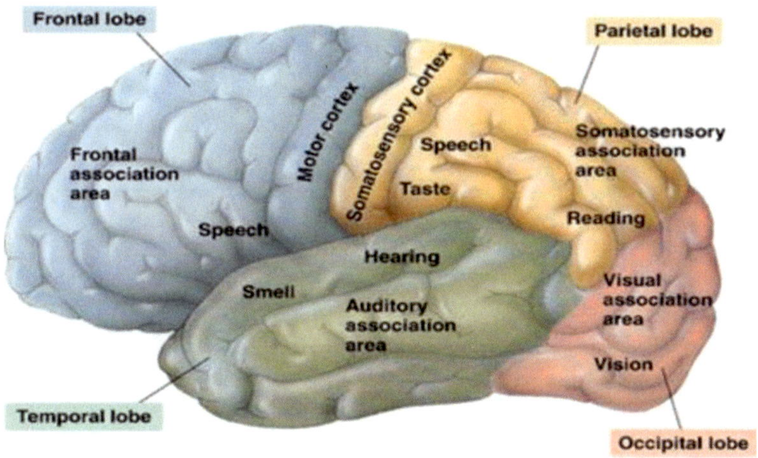

The Frontal Lobe

The frontal lobe is an area in the brain of mammals, located at the front of each cerebral hemisphere and positioned anterior to the parietal lobe and superior and anterior to the temporal lobes. (77*) It is separated from the parietal lobe by a space between tissues called the central sulcus, and from the temporal lobe by a deep fold called the lateral (Sylvian) sulcus .(78) The precentral gyrus (79), forming the posterior border of the frontal lobe, contains the primary motor cortex, which controls voluntary movements of specific body parts.

The frontal lobe contains most of the dopamine-sensitive neurons in the cerebral cortex. The dopamine system is associated with reward, attention, short-term memory tasks, planning, and motivation. Dopamine tends to limit and select sensory information arriving from the thalamus to the fore-brain. A reduction in dopamine activity in the prefrontal cortex is related to poorer performance and inefficient functioning of that brain region during working memory tasks, and to slightly increased risk for schizophrenia. (80)

The executive functions of the frontal lobes involve the ability to recognize future consequences resulting from current actions, to choose between good and bad actions, override and suppress socially unacceptable responses, and determine similarities and differences between things or events.

The frontal lobes also play an important part in retaining longer term memories which are not task-based. These are often memories associated with emotions derived from input from the brain's limbic system. (81) The frontal lobe modifies those emotions to generally fit socially acceptable norms.

Direct damage to the Frontal Lobe or interruption of communication can be associated with:

- Loss of simple movement of various body parts

- Inability to plan a sequence of complex movements, such as making coffee (Sequencing).

- Loss of spontaneity in interacting with others.

- Loss of flexibility in thinking.

- Persistence of a single thought (Perseveration).

- Inability to focus on task (Attending).

- Mood changes (Emotionally Labile).

- Changes in social behavior.

- Changes in personality.

- Difficulty with problem solving.

- Inability to express language (Broca's Aphasia).

The Parietal Lobe

The parietal lobe is a part of the brain positioned above the occipital lobe and behind the frontal lobe. (82*) The parietal lobe plays important roles in integrating sensory information from various parts of the body, knowledge of numbers and their relations, and in the manipulation of objects. Its function also includes processing information relating to the sense of touch. Portions of the parietal lobe are involved with visuospatial processing. (83) Although multi-sensory in nature, the posterior parietal cortex is often referred to by vision scientists as the dorsal stream of vision. This dorsal stream has been called both the 'where' stream (as in spatial vision) and the 'how' stream (as in vision for action). The posterior parietal cortex (PPC) receives somatosensory and/or visual input, which then, through motor signals, controls movement of the arm, hand, as well as eye movements.

The Parietal lobe is divided into two hemispheres — left and right. The left hemisphere is involved in symbolic functions in language and mathematics, meanwhile, the right hemisphere is specialized to carry out images and understanding of maps, i.e., spatial relationships. When damage occurs to the right hemisphere there is loss of imagery, visualization of spatial relationships and neglect of left-sided space and left side of the body. Damage to the left hemisphere will result in problems in mathematics, long reading, writing, and understanding symbols. The parietal association cortex enables individuals to read, write, and solve mathematical problems. The sensory inputs from the right side of the body go to the left side of the brain and vice-versa. Additionally, both the left and right parietal systems play a determining role in self-transcendence (84), the personality trait measuring predisposition to spirituality.

Direct damage to the Parietal Lobe or interruption of communication can be associated with:

- Inability to attend to more than one object at a time.
- Inability to name an object (Anomia).
- Inability to locate the words for writing (Agraphia).
- Problems with reading (Alexia).
- Difficulty with drawing objects.
- Difficulty in distinguishing left from right.
- Difficulty with doing mathematics (Dyscalculia).
- Lack of self-awareness and/or surrounding space (Apraxia).
- Inability to focus visual attention.
- Difficulties with eye and hand coordination.

The Temporal Lobe

The temporal lobe is a region of the cerebral cortex that is located beneath the Lateral fissure (Sylvian) on both cerebral hemispheres of the mammalian brain. The temporal lobes are involved in functions that control the retention of visual memories; processing of sensory input; comprehending language; storing new memories; emotion and deriving meaning from all forms of input data. (85*)

The medial temporal lobes are thought to be involved in encoding into declarative long term memory. (86) The medial temporal lobes include the hippocampus (87), which plays a key role in the formation of explicit long-term memory (88) modulated by the amygdala (89); therefore damage to this area can result in impairment in new memory formation leading to permanent or temporary anterograde amnesia. (90)

The areas associated for vision in the temporal lobe interpret the meaning of visual stimuli and establish object recognition. The ventral portions of the temporal cortices appear to be involved in high-level visual processing of complex stimuli such as faces (fusiform gyrus) (91) and scenes (parahippocampal gyrus). (92) Anterior parts of this ventral stream (93) for visual processing (94) are involved in object perception and recognition.

Adjacent areas in the superior, posterior and lateral parts of the temporal lobes are involved in high-level auditory processing. The temporal lobe is involved in primary auditory perception (95), such as hearing and holds the primary auditory cortex. (96) The superior temporal gyrus (97) includes an area where signals from the ear first reach the cerebral cortex and are processed by the primary auditory cortex in the left temporal lobe. The left temporal lobe holds the primary auditory cortex which is important for the processing of semantics in both speech and vision in humans. Wernicke's area (98), which spans the region between temporal and parietal lobes, plays a key role in speech comprehension. The left temporal lobe encases the primary auditory cortex, which goes beyond low-level perception but, extend to comprehension, naming, verbal memory (99) and other language functions.

Direct damage to the Temporal Lobe or interruption of communication can be associated with:

- Difficulty in recognizing faces (Prosopagnosia).

- Difficulty in understanding spoken words (Wernicke's Aphasia).

- Difficulty with verbal ID of objects.

- Short term memory loss.

- Interference with long term memory.

- Alteration in Libido and Sexual Behavior.

- Inability to categorize objects (Categorization).

- Right lobe damage can cause persistent talking.

- Increased aggressive behavior.

The Occipital Lobe

The occipital lobe contains the primary visual cortex and is the visual processing center of the mammalian brain containing most of the anatomical region of the visual cortex. (100*) The primary visual cortex is

Brodmann area 17 (101), commonly called V1 (visual one). Human V1 is located on the medial side of the occipital lobe within the calcarine sulcus; the full extent of V1 often continues onto the posterior pole of the occipital lobe. V1 is often also called striate cortex because it can be identified by a large stripe of myelin, the Stria of Gennari. (102) Visually driven regions outside V1 are called extrastriate cortex that are specialized for different visual tasks, such as visuospatial processing, color discrimination and motion perception. (103)

If one occipital lobe is damaged, the result can be homonymous hemianopsia vision loss from similarly positioned "field cuts" in each eye. Occipital lesions can cause visual hallucinations. Lesions in the parietal-temporal-occipital association area are associated with color agnosia, movement agnosia, and agraphia. Damage to the primary visual cortex which is located on the surface of the posterior occipital lobe, can cause blindness due to the holes in the visual map on the surface of the visual cortex that resulted from the lesion(s). Direct damage to the Occipital Lobe or interruption of communication can be associated with:

- Defects in vision (Visual Field Cuts).
- Difficulty with locating objects in environment.
- Difficulty with identifying colors (Color Agnosia).
- Production of hallucinations.
- Visual illusions — inaccurately seeing objects.
- Word blindness — inability to recognize words.
- Difficulty in recognizing drawn objects.
- Inability to recognize the movement of object.
- Difficulties with reading and writing.

The Cerebellum

The cerebellum (the "real little brain") is a region of the brain that plays an important role in motor control. (104) It may also be involved in some cognitive functions such as attention and language, and in regulating fear and pleasure responses (105), but its movement-related functions are the most solidly established. The cerebellum does not initiate movement, but it contributes to coordination (106), precision, and accurate timing. It receives input from sensory systems of the spinal cord and from other parts of the brain, and integrates these inputs to fine tune motor activity. Because of this fine-tuning function, damage to the cerebellum does not cause paralysis, but instead produces disorders in fine movement, equilibrium, posture, and motor learning.

In terms of anatomy, the cerebellum has the appearance of a separate structure attached to the bottom of the brain, tucked underneath the cerebral hemispheres. The surface of the cerebellum is covered with finely spaced parallel grooves, in striking contrast to the broad irregular convolutions of the cerebral cortex. These parallel grooves conceal the fact that the cerebellum is actually a continuous thin layer of tissue (the cerebellar cortex), tightly folded in the style of an accordion. Within this thin layer are several types of neurons with a highly regular arrangement, the most important being Purkinje cells and granule cells. (107[1])

The strongest clues to the function of the cerebellum have come from examining the consequences of damage to it. Animals and humans with cerebellar dysfunction show, above all, problems with motor control, on the side of the body ipsilateral to the damaged cerebellum. They continue to be able to generate motor activity, but it loses precision, producing erratic, uncoordinated, or incorrectly timed movements. A standard test of cerebellar function is to reach with the tip of the finger for a target at arm's length: A healthy person will move the fingertip in a rapid straight trajectory, whereas a person with cerebellar damage will reach slowly and erratically, with many mid-course corrections. Deficits in non-motor functions are more difficult to detect. Thus, the general conclusion reached decades ago is that the basic function of the cerebellum is not to initiate movements, or to decide which movements to execute, but rather to calibrate the detailed form of a movement. (108)

Direct damage to the Cerebellum or the interruption of communication can be associated with:

- Loss of ability to coordinate fine movements (Ataxia).

- Loss of ability to walk.

- Inability to reach out and grab objects.

- Tremors.

- Dizziness (Vertigo).

- Slurred Speech (Scanning Speech).

- Inability to make rapid movements.

- Negative Romberg's Sign with Ataxia.

The Limbic System

The limbic system (LS) is a group of interconnected cortical and subcortical structures dedicated to linking visceral states and emotion to cognition and behavior. The cortical components of the limbic system include areas separated into limbic and paralimbic zones. The subcortical limbic structures include the amygdala, mammillary bodies, hypothalamus, some thalamic nuclei and the ventral striatum.

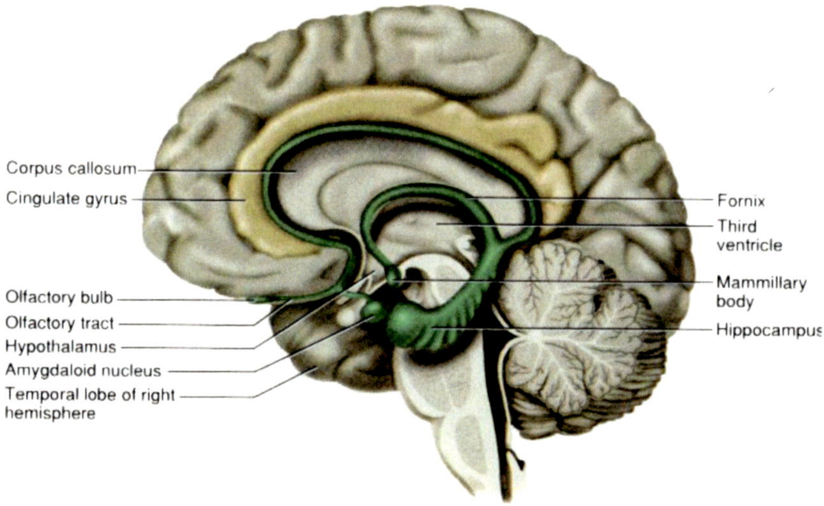

Together they play a concerted role in the regulation and integration of cognition, affect, sensory perception, biological behavior, and autonomic, immunological and endocrine functions. They set the level of arousal and are involved in motivation and reinforcing behaviors. Many of these areas are critical to particular types of memory. (109[1]) A brief description of the major structures follows.

The Hypothalamus

The hypothalamus is a small part of the brain located just below the thalamus on both sides of the third ventricle. It sits just inside the two tracts of the optic nerve, and just above the pituitary gland.

The hypothalamus is one of the busiest parts of the brain, and is mainly concerned with homeostasis (110a); the process of returning something to an established "set point." It is responsible for regulating your hunger, thirst, response to pain, levels of pleasure, sexual satisfaction, anger and aggressive behavior. It also regulates the functioning of the autonomic nervous system (110b), including pulse, blood pressure, breathing, and arousal in response to diverse emotional circumstances.

The hypothalamus receives inputs from a number of sources; from the vagus nerve (110c), it gets information about blood pressure and the distension of the gut. From the reticular formation in the brainstem, it gets information about skin temperature. From the optic nerve (110d), it gets information about light and darkness. From specialized neurons lining the ventricles, it gets information about the contents of the cerebrospinal fluid, including toxins that lead to vomiting. And from the other parts of the limbic system and the olfactory nerves (110e), it gets information that helps regulate eating and sexuality. The hypothalamus also has some receptors of its own, that provide information about ion balance and temperature of the blood.

As an aside, the hypothalamus has been found to use the increasing serum levels of Leptin (111) to decrease one's appetite. Leptin is mostly produced in the body's white fat cells (White Adipose Tissue) that is a primary source of healthy stores of energy. As the level of Leptin increases the hypothalamus is responsible to signal "stop eating" (Satiation Center). Apparently, this system is broken in many of us.

The hypothalamus sends instructions to the rest of the body in two ways. The first is to the autonomic nervous system allowing the hypothalamus to have ultimate control of things like blood pressure, heart rate, breathing, digestion, sweating, and all the sympathetic and parasympathetic functions. (112) The second is by way of trophic hormone signals sent to the anterior pituitary gland through the hypophyseal portal system and to the posterior pituitary gland through long axons.

Type 2 diabetes mellitus results from the complex association of insulin resistance and pancreatic beta-cell failure. Recently, inflammation of the hypothalamus has been found to increase the occurrence of insulin resistant type II diabetes. (113*)Many of the neural inputs that control Beta cell activity are generated in the hypothalamus. (114) Therefore, the development of Insulin Resistance (Metabolic Syndrome) Diabetes can develop post-TBI when the hypothalamus is damaged.

Of great importance to the premise of this book, is the fact that the hypothalamus controls the release of life-maintaining and promoting hormones via its neural and chemical connection to the pituitary gland. It is the interruption of this control that lead to the development of both insufficiencies and deficiencies of our hormones, a topic to be developed in Chapter 4: Neuroendocrinology.

Thalamus

The thalamus has a multitude of functions acting as a way-station or switchboard of information. It provides switching and relay capacity between subcortical areas and the cerebral cortex. In particular, every sensory system (save the olfactory system) includes a thalamic nucleus that receives sensory signals and sends them to the associated primary cortical area. For the visual system, for example, inputs from the retina are sent to the lateral geniculate nucleus (115a) of the thalamus, which in turn projects to the primary visual cortex (115b) in the occipital lobe. The thalamus is believed to both process sensory information as well as relay it—each of the primary sensory relay areas receives strong "back projections" from the cerebral cortex. Similarly the medial geniculate nucleus (116) acts as a key auditory relay between the inferior colliculus (117) of the midbrain and the primary auditory cortex, and the ventral posterior nucleus (118) is a key somatosensory relay (119), which sends touch and proprioceptive (120) information to the primary somatosensory cortex. (121)

The thalamus also plays an important role in regulating states of sleep and wakefulness. Thalamic nuclei have strong reciprocal connections with the cerebral cortex, forming thalamo-cortico-thalamic circuits (122) that are believed to be involved with consciousness. The thalamus plays a major role in regulating arousal, the level of awareness, and activity. Damage to the thalamus can lead to permanent coma.

Hippocampus

The Hippocampus consists of two "horns" that curve back from the amygdala. It appears to be very important in converting things that are "in your mind" at the moment (in short-term memory) into things that you will remember for the long run (long-term memory). If the hippocampus is damaged, a person cannot build new memories and lives instead in a strange world where everything they experience just fades away, even while older memories from the time before the damage are untouched. (123[1])

Amygdalas

The amygdalas are two almond-shaped masses of neurons on either side of the thalamus at the lower end of the hippocampus. When it is stimulated electrically, animals respond with aggression. And if the amygdala is removed, animals get very tame and no longer respond to things that would have caused rage before. But there is more to it than just anger. When removed, animals also become indifferent to stimuli that would have otherwise have caused fear and even sexual responses. (124*)

Summary

Traumatic brain injury (TBI) induces secondary molecular changes that lead to neuronal death, microglial activation, inflammation, and reactive astrogliosis. (125) Collectively, these alterations contribute to tissue loss, as well as glial scar formation, which may serve to impair recovery and alter important connective pathways between different regions, nuclei, and centers in the brain. (126) The magnitude of the neurotrauma will regulate, for the most part, the perseverance of who we were prior to the trauma.

Damage to the brain's ability to convey information from somatosensory systems to emotional and cognitive processes can lead to a number of affective disorders of mood, anger, aggression, agitation, and fear. The unifying relationship is in the brains ability to appropriately conduct the direct and indirect neuroelectrical and neurochemical impulses down interconnecting pathways that link interpretation, responsiveness, and execution of thoughts.

Reactive (responding to a threat) and instrumental aggression (a pre-emptive response in anticipation of a threat) are examples of how a good system can go bad. Damage to the frontal cortices and/or amygdala can lead to disruption of connectivity between areas which adjudicate the level of personal threat and provide an appropriate response. A healthy response to a pedestrian walking towards you on a busy street might be; to just walk past them or even to say hello. While under conditions of damage secondary to TBI, the pedestrian might be perceived as a threat thereby being verbally or physically accosted. (127)

This chapter has offered on a microscopic level, the cellular components of the brain that develop, propagate, and modulate electrochemical impulses to, from, and between emotional and motor areas of the different lobes. We have addressed on the macroscopic level the roles that each lobe and region of the brain plays in providing us with normal functioning. In as short as the blink of an eye, these can be lost — leaving the host with a diminished functional capacity. Recognition of the areas of damage is only an academic exercise that allows for our abilities as clinical practitioners to test our acumen. The real challenge here is in the subsequent steps in which we take, that will provide the patient with notable improvement and leave us with the satisfaction of knowing we made a difference. The continuation of providing traditional approaches will afford us no change since we will continue to obtain traditional outcomes.

Chapter 3: Neuropathology in TBI

"This is only the tip of the iceberg; just a small indication of a larger possibility."

— Anonymous

Introduction

Trauma to the hypothalamic-pituitary axis (HP) is underestimated in most cases of mild, non-penetrating, traumatic brain injury (mTBI). (1) Frequently, as the initial symptoms associated with the physical component of trauma fades, an underlying and insidious process takes on a more dominant role that can take decades to become clinically evident. (2) Many times, the acute symptoms are not due to the physical trauma, but from activation of disruptive biochemical pathways within the brain. (3) Recent data suggests that pituitary hormone deficiency is not infrequent amongst moderate and severe TBI survivors with as many as 40 to 50 percent of these patients reported to develop some degree of pituitary dysfunction. (4, 5) While in mTBI, the reports have varied from 23 percent to 84 percent of cases having from one or more hormone deficiencies. (6)

It has been the popular perception that the causative factor for hormonal deficiencies and more frequently, insufficiencies in TBI is due to direct trauma to the pituitary gland, its stalk or its blood supply. (7[1]) Based upon high-resolution MRI studies using a 3.0 Tesla coil, only 14 percent of the mTBI cases showed evidence of pituitary gland involvement (8) leaving other mechanisms as causative factors for hormonal dysregulation. (9, 10, 11) It is the contention of this author that traumatic brain injury can cause a number of destructive pathways to be initiated that can lead to the ultimate dysregulation of hormones (neurosteroids and neuroactive steroids). Furthermore, it is this dysregulation within the central nervous system that creates the clinical presentation that is ultimately treated with a superficial approach frequently consisting of mood altering medication.

In the years since, Millennium-TBI has addressed the underlying hormonal and oxidative stress conditions that lead to mood and cognitive alterations, many of the patients were able to stop those medications that only mask the symptoms doing little for true recovery. Only with an understanding of the diffuse environmental changes that occur to the traumatically injured brain parenchyma, examining both the cellular and subcellular responses evoked by TBI to neurons and their axonal extensions, can a more adept treatment protocol be provided that addresses what is broken and not just mask the symptoms.

Macro-traumatic Brain Injury

The primary phase of brain injury is mechanical in nature where cerebral contusions, intracerebral hemorrhages, subarachnoid hemorrhages, subdural hematomas, and edema are its hallmark. (12) On a microscopic level, the forces of injury can cause "shearing" of axons due to the density differences between the margins of the white and gray matter making up the brain. The gray matter, representing the neuronal bodies, is denser than the white matter, which is made up of long axons emanating from these neurons. (13*) Sudden impact forces whether due to a physical object or blast waves from an IED, imparts momentum to the calvarium causing the gray matter to move faster than the white matter, causing shearing of axons and any associated capillaries at the margin between the white and gray matters. This is referred to as Diffuse Axonal Injury (DAI) and is the principle pathology in 40 to 50 percent of TBI hospitalized patients as well as a major contributing factor for loss of consciousness (LOC) and interruption of communication between different lobes within the brain. (14*)

Biomechanical impact associated with blunt trauma tends to be associated with damage to the gray matter, while a diffuse impact (blast trauma, IED) is associated with injury to the white matter. In this instance, it appears that rotational forces caused by explosions, coup-counter-coup type of injuries are distinct causes of shearing force injury to axons. (15*)

Although the Glasgow Coma Score (GCS) is predictive of neurological consequences in moderate to severe TBI (16), in mild TBI (GCS above 13 without loss of consciousness) subsequent neurological aberrations can be ascribed to the precipitation of neurochemical cascades leading to the processes of apoptosis, necrosis, autophagy, or parthanatos with subsequent neuronal death. (17)

Micro-traumatic Brain Injury

Acute cellular damage at the time of primary injury yields increased production of reactive oxygen species (ROS) due to excitotoxicity and exhaustion of the endogenous antioxidant system (18) within the brain. The growing oxidative stress induces peroxidation of cellular and vascular structures, protein oxidation, cleavage of DNA, and inhibition of the mitochondrial electron transport chain on top of release of pro-inflammatory cytokines (IL-1β, TNF-α, and IL-6), all adding to create an expanding toxic environment (non-neuropermissive environment) with collateral damage to neighboring and remote neurons. (19) The magnitude of these two processes, mechanical (primary) and neurochemical (secondary), will dictate the ultimate neurological outcome in the TBI patient as well as the effects upon cognition, personality, physiology, and physical aspects that all need to be addressed for protection of the individual's quality of life (QOL).

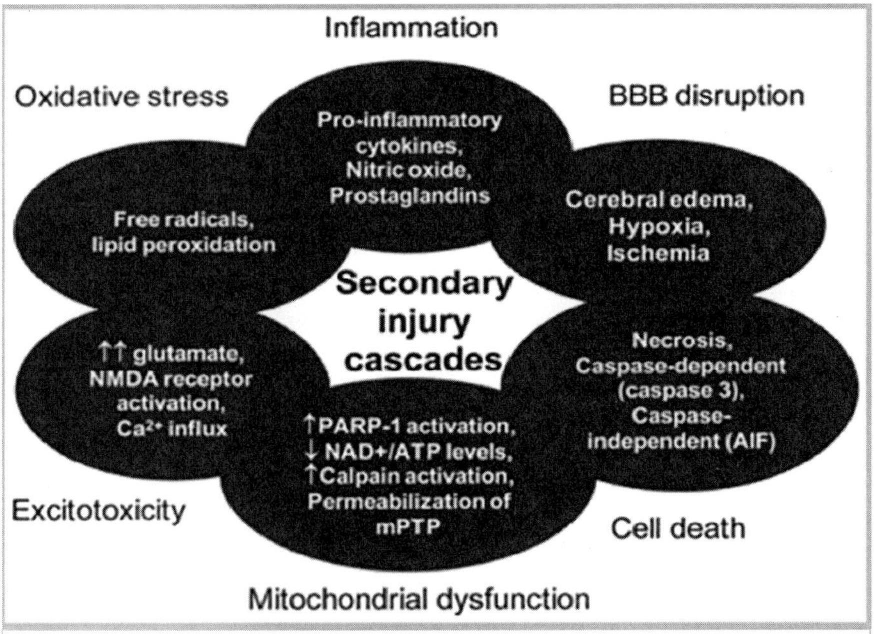

Image 3.1: Secondary injury cascades creating the non-permissive environment decreasing the capacity of neurons to repair, regenerate and communicate. Control of each of these events can foster a Neuropermissive environment with recovery.

During the secondary phase of injury, neuronal and glial cell death, and traumatic axonal injury, due to shearing, all contribute to the neuropathology that becomes the clinical presentation of the patient. As the initial area of injury expands, collateral damage and death of additional neurons and oligodendrocytes contribute to the overall neuropathology associated with traumatic brain injury. It has been observed that neuronal death is associated with focal injuries, while death of oligodendrocytes is a hallmark of diffuse brain trauma. (20*)

Dying neuronal cells exhibit either an apoptotic of a necrotic morphology. Apoptotic and necrotic neurons have been identified within the contusion zone(s) in the acute post-traumatic injury period as well as in regions remote to the site of impact injury within days or weeks after trauma. Degenerating oligodendrocytes and astrocytes have been observed within injured white matter tracts with progression that can persist for months or even years. (21)

Furthermore, accumulating information from a number of studies is defining a pattern of injury between the gray and white matter and their associated cellular portions. Biomechanical impact associated with blunt trauma tends to be associated with damage to the gray matter, while a diffuse impact (blast trauma) is associated with injury to the white matter. In this instance, it appears that rotational forces caused by explosions, coup-counter-coup type of injuries are distinct causes of shearing force injury (22) to axons.

Additionally and subsequent to (blast) trauma, swollen axons in the white matter undergo degeneration or axotomy (23) which is associated with oligodendrocytic death. Aside from trauma, oligodendrocytic death can be induced by reactive microglia (24) and astrocytes that are present in the traumatized white matter. (25*)

It is generally accepted that there is an inflammatory shift in the balance of neurochemistry between pro- and anti-apoptotic protein production (cytokines and cytokinins) known to regulate mechanisms underlying apoptotic cell death. (26) Additionally, findings of post-TBI auto-antibodies to both hypothalamus and pituitary gland offers a further understanding of how insidious and progressive the pathological processes are in TBI. (27, 28)

Regional cell death patterns following TBI suggest that there is an inherent susceptibility to trauma in that there is commonly neuronal loss in the cortex; hippocampus, cerebellum, and thalamus regardless of the focus of the primary trauma. (29) Bilateral loss of hippocampal neurons has been seen in 85 percent of fatal head injury cases as early as 48hrs post trauma. In the early post-traumatic period injured neurons in the contusion become swollen, and then they shrink, become eosinophilic, with pyknosis of the nuclei. Electron microscopic (EM), studies show a generalized swollen appearance to the cell with swollen mitochondria, vacuolated cytoplasm and pyknotic nuclei suggestive of necrosis. (30)

While excitatory amino acids accumulate (excitotoxins like glutamate and aspartate), there is also an increase in intracellular calcium and free radicals that studies have indicated can activate Intrinsic Caspase pathways that can cause neuronal cells to undergo apoptosis. (31*) Transient rises in the cytoplasmic concentration of calcium ions serve as second messenger signals that control many neuronal functions (32*) as well as increases damage to both endoplasmic reticula and mitochondria.

The appreciation of a delayed or chronic component to the post-traumatic period has been based upon the finding of a time-dependent increase in the volume of degenerating neurons in cortical lesions. This can account for a patient's slow progression of neurological deficits and changes in radiographic studies over time. (33)

The Non Neuro-permissive Environment

Oxidative Stress

A cardinal and damaging event that occurs in all forms of TBI (including surgery, stroke, Alzheimer's disease, radiation exposure, and chemotherapy), is that of oxidative stress (OS). OS is represented by the production of free radicals from impaired mitochondrial metabolism, an overwhelmed endogenous antioxidant system, and exacerbated by a number of inflammatory byproducts (heme degradation, nitric oxide, nitriles and a slew of other chemicals all categorized as reactive oxygen species (ROS) and reactive nitrogen species (RNS). (34*)

In order to understand the mechanism by which mild neurotrauma (mTBI) can precipitate an acute loss of neuronal functioning followed by a protracted neurodegenerative course over many years (35), we must look closely at the intracellular cascades or "death marches" that can be triggered by ROS and RNS as well as proinflammatory chemistry; those reactive products that become deadly. Once you become familiar with these mechanisms your treatment options will become plentiful.

Under conditions precipitated by TBI, the mitochondria attempt to generate more energy (ATP) either in compensation for the loss of energy production from other cells or under the reactive stimulation by toxic elements (calcium, hypoxia, and hypoglycemia). The net effect is that there is an increased demand for energy with a concomitant loss of the endogenous antioxidant mechanisms to deal with rising ROS causing oxidative stress to loom. Oxidative stress occurs within 30 minutes after TBI and may account for the early mitochondrial dysfunction following injury. (36[1])

Within hours of traumatic brain injury, both the intra- and extracellular environments are overwhelmed by rising levels of neurotoxic substances from reactive oxygen species, interleukins (37), caspases (38), calpain, cytokines, calcium, excitotoxic glutamate, proteases, kinases(39), nitric oxide, endonucleases (40), and more. Many of these are constituents of a healthy brain that is also endowed with a number of robust mechanisms to deal with vacillations in their levels in order to maintain a fit and healthy environment (pro-neuron). Unfortunately, insults to the brain causing ischemia, hemorrhage, anoxia, and hypoglycemia can tip the balance in favor of creating a toxic non-permissive environment where neurons are lost. (41)

Under normal activities of daily living, oxygen itself an oxidant containing two unpaired electrons, is used by mitochondria to generate the energy molecule ATP. The mitochondria are the main source of ROS although other endogenous sources of ROS in the brain include enzymatic processes in which ROS are generated directly or indirectly (e.g., monoamine oxidase, nitric oxide synthase, and cyclooxygenase) from cells such as activated neutrophils. (42*)

The direct-acting group contains proteins such as superoxide dismutase (43), catalase, and peroxidase, which can remove hydrogen peroxide, the product of the dismutation reaction. (44) Under normal conditions, the more the brain tissue is exposed to oxidative stress the more efficient and complex is its antioxidant defense system. Hence, the brain, which is particularly vulnerable to oxidative damage, possesses an extremely efficient antioxidant activity. (45)

$$O_2- + H_2O \rightarrow H_2O_2 + O_2^{\circ -}$$

Image 3.2: Production of superoxide radical from oxygen and water.

The generation of mitochondrial ROS is a consequence of oxidative phosphorylation (46), a process that occurs in the inner mitochondrial membrane and involves the oxidation of NADH to produce ATP. However, during mitochondrial electron transport, a one-electron reduction of O_2 results in superoxide anions ($O_2^{\circ -}$). Studies on isolated mitochondria in the presence of a high, non-physiological concentration of oxygen estimated that mitochondria convert one to two percent of the oxygen molecules consumed into $O_2^{\circ-}$. Superoxide anion is detoxified by the mitochondrial manganese superoxide dismutase (SOD) (47) to yield hydrogen peroxide (H_2O_2), which is then converted to H_2O by catalase. (48)

$$O_2^- + O_2^- + H_2^+ \rightarrow H_2O_2 + O_2$$

Image 3.3: Production of hydrogen peroxide from super oxide radicals.

Recent studies on the time course of mitochondrial failure during the first 72 hours after TBI revealed that mitochondrial respiratory dysfunction, as a result of changes in oxidative phosphorylation, occurred simultaneously with the appearance of oxidative markers and were sustained for up to 72 hours. (49) It was also demonstrated that, after TBI, cortical mitochondria displayed progressive (three to twelve hours) structural damage consisting of swelling and breakage of the outer membranes due to the reactive nitrogen species ONOO-(peroxynitrite), the product of the reaction between NO radical and superoxide radical, during post-traumatic mitochondrial dysfunction. (50)

The pathophysiological cascade induced after TBI is initiated by an excitotoxic process triggered by excessive glutamate release. Glutamate is the major mediator of excitatory signals in the CNS and is involved in most aspects of normal brain function including cognition, memory, and learning. (51)

Following head injury, increasing levels of extracellular glutamate cause over-stimulation of metabotropic (52) and ionotropic (53) receptors that may result in secondary events leading to neuronal cell death. The ionotropic receptors regulate the opening of ion pores for the movement of Ca+, Na+, and K+ while the metabotropic receptors use a second messenger system based upon binding sites on the cell membrane. Activation of metabotropic receptors causes mobilization of calcium from internal stores found in the endoplasmic reticulum (54) and mitochondria. A sudden rise in cytoplasmic calcium will trigger caspase-12 activation leading to some degree of apoptotic cell death, necrosis and autophagy.

Oxidative stress relates to the generation of reactive oxygen species (oxygen free radicals and associated entities including superoxides, hydrogen peroxide, nitric oxide, and peroxynitrite) in response to TBI. The excessive production of reactive oxygen species due to excitotoxicity and exhaustion of the endogenous antioxidant system (e.g., superoxide dismutase, glutathione peroxidase, and catalase) induces peroxidation of cellular and vascular structures, protein oxidation, cleavage of DNA, and inhibition of the mitochondrial electron transport chain. Although these mechanisms are adequate to contribute to immediate cell death, inflammatory processes and early or late apoptotic programs are induced by oxidative stress. (55) Once created this non-neuropermissive environment (NNPE) promotes the progressive loss of neurons, glia and the inhibition of repair mechanisms. (56)

Inflammation

The impact of oxidative stress on the cerebral environment can be catastrophic due to the loss of cellular integrity. Lipid peroxidation alters the neuronal cell membrane allowing for disruption of the ion-gated channels and their ATP dependent transport. Loss of transport regulation allows for ions to pass into the cytoplasm leading to the initiation of caspases, calpain, and the rise in cytokines (IL-1β), culminating in cell death. (57) The rate and extent of this process, based upon the magnitude of trauma, will dictate the type and extent of the four cellular responses; necrosis, apoptosis, autophagy, and parthanatos.

Inflammation, although initiated by a combination of factors (hypoxia, hypoglycemia, ischemia, oxidative stressor, and autoimmunity) has at its core an immunologic response that is designed to protect by ultimately minimizing damage. Microglia, are the macrophages of the central nervous system (CNS), are ubiquitously distributed in the CNS, being the first elements that react to the pathophysiological stimuli; thus, they participate in all brain pathologies, either chronic or acute. (58*) In response to these different triggers, microglia change shape, motility, expression of innate and adaptive immune molecules and function; they release various cytokines, chemokines, reactive oxygen species, and prostaglandin metabolites, bringing a major and direct contribution to neuroinflammation and thereby promoting neurodegeneration. (59*)

Cytokines and chemokines representing the pro-and anti-inflammatory limbs of the immune system (TH1 and TH2) are constantly battling for homeostasis under normal situation being influenced by epigenomic and genomic factors. (60) Impacted by mTBI, the immune system favors a more inflammatory condition brought on by the body's innate and automated directives to survive. In this process, cells are removed that are perceived to be damaged beyond repair (apoptosis) or leaking calcium (endoplasmic reticula and mitochondria) to be engulfed in autophagosomes where they are digested to their elemental components for use elsewhere. (61*)

Fragmented cells, lipid peroxidation, or an altered pH can cause damage to proteins rendering them "foreign" thereby precipitating an auto-immune response such as that which would happen with Neisseria meningitides. Activated microglia respond to this perceived incursion by mounting a defensive line with additional chemistry (cytokines) that only increase the oxidative stress and state of inflammation.

Astrocytes are responsible for supporting neurons, promotion of myelin production (62), modulation of electrical and chemical transmissions, regulation of ion transport, and metabolism of neurosteroids. (63) Research has shown that TBI patients develop autoantibodies directed primarily against glial fibrillary acidic protein (GFAP) and its breakdown products (BDP). GFAP is an intermediate filament protein specifically localized to the cytoskeleton of mature astrocytes, the most abundant cell type in the central nervous system. TBI patients showed an average 3.77 fold increase in anti-GFAP autoantibody levels from early (zero to one days) to late (seven to ten days) times post injury. Changes in autoantibody levels were negatively correlated with outcome as measured by GOS-E score at six months, suggesting that TBI patients with greater anti-GFAP immune-responses had worse outcomes. (64)

Excitotoxicity

Excitotoxicity is a process resulting from the overstimulation of glutamate receptors. Three types of ionotropic glutamatergic receptors (65) are activated by this over abundant state: N-methyl-D-aspartate (NMDA) receptor, 2-amino-5-methylisoxazol propionic acid receptor (AMPAR), and kainic acid receptor (KA). (66) When activated, AMPAR leads to the entry of Na+ into the cell contributing to membrane depolarization. Intracellular water increases inducing cellular swelling. When activated, NMDA receptor promotes the entry of Na+ and Ca^{2+} into the cell contributing to membrane depolarization and to activation of Ca^{2+} -dependent enzymes. When activated, the KA receptor can increase the epileptogenic occurrence of seizures. (67) Furthermore, the threshold at which kainic acid receptor stimulation can produce seizure activity is decreased under conditions characterized by a decline in endogenous levels of the neurosteroid Allopregnanolone. (68)

The important role that calcium plays in cell death has been under investigation for over ten years. Calcium overload can trigger many downstream neurotoxic cascades, including the uncoupling of mitochondrial electron transfer from ATP synthesis, and the activation and overstimulation of enzymes, such as calpains, protein kinases, endonucleases, and nitric oxide synthetase. (69) Additionally, imaging techniques have shown that astrocytes exposed to increased cytoplasmic Ca^{2+} release the excitatory neurotransmitter glutamate which augments the neurotransmitter released by the neuron. (70)

Studies have suggested that calcium-mediated cell death following neurotrauma was the "final common pathway." The increase in cytosol calcium, from either or both extracellular and intracellular sources, leads to the activation of calcium activation dependent proteases called calpains. (71) These have been implicated in the pathogeneses of TBI and the means by which neuronal death occurs. Activation of calpains leads to proteolysis of a number of intracellular proteins such as cytoskeletal proteins (72) only in cells that are involved in the direct areas of neurotrauma or those neurons and cells adjacent to the trauma site. In vitro studies suggest that low levels of intracellular calcium may initiate apoptotic pathways while a high elevated intracellular level may initiate necrosis. Additionally, activation of calpain may preferentially be associated with necrotic more than apoptotic cell death. (73*)

Cell Death Mechanisms

Apoptosis (programmed cell death) represents a highly sophisticated and organized mechanism by which cells are put to death and their remnants neatly collected and removed avoiding inflammation and collateral damage. (74*) On the other hand, necrosis is a messy process leaving inflammation and collateral damage to healthy neighboring cells (and tissues). (75) These two major types of cell death are joined by a third mode, autophagy, which is characterized by a process in which cells digest their own organelles (endoplasmic reticulum, mitochondrion, and Golgi bodies) and structural proteins (cytoskeleton and cytosolic macromolecules) cannibalizing their structural components to build newer organelles or to effect cell repair. (76) This is seen as a cellular conservation effort when energy stores or the ability to produce adequate

ATP is in jeopardy, like during starvation. This process is not associated with local inflammation and does not affect its neighbors.

	Necrosis	Apoptosis	Autophagy	Parthanatos
Nucleus Fragmentation	No	Yes	No	Yes
Chromatin Condensation	No	Yes	No	Yes
Apoptotic Bodies	No	Yes	No	No
Cytoplasmic Vacuolation	Yes	No	Yes	No
Organelle Degradation	Yes	No	Yes	No
Mitochondrial Swelling	Yes	Late	Variable	-
Cytoplasmic Swelling	Yes	No	No	No
Caspase Activity	No	Yes	No	No
PARP	Active	Cleaved	No`	Yes
Cathepsin B	No	No	Yes	?
Bcl-2 Protein	No	Yes	No	No
Death Associated Protein	Yes	Yes	Yes	-

Table 3.1: Cellular survival after trauma is based upon the cells ability to initiate self-preservation mechanisms. Severe cellular damage initiates necrosis while apoptosis and parthanatos deal with moderate damage leaving Autophagy to remove damaged organelle.

Apoptosis, necrosis, and autophagy can each be initiated or modulated by a number of complex control mechanisms that have the ability to crosstalk allowing for the potentiality that each cell-death mechanism can overlap. (77) It is believed that through crosstalk these three mechanisms can arbitrate which one will dominate based upon extracellular signaling.

Moreover, and to confuse issues even more, another cell death mechanism has been described called parthanatos which involves crosstalk between the nuclear polymerase-1 (PARP-1) and mitochondrial apoptosis-inducing factor (AIF). The release of AIF from oxidative stressed mitochondria provides the trigger for turning a repair molecule (PARP-1) into another death messenger. (78) Table 3.1 shows the major comparative differences and similarities amongst the four cellular death mechanism.

As you will learn our previous appreciation of necrosis was one of an uncontrolled process of cell death. Recent research now paints the picture where necrosis is also form of "programmed cell death" where rapid cellular destruction and inflammation are its goal.

Apoptosis (Cell Death Type I)

Aside from a rudimentary 2-dimensional description of this classical process of "programmed cell death", it is nearly impossible to provide clarity of understanding without dividing this process into its subdivisions. Then, at the end we can reconstruct the process putting each subdivision into place so that the incredible complexity of the process of secondary brain injury can be better understood. Personally, each time I reread the many articles used to write this chapter I find myself "spacing out" and visualizing the process as two basketball teams with five balls on the court; nearly impossible to follow the game.

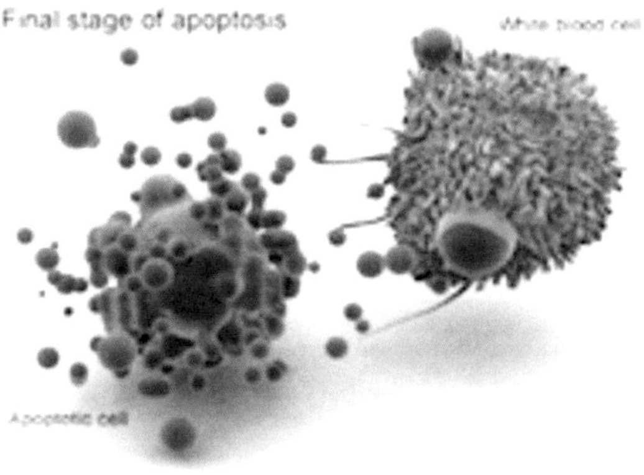

There appear to be three major factors that influence the degree and duration of cellular damage precipitated by one; edema leading to vascular compromise resulting in regional ischemia, hypoxia and hypoglycemia, two; the genetic makeup of the individual regulating either an over-expression or under-expression of pro- or anti-apoptotic proteins, and third; the cross-talking that occurs amongst the four means of cell death including necrosis, autophagy, and parthanatos. (79, 80)

At this point, regardless of the mechanism, the endpoint of neuronal apoptosis after brain injury is the systematic fragmentation of cellular DNA and the collapse of nuclear structure, followed by the formation of membrane wrapped apoptotic bodies that are subsequently cleared by macrophages/microglia signaled by phosphatidylserine's (PS) exposure on the cell membrane surface. (81) The resulting affect is a progressive loss of brain volume and function.

Identification of cellular apoptosis is made possible by the TUNEL technique, a staining process that identifies internucleosomal DNA strand breaks. Following an acute neurological event, neurons and oligodendrocytes display a positive TUNEL test indicating apoptosis has occurred. Researchers have established that neural cell apoptosis is an integral part of TBI and that there exists a biphasic increase in the number of apoptotic cells in the cortex and a delay in appearance of apoptotic cells in the thalamus at one week post injury. Furthermore, TUNEL positive cells, predominantly in the white matter of patients with TBI were observed up to twelve months post-injury. (82)

The process of apoptosis, also called Type-1 Cell Death, can occur by multiple pathways that may be independent although, crosstalk between the different pathways can and does occur. In broad terms, neuronal apoptosis can be separated into two pathways, one involving the activation of a family of cysteine proteases termed ‘Caspases’ (Caspase-3, Caspase-8, and Caspace-9), and therefore, caspase-dependent, and the other involving the caspase-independent release of apoptotic factors from mitochondria (apoptotic inducing factor (AIF), and Cytochrome c). (83)

Tissue trauma triggers a series of molecular events leading to a sudden elevation in neuronal calcium, which has been associated with the activation of a number of calcium-dependent enzymes such as phospholipases, kinases, phosphatases, and proteases. Within the proteases is the family of Caspases, a group of cysteine proteases. The Caspase family proteases include 14 currently identified members that are synthesized as pro-enzymes or zymogens. (84) In a multi-tiered process a group of Initiator Caspases (caspase-8, -9, and -10) must be activated so that they themselves can activate the final apoptotic pathway under the control of the ‘executioners’; Caspase-3, -6, and -7 leading to irreversible cell death. (85*)

Caspase-dependent Apoptosis

Caspase-dependent apoptosis (CDA) can occur via an extrinsic or intrinsic pathway. The extrinsic pathway involves cell surface receptors present on neurons, as well as other cell types. The coupling of cell surface tumor necrosis factor (TNF) with its extracellular TNF-receptor or the Fas receptors with its extracellular Fas ligand causes the receptors to broach the cell surface to form complexes with intracellular signaling molecules: TNF receptor associated death domain protein (TRADD) and Fas-associated protein with death domain (FADD). These death-inducing signaling complexes then bind and induce the activation of caspase-8. Caspase-3 is subsequently cleaved and activated by these initiator Caspases, whereupon the process of apoptosis is now irreversible. (86*)

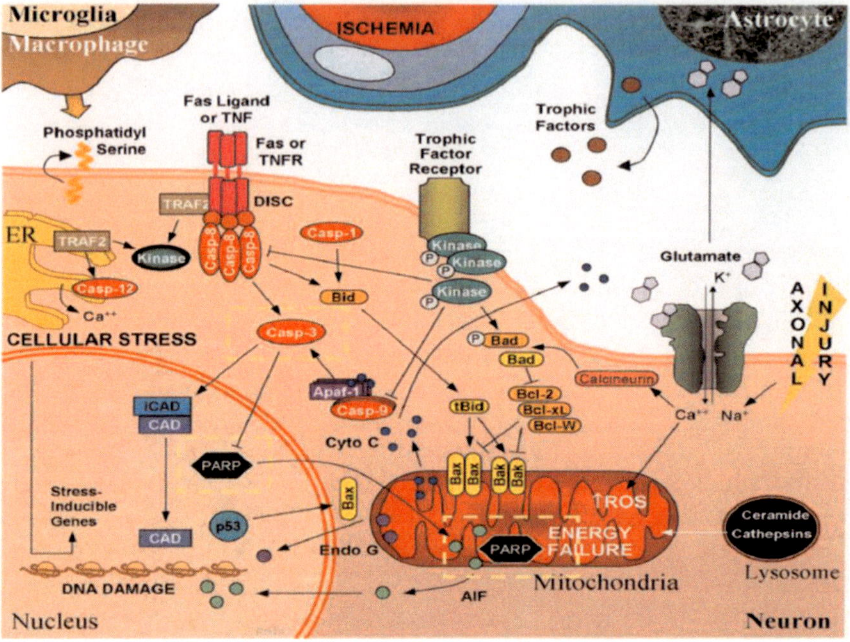

Figure 3.1: Simplified schematic by Zhang et al, representation of the initiation and regulation of neuronal apoptosis after traumatic brain injury (TBI). Pathologic mechanisms triggering apoptosis after TBI include ischemia, oxidative stress, energy failure, excitotoxicity, axonal injury, trophic factor withdrawal, ER stress, and/or death receptor-ligand binding (like TNF, Fas). Execution of apoptosis involves the caspase cascade and/or release of apoptogenic factors from organelles such as mitochondria and lysosomes. Ultimately DNA fragmentation, cytoskeletal disintegration, and externalization of membrane phosphatidylserine occurs, signaling macrophages and microglia to engulf cellular debris.

In the Extrinsic Pathway, damage to neighboring neurons with release of organelle and cytoplasmic proteins, triggers the brain's immune system microglia cells to respond. The microglia produce TNF alpha (TNFα) which acts as the ligand for the TNF cell surface receptors. Once the association has been made the surface Fas-FasL or TNFα-TNFL enters the cell and activates Caspase-8, an initiator caspase. Once Caspase-8 is activated, the messenger of death, Caspase-3 is cleaved and precipitates apoptosis. (87)

When the Intrinsic Pathway is initiated by stress on cellular organelles (oxidative stress, excessive calcium, hypoxia, and hypoglycemia), including mitochondria and endoplasmic reticulum (ER), caspase-dependent apoptosis can be triggered by the mitochondrial release of cytochrome *c* induced after mitochondrial membrane depolarization and formation of mitochondrial permeability transition pores brought on by the oxidative stress. (88) Cytosolic Cytochrome *c* interacts with apoptotic protease activating factor-1 (APAF-1), ATP, and pro-caspase-9 to form a complex termed an 'apoptosome', which in turn activates caspase-3. (89)

Recent data indicate that after being released from mitochondria, cytochrome *c* can translocate to the endoplasmic reticulum to block the inositol trisphosphate receptor (90), amplifying calcium signaling and the release of cytochrome *c* from mitochondria. Endoplasmic reticulum stress, including the disruption of ER calcium homeostasis and accumulation of excess proteins, induce apoptosis by the activation of ER-localized caspase-12. The ER-stress-related activation of caspase-12 has been detected in experimental models of neurodegenerative disease and TBI, although in humans caspase-12 seems to have a role in inflammation but not in apoptosis. (91*)

	Caspase-dependent	**Caspase-independent**
Nucleus	Cleavage of caspase, nuclear fragmentation, chromatin condensation.	Partial chromatin condensation, chromatin marginalization, nuclear shrinkage without fragmentation.
Mitochondrion	MOMP, cleavage of caspase, rapid loss of membrane potential.	MOMP, swollen cristae, gradual loss of membrane potential.
Cytoplasm	Cleavage of caspase, increased Ca^{2+}, protein cross-linkage, condensation.	Many autophagosomes, ribosome clumping, cytoplasmic vacuolation.
Plasma membrane	Cleavage of caspase, regional loss of membrane phospholipids, membrane blebs,	Irregular membrane.

Table 3.2: Two apoptotic mechanisms: Caspase-dependent and Caspase-independent morphological differences. MOMP = mitochondrial opening membrane permeability (pore).

Caspase-independent Apoptosis (CIA)

Mitochondrial dysfunction associated with the loss of Ca^{2+} homeostasis and enhanced cellular oxidative stress have long been recognized to play a major role in cell damage associated with excitotoxicity, a process resulting from the overstimulation of glutamate receptors (NMDA). (92) Sustained Ca^{2+} influx through glutamate receptor channels is thought to represent a common pathway of neuronal cell death. Excess levels of glutamate in the CNS can result in elevated intracellular Ca^{2+} levels, which in turn cause a rise in the Ca^{2+} concentration in sensitive organelles such as mitochondria and the endoplasmic reticulum. Additionally, when Ca^{2+} is taken up by mitochondria it can physiologically increase ATP generation by activating matrix dehydrogenases thereby promoting ROS generation. (93)

Calcium is known to activate several intracellular enzymes, such as phospholipase A2 (94), NOS, xanthine dehydrogenase (95), calcineurin (96), and endonucleases, many of which can provoke the generation of endogenous ROS. (A comment on Calcineurin; it is linked to receptors for several brain chemicals including NMDA, dopamine and GABA. (97) An experiment with genetically altered mice that could not produce calcineurin showed similar symptoms as in humans with schizophrenia: impairment in working memory, attention deficits, aberrant social behavior, and several other abnormalities characteristic of schizophrenia.) (98)

Progressive damage to the mitochondrial integrity by free radicals can lead to the activation of a family of proteins called BCl-2. (99) Within this family are a number of pro- and anti-apoptotic members (pro-[Bax, Bad, Bid, Bcl_{xs}], anti-[Bcl-2, $Bclx_{L}$]) that regulate mitochondrial membrane permeabilization (MMP). Preceding the initiation of apoptosis, there is an increase in the permeability of the mitochondrial membrane with the release of Cytochrome c into the cytosol then translocates to the nucleus precipitating apoptosis. (100)

Another form of CIA is regulated by mitochondrial apoptotic inducing factor (AIF). Normally residing in the intermembrane mitochondrial space, where it performs an oxidoreductase function, AIF becomes an active initiator of apoptosis when it is released to the cytosol; it then translocates to the nucleus and triggers chromatin condensation. (101)

Autophagy (Cell Death type II)

Autophagy, also called Type 2 non-apoptotic cell death, is characterized by the sequestration of cytoplasmic material in vacuoles that subsequently merge with lysosomes for degradation. Considered a process of self-destruction, it does not obligate the cell to death, but can be used as a mechanism to protect the cell from death. In conditions of oxidative stress resulting from hypoxia, ischemia, chemical toxins (chemotherapeutic agents), ionizing radiation, and nutritional starvation autophagy can remove damaged organelles and provide additional ATP generated by catabolism of cellular macromolecules (carbohydrates, protein, fats, and nucleic acids) for the repair or replacement of those organelles. (102*)

Two modes of autophagy have been identified, microautophagy and macroautophagy. These two modes differ with respect to the pathway by which cytoplasmic material is delivered to the lysosome but share in common the final steps of lysosomal degradation of its content with eventual recycling of the degraded material. Microautophagy involves the engulfment of cytoplasm directly at the lysosomal surface, by invagination, protrusion, and/or septation of the lysosomal limiting membrane, endocytosis. (103) In contrast, macroautophagy involves the formation of cytosolic double-membrane vesicles that sequester portions of the cytoplasm. (104). Fusion of the completed vesicle, an autophagosome (105), with the lysosome results in the delivery of an inner vesicle or autophagic body into the lumen of the degradative compartment .(106)

In conditions related to traumatic brain injury, oxidative stress in the form of free radical damage, leading to leakage of mitochondrial Cytochrome c, loss of intracellular calcium homeostasis from both mitochondria and endoplasmic reticulum, triggers the Autophagy (ATG) gene. (107) This is a form of damage control; otherwise, proteins liberated from damaged organelles, such as mitochondrial Cytochrome c, have the potential of precipitating any one of number of apoptotic processes (caspase - dependent (CDA) and caspase-independent apoptosis (CIA)). Therefore, mechanisms that can appropriately avert ultimate cell death, favor conservation of tissue homeostasis and cellular energy. (108)

Necrosis (Cell Death type III)

Over the past decade, it has become evident that in certain conditions, necrosis is the result of a strictly regulated interplay of signaling events which are initiated by a diverse range of stimuli. In most cell lines, death receptor ligands (FAS/TNF) activate apoptosis rather than necrosis as the default cell death pathway. However, if the caspase activation pathway is hampered, necrotic cell death ensues instead, acting as a kind of back-up cell death pathway. (109)

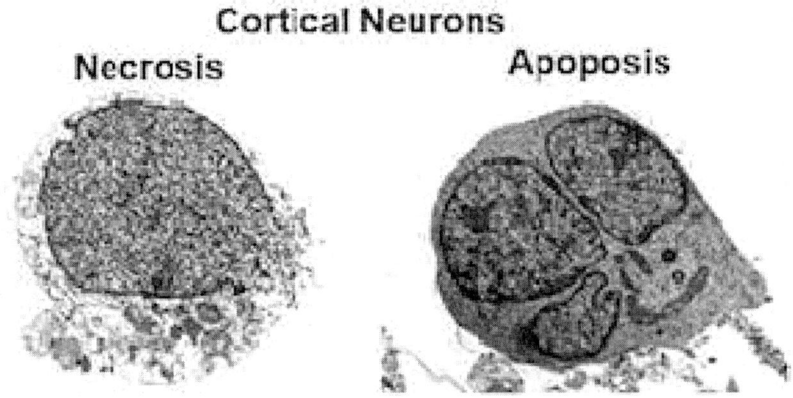

Ueda H, etal., J Cell Biol. 2007 Mar 12;176(6):853-62 PMID: 17353341

This has in fact been proven by the use of designer drugs that selectively block apoptotic and autophagic pathways leaving the only pathway to necrosis unimpeded. The end result is an organized procession of necrosis characterized morphologically by vacuolation of the cytoplasm, breakdown of the plasma membrane and an induction of inflammation around the dying cell attributable to the release of cellular contents and pro-inflammatory molecules into the environment. Cells that die by necrosis frequently exhibit changes in nuclear morphology but not the organized chromatin condensation and fragmentation of DNA that is characteristic of apoptotic cell death. (110)

It has become increasingly clear that necrosis and apoptosis share biochemical networks. The final form of a cell's death is highly dependent on its physiologic context at the time when the death signal is received. Linking the term "programmed" to the word "necrosis" implies that cellular signaling pathways initiate necrosis in response to specific cues rather than "by accident". Programmed necrosis may not simply be a backup when apoptosis fails, but has a biological function under conditions where an immune reaction to the dying cell is desirable, such as in microbial infection. (111)

Necrosis has been observed during ischemia/ reperfusion which contributes to excitotoxicity, which may be involved in stroke, traumatic brain injury, and neurodegenerative disorders. (112)

Parthanatos

Within the nucleus, the poly-(ADP-ribose) polymerase-1 (PARP-1) enzyme uses nicotinamide adenine dinucleotide (NAD+) as a cofactor for ADP-ribosylation of amino acids and proteins for the purpose of DNA repair. Oxidative stress can cause excessive DNA damage results in hyperactivation of PARP-1 and precipitation of necrotic cell death called "parthanatos", a form of caspase-independent cell death that is distinct from apoptosis and necrosis in being dependent on the release of apoptosis-inducing factor (AIF) from mitochondria. (113)

During excessive PARP-1 activation, depletion of NAD^+ occurs as it is used to catalyzing the hydrolysis of NAD^+ into nicotinamide and poly (ADP- ribose) (PAR), leading to ATP depletion, irreversible cellular energy failure, and necrotic cell death. (114*) This process involves a pathogenic role of PARP-1 which is generated in the nucleus and translocates to the mitochondria to mediate AIF release following lethal PARP-1 activation. AIF has a high-affinity poly (ADP-ribose) (PAR)-binding protein and that PAR binding to AIF is required for parthanatos both in vitro and in vivo. AIF binds PAR at a site distinct from AIF's DNA binding site, and this interaction triggered AIF release from the cytosolic side of the mitochondrial outer membrane. PAR polymer itself is toxic to cells. Thus, PAR polymer signaling to mitochondrial AIF is the key event initiating the deadly crosstalk between the nucleus and the mitochondria in parthanatos. (115, 116)

Mitochondrial dysfunction

Mitochondrial dysfunction has been discussed thoroughly throughout this chapter with emphasis on reactive oxygen species, calcium overload, AIF, caspase-independent apoptosis, autophagy and parthanatos. Again, each of these negative influences on mitochondrial functioning are rooted in the production or effects of free radicals. Therefore, in addressing treatment, it is hopefully obvious that an aggressive approach with a number of potent antioxidants will be needed to counter the present and future damage.

Blood Brain Barrier disruption

The homeostasis of the central nervous system's environment is maintained by the blood-brain barrier (BBB), which separates the brain from the systemic blood circulation. The cerebral capillaries are organized such that the brain is protected from blood-borne compounds (organisms, toxins, chemicals, antibodies, and antigens), since a strict homeostasis of the neuronal environment and an intact barrier are essential for optimal brain functioning. However, during various neurological diseases as well as neurotrauma the permeability of the BBB may be altered.

The cerebral vasculature plays a crucial role in oxygen and nutrient delivery to the brain, which is noted to have the highest metabolic demand receiving 20 percent of the cardiac output. (117) Moreover, it has a vital function in maintaining a stable ionic environment and protecting against passage of neurotoxic substances into the brain during development and function. Brain endothelial cells are especially suited for these functions providing a selective physical barrier having a specialized structure in the CNS consisting of capillary beds based on endothelial cell tight junctions, with no endothelial fenestrae, and expression of specific membrane transporters, thus ensuring homeostasis and proper functioning of the brain. (118)

In traumatic brain injury, local and peripheral production of inflammatory cytokines such as, TNF-α and IL-6, lead to the loss of integrity of the tight junctions (119) by stimulating the expression of matrix metalloproteinases (MMPs), a gene family of extracellular matrix enzymes which degrade junction proteins and change the permeability of the BBB. (120) Once the selective permeability of the BBB is lost, peripherally circulating compounds gain unrestricted access to the brain parenchyma furthering damage. Therefore, it is imperative during the acute course of care that support be given to maintain an intact BBB. Progesterone and more so its metabolite allopregnanolone have been shown to down-regulate the production of TNF and IL-6 from peripheral mononuclear lymphocytes, and osteoblast and centrally by glial cells (astrocytes, oligodendrocytes and microglia).

Summary

Traumatic brain injury has been a reluctant mistress keeping her attire loose enough to avoid clear definition. Nonetheless, we have been able to piece together many of her attributes in terms of sequelae that follow the initial impact of primary damage followed by the secondary neurochemical cascades.

The onset of temporal waves of neuronal destruction are based upon a blend of four fairly well defined cellular processes – Apoptosis, Necrosis, Autophagy and Parthanatos – whose intentions are based upon reactivity to both primary and secondary insults (contusion, neuronal shearing, hemorrhage, ischemia, hypoxia, hypoglycemia, ionizing radiation, excitotoxicity, and release of traumatic cellular debris).

It appears that the underlying and unifying factor found in each of these mechanisms is the ultimate production of free radicals and the loss of calcium and ionic homeostasis. Free radicals represented by both ROS and RNS create damage to the cerebral environment starting at the site of primary injury and radiating out to encompass the entire brain. (121*) As the oxidative stress of these free radicals rise, our endogenous antioxidant protective system becomes overwhelmed and fails initiating the presence of a non neuropermissive environment (NNPE).

Lipid peroxidative damage caused by free radicals, leads to loss of cellular membrane integrity with an impact on ionic pumps allowing for the uncontrolled passage of calcium, potassium, sodium and chloride into the cytosol. Rising levels of intracellular calcium are initially buffered by endoplasmic reticula, but eventually they become overloaded and leak calcium back into the cytosol. Calcium can directly activate Caspase-12 (122) as well as up-regulate mitochondrial production of ATP at a risk of production of more ROS and the leakage of Cytochrome c (123) which translocates to the nucleus as a messenger of death.

Injury to the central nervous system (CNS) generally leads to severe and persistent functional deficits and it has been proposed for a long time that neurons in adult mammalian CNS fail to regenerate after injury. (124) It is now known that the failure of adult axons to regenerate is not exclusively due to neurons' intrinsic and irreversible lack of regenerative ability, but is largely attributable to the presence of an inhibitory and non-permissive environment. (125) Thus, adult neurons are not only able to sprout new axonal or dendritic branches in response to various changes of their environment, but also have a genuine endogenous ability to regenerate after lesion formation.

Taking all this information into consideration would allow us to approach the initial and long-term treatment of survivors of TBI with medication and supplements that address the underlying processes that fail to abate on their own. The need to transform the post-TBI non-permissive environment into one that fosters the regeneration and repair of neurons is crucial to rehabilitation.

The literature, as well as our clinical experience at the Millennium-TBI shows the beneficial outcome from a combination of neurosteroids, neuroactive steroids and a combination of free radical scavengers. This approach taken in concert will afford the possibility of reversing the pervasive NNPE with the down-regulation of cytokines, chemokines, and oxidative stressors while embellishing a neuroprotective and neuropermissive environment that can lead to neuroregeneration, synaptogenesis, stabilization of myelin, and improved neurocommunication (GABA, SIGMA, NMDA, and AMPA receptors). What the patients are experiencing is an improvement in neurobehavior and neurofunction without the need for many of their previous medication.

Chapter 4: Neuroendocrinology in TBI

"There is a thread in the Universe's sanity (or insanity) that ties many of us together on paths that make no sense until the magnitude of forces clears from the air and then, there is sense!"

— Anonymous

Introduction

Neuroendocrinology is the study of what is most definitely a complex set of neurochemical and neurohormonal interactions between the nervous and endocrine systems; both centrally and peripherally. Our understanding of the regulatory influences of neurotransmitters (1) (cholinergic, adrenergic, dopaminergic) on hormone regulation, and vice-versa, has expanded significantly to allow us to see the biological features involved in how cells in these two systems communicate. The occurrence of neurotrauma (TBI) undermines this relationship and conceivably becomes the mechanism responsible for regulating the associated morbidity and mortality. (2)

Neuroendocrinology arose from the recognition that the brain, especially the hypothalamus, controls the secretion of pituitary trophic hormones, and has further expanded to include investigation of the numerous interconnections between the endocrine and nervous systems. Thereby, one of the most important functions of the hypothalamus is to link the nervous system to the endocrine system via the pituitary gland and together they act to regulate the physiological processes of the entire human body. (3)

The regulation of pituitary function by the hypothalamus is the primary means by which the body maintains the dynamic equilibrium or homeostasis of our hormones. Involved in this complex system are the hypothalamus, pituitary, and peripheral target tissues that utilize a feedback mechanism to assure that each hormone is optimized for the momentary needs for ideal bodily functioning. (4)

Both environmental and physiological factors can influence hormonal regulation as is often seen in situations of stress. Most prominent is the elevation of corticotrophin-releasing hormone (CRH) which leads to the down-regulation of pituitary trophic hormones LH, FSH, GH, and TSH causing associated deficiencies in their associated peripheral hormones responsible for maintaining cellular and organismal health; as can be exemplified by runner's amenorrhea. (5)

Traumatic injury to the head poses a significant risk to pituitary function in view of the gland's bony encasement within the sella turcica. The frequency and pattern of endocrine dysfunction amongst patients with traumatic brain injury implies a disruption in communication between nervous and endocrine systems. (6[L])

Amongst the many problems precipitated by the initial injury (orthopedic, cognitive), chronic neurobehavioral problems and quality of life complaints plague many patients with traumatic brain injury, which are often similar to those of patients who have adult-onset hormone deficiencies. Hypothalamic-pituitary dysfunction, however, is rarely considered as a cause of the above problems. Instead it is the primary injury to the brain injury and secondary cerebral insults (edema and ischemia) that are considered as causes. (7)

A core concept that will be repeated throughout this chapter is this delicate relationship between hypothalamic control of pituitary hormones and the disruption of a self-mediated balance affecting neurobehavioral functioning. It is not only my belief, but the belief of many published research clinicians who note the association of depression, anxiety, paranoia, psychoses, and substance abuse that if left unchecked, raising the risk for suicide, when hormonal dysfunction exists (see Chapter 7).

In my attempt to be complete and comprehensive in the writing of this chapter, I have found that the basic and standard representation of Neuroendocrinology consists of a lengthy discussion of the hypothalamic-pituitary interactions and how they influence weight, temperature, reproduction and so forth. But, I have decided, instead, to focus on the area of neurosteroids and neuroactive steroids, since they are a significant part of our treatment protocols — and are precisely what has been frequently been omitted. So, I will refer you to *The Textbook of Endocrinology* by Williams and Williams as an excellent reference for more in-depth educational points while I skim the surface here.

The Hypothalamic-Pituitary Connections

Hypothalamus (S[1])

The main function of the hypothalamus is homeostasis and includes regulation of blood pressure, body temperature, fluid and electrolyte balance, circadian rhythm issues, and body weight. These are maintained at optimal values based upon what is referred to as "set points" by the regulation of three interrelated functions: endocrine secretions, autonomic nervous system tone, and emotional status. Additionally, each of these factors acts within a feedback mechanism to finely regulate the magnitude of their individual influence on hypothalamic functioning. (8[1])

The hypothalamus is a part of the diencephalon (9), which integrates the nervous system into the functioning of the endocrine system. The hypothalamus controls the release of posterior pituitary hormones (neurohypophysis) by direct neuronal stimulation via the infundibulum (10), and that of the anterior pituitary gland via dependence upon the portal plexus (a vascular conduit) that carries hypothalamic releasing factors to the anterior pituitary. (11)

The hypothalamus lies below and in front of the thalamus (12). It forms the floor and lower walls of the third ventricle (13). External landmarks of the hypothalamus are the optic chiasm; the tuber cinereum, with its infundibulum extending to the posterior lobe of the hypophysis; and the mammillary bodies lying between the cerebral peduncles.

The right and left sides of the hypothalamus each have a medial hypothalamic area that contains many nuclei and a lateral hypothalamic area that contains fiber systems and diffuse lateral nuclei. It is through these pathways that the hypothalamus relays afferent and efferent signals. The hypothalamus receives (afferent) inputs from limbic structures, thalamus and cortex, visceral and somatic afferents, and osmoreceptors, which permit monitoring of the circulation. (14)

Hypothalamic Nuclei	Function
Medial Pre-optic Nucleus	Regulates the release of GnRH from the adenohypophysis. Contains the sexual dimorphic nucleus which releases GnRH, differential development between sexes is based upon in utero testosterone levels.
Supraoptic Nucleus	Oxytocin and Vasopressin release.
Paraventricular Nucleus	TRH, CRH, Oxytocin, and Vasopressin release.
Anterior Hypothalamic Nucleus	Thermoregulation, panting, sweating, and Thyrotropin inhibition.
Suprachiasmatic Nucleus	Vasopressin release and Circadian rhythm.
Lateral Nucleus	Thirst and hunger (Leptin).
Dorsomedial Hypothalamic Nucleus	Blood pressure, heart rate, and GI stimulation
Ventromedial Nucleus	Satiety and neuroendocrine control.
Arcuate Nucleus	Growth hormone releasing hormone, feeding and dopamine regulation.

Table 4.1: Hypothalamic nuclei responsible for integration of hormonal homeostasis and the nervous system.

Efferent signals are generated and influence the hypothalamic nuclei contained within either the magnocellular system (MC) (15) or the parvocellular neurosecretory (16) system (PCN) to regulate pituitary function. The MC system contains the supraoptic nuclei (SON), which synthesize oxytocin and the paraventricular nuclei (PVN) that synthesizes vasopressin (ADH). These are long neurons that descend into the posterior pituitary to directly release their tropic hormones. The PCN system contains the ventromedial nucleus whose axons converge toward the pituitary stalk approximating themselves close to the primary plexus of the portal system of the median eminence where their secretions of hypophysiotropic factors (GHRH, TRH, CRH, and GnRH) are taken up to influence the release of anterior pituitary hormones. (13)

Another important hypothalamic area is the arcuate nucleus (14) representing an aggregation of neurons in the mediobasal hypothalamus, adjacent to the third ventricle and the median eminence. The arcuate nucleus contains both neuroendocrine and centrally-projecting neurons. The neuroendocrine neurons have nerve endings in the median eminence that release dopamine (14b) into the hypophyseal portal blood; the "tuberoinfundibular dopamine" (TIDA) neurons. These TIDA neurons are inhibited by the stimulus of suckling. Dopamine released from their nerve endings at the median eminence is transported to the anterior pituitary gland, where it regulates the secretion of prolactin. Dopamine inhibits prolactin secretion, so, when the TIDA neurons are inhibited, there is increased secretion of prolactin, which stimulates lactogenesis (milk production). (15)

Prolactin acts in a short-loop negative feedback manner to decrease its levels by stimulating the release of dopamine. Dopaminergic neurons of the arcuate nucleus also inhibit the release of gonadotropin-releasing hormone (GnRH) (16), explaining in part why lactating women experience oligomenorrhea or amenorrhea, while in men it can reduce testosterone production from the Leydig cells.

Secreted Hormone	Abrev.	Produced by	Effect
Thyrotropin releasing hormone (prolactin releasing hormone)	TRH (PRH)	Parvocellular Neurosecretory cells	Stimulates TSH and Prolactin release from AP.
Dopamine (Prolactin Inhibiting Factor)	DA or PIF	Neurons of the Arcuate Nucleus	Inhibits Prolactin release from AP
Growth hormone releasing hormone	GHRH	Neurons of the Arcuate Nucleus	Stimulates GH release from AP
Somatostatin (Somatotropin Release Inhibiting factor)	SSS or SRIF	Neurons of the Periventricular nucleus	Inhibits GH and TSH release from AP
Gonadotropin Releasing hormone	GnRH	Neurons of the Preoptic Area	Stimulates FSH and LH release from AP.
Cortotropin Releasing Hormone	CRH	Parvocellular Neurosecretory Cells	Stimulates ACTH release from the AP, and inhibits LH, GH, LH and FSH release.
Oxytocin		Magnocellular Neurons	Stimulates uterine contractions and lactation.
Vasopressin (ADH)	ADH	Magnocellular Neurons	Increases water reabsorption and decreases water loss from kidneys.

Table 4.2: Hypothalamic hormones.

Males who develop galactorrhea (low testosterone levels with loss of libido after a TBI) should be evaluated for both pituitary trauma and a pituitary adenoma. When trauma to the hypothalamus interrupts the production of Prolactin Inhibitory Factor (dopamine), the lactotrophs are free to produce prolactin.

Somatostatin (SRIF) is produced by neuroendocrine neurons of the periventricular nucleus of the hypothalamus. These neurons project to the median eminence, where somatostatin is released from neurosecretory nerve endings into the hypothalamo-hypophysial system through neuron axons. (17) Somatostatin is then carried to the anterior pituitary gland, where it inhibits the secretion of growth hormone from somatotrope cells (and TSH). The somatostatin neurons in the periventricular nucleus mediate negative feedback effects of growth hormone on its own release.

The somatostatin neurons respond to high circulating concentrations of growth hormone and somatomedins (IGF-I and II) by increasing the release of somatostatin, so reducing the rate of secretion of growth hormone.

Additionally, SRIF was found to be responsible for influence over the pituitary gland, immune responses, and neurobehavior. Therefore, damage to this area can lead to an uncontrolled elevation in growth hormone production due to the loss of negative feed-back (18), changes in immunity, and emotional consequences. (19)

Another major symptom associated with TBI is chronic daytime fatigue (CDF) or sleepiness. In about 1997, there was found within the lateral hypothalamus a cluster of neurons responsible for the production of the wake-promoting neuropeptide orexin (hypocretin). (20) Of the billions of cells found in the brain there are only 10,000 to 20,000 of orexin secreting neurons. The region of the hypothalamus containing these orexin secreting neurons was previously known to be important in the stimulation of feeding (orexin = appetite; Greek). It appears that an extensive loss of these neurons is associated with the syndrome of narcolepsy (21), and varying degrees of neuronal loss is seen in Parkinson's disease (22) and in traumatic brain injuries. (23*) Therefore, the development of both diminished appetite and CDF can conceivably be attributed to damage to these neurons deep within the hypothalamus.

So far, two differing forms of Orexin have been identified and labeled Orexin-A and -B. In the acute phase of TBI, the CSF level of Orexin-A is noted to be reduced and has been documented to persist low for more than six months. These individuals complain of fatigue, sleepiness, and cognitive impairment. Testing for Orexin-A is presently only available by spinal tap with a serum blood test unavailable. (24*)

The Pituitary Gland

The pituitary gland, typically weighing less than one gram and measuring approximately eight mm by ten mm, is located within the sella turcica in the base of the skull. It is separated from the suprasellar cistern by the diaphragma sella and is joined to the hypothalamus by the infundibulum, which inserts on its superior surface.

The adenohypophysis (anterior) and neurohypophysis (posterior) receive their blood supply primarily from the internal carotid arteries. The long hypophyseal portal vessels arise from branches of the internal carotid artery (superior hypophyseal arteries) and anterior Circle of Willis above the diaphragma sella, travel down the infundibulum and provide the anterior pituitary gland with 70 to 90 percent of its blood supply (Figure 4.2).

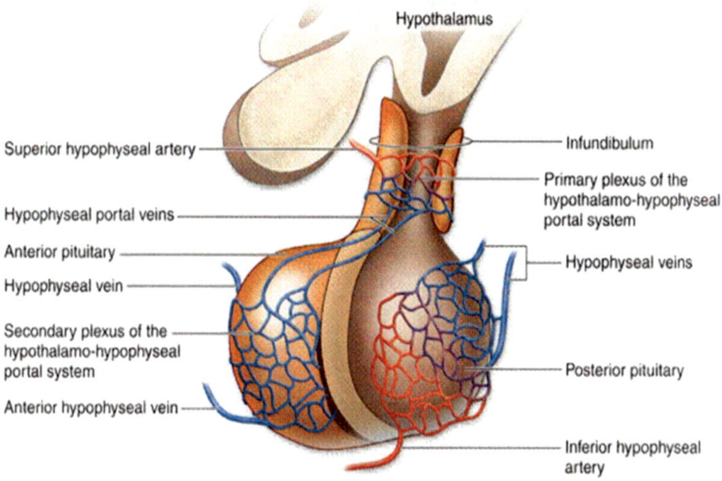

Figure 4.2: The Hypothalamo-hypophyseal portal system is a delicate network of blood vessels providing a conduit by which releasing hormones and trophic hormones can be disseminated.

Hypothalamic releasing hormones are carried by this vascular system to the anterior pituitary. The cellular distribution in the pituitary gland supplied by the long hypophyseal veins includes the somatotroph (lateral wings of the gland) and the gonadotroph (peripheral parts of the gland). The short hypophyseal portal veins arise from branches of the intracavernous internal carotid artery, the inferior hypophyseal arteries that enter the sella from below the diaphragma sella, and together provide less than 30 percent of its vascular supply, predominantly in the medial portion of the gland. The posterior lobe receives its blood supply through the inferior hypophyseal arterial branches.

Anterior Pituitary

Of all the glands in the body it is the "Master Gland", the pituitary that controls our hormonal milieu. The anterior pituitary, or adenohypophysis, plays a central role in the regulation of endocrine function through the production and release of tropic hormones. The function of the anterior pituitary, and thereby the production of tropic hormones, is under hypothalamic regulation by the hypophysiotropic neuropeptides released in the median eminence. The tropic hormones produced by the anterior pituitary are released into the systemic circulation, from where they reach their target organs to produce a physiologic response, most frequently involving the release of a target organ hormone. The hormones produced by the target organs affect anterior pituitary function as well as the release of hypophysiotropic neuropeptides, maintaining an integrated feedback control system of endocrine function.

Secreted	ID	From	Effect
Growth Hormone (Somatotropin)	GH	Somatotrophs	Stimulates growth and cell reproduction. Stimulates Insulin-like growth factor 1 release from liver
Thyroid-Stimulating Hormone (Thyrotropin)	TSH	Thyrotrophs	Stimulates thyroxine (T4) and triiodothyronine (T3) synthesis and release from thyroid gland. Stimulates iodine absorption by thyroid gland
Adrenocorticotropic hormone (Corticotropin)	ACTH	Corticotrophs	Stimulates corticosteroid (glucocorticoid and mineralcorticoid) and androgen synthesis and release from adrenocortical cells .
Follicle-stimulating hormone	FSH	Gonadotrophs	In females: Stimulates maturation of ovarian follicles in ovary In males: Stimulates maturation of seminiferous tubules, spermatogenesis, production of androgen-binding protein from Sertoli cells of the testes.
Luteinizing hormone	LH	Gonadotrophs	In females: Stimulates ovulation and formation of corpus luteum In males: Stimulates testosterone synthesis from Leydig cells.
Prolactin	PRL	Lactotrophs	Stimulates milk synthesis and release from mammary glands Mediates sexual gratification

Table 4.3: Anterior Pituitary Hormones and their effects in humans.

Posterior Pituitary

The neurohypophysial hormones form a family of structurally and functionally related peptide hormones. Their main representatives are oxytocin and vasopressin. They are named for being secreted by the neurohypophysis, i.e., the posterior pituitary gland (hypophysis refers to the pituitary gland), itself a neuronal projection from the hypothalamus. Most of the circulating oxytocin and vasopressin hormones are synthesized in magnocellular neurosecretory cells of the supraoptic nucleus and paraventricular nucleus of the hypothalamus. They are then transported in neurosecretory granules along axons within the hypothalamo-neurohypophysial tract by axoplasmic flow to axon terminals forming the pars nervosa of the posterior pituitary where they are stored in Herring bodies waiting to be released into the circulation on the basis of hormonal and synaptic signals.

Vasopressin and oxytocin are also synthesized in the parvocellular neurosecretory cells of the paraventricular nucleus of the hypothalamus, which project to the median eminence, where they are transported and secreted into the hypophyseal portal system to stimulate the anterior pituitary. Thus, they can also be considered as hypophysiotropic hormones.

Head trauma presents a substantial risk to pituitary function because of the gland's encasement within the sella turcica, its delicate infundibular hypothalamic structures, and its vulnerable vascular supply. Therefore, mechanical compression from injury or pituitary gland swelling may play a part in diffuse vascular injury (DVI). The long hypophyseal portal vessels and the pituitary stalk are thought to be particularly vulnerable to mechanical trauma, low cerebral blood flow, brain swelling, and intracranial hypertension. (25*) The first study that showed traumatic infarction of the anterior pituitary gland was conducted by Daniel half a century ago when they studied fatal head injuries. A decade later, larger studies by Ceballos, Kornblum and Fisher showed similar findings. (26*)

In addition, Benvenga commented on the peculiar vascularization of the pituitary, noting that the peripheral layer of anterior pituitary cells under the capsule receives arterial blood from the capsule, and not from the two systems of portal veins. Therefore, these cells and those in a small area close to the posterior lobe are the only surviving cells in cases of pure anterior lobe necrosis. Interestingly, severed portal vessels can regenerate, which may explain the occasional report of recovery from anterior pituitary insufficiency that is a complication of head trauma. (27)

The stress of critical illness has serious effects on the acute functioning of all anterior pituitary hormonal axes. Euthyroid syndrome (low thyroid-stimulating hormone [TSH], low T3 and high rT3) occurs commonly in critically ill patients. The gonadotropic axis is also suppressed, with acute lowering of gonadal hormones. (28)

What we are encountering is that the clinical manifestations of TBI vary widely depending on the type, site, and severity of the precipitating injury, including direct or indirect injury to the hypothalamus and pituitary. In addition, any of the hormones produced by the anterior or posterior pituitary can be affected by TBI whether the insult is mild, moderate or severe.

The association of traumatic brain injury with hypopituitarism might appear to us as being just a decade old, but was actually first reported by Cyran in 1918. Nonetheless, the number of articles being published finally relating the insult of trauma on the regulatory functions of the Hypothalamus is in the thousands. In fact, a search by Google Scholar using the terms Trauma, Hypopituitarism, and Hypothalamus generated 3,700 articles since the year 2000; a good number to consider as well as their content and support for these facts.

Neurosteroids and Neuroactive Steroids

Whenever we speak in terms of hormones, we are generally referring to those produced by the peripheral glands (neuroactive steroids) and not those made in the brain (neurosteroids). In my estimation, it will be the neurosteroids that will be shown to have an essential role in the regeneration and repair of traumatic brain injuries. Additionally, their role in the modulation of neurotransmission will be found to either single-handedly improve neuropsychiatric problems, or be helpful as adjuvants to enhance a lower dose regimen of traditional therapies.

The remainder of this chapter will address the role of these neurosteroids as an exciting new approach to recovery from neurotrauma, regardless of its cause. Their scope and breath of influence over the brain and rest of the body is overwhelming at best but hopefully palatable herewith.

Robel and Baulieu in 1985 reported on steroids directly synthesized within the CNS, either de novo from cholesterol or by in situ metabolism of circulating steroid precursors, designating them by the generic term neurosteroids. By 1992, a number of reports came out with growing evidence that neurosteroids play an important role as endogenous modulators of neuronal function and behavioral processes, and that alterations of neurosteroid concentrations may contribute to the pathology of neuronal disorders. (29)

At present, the best known role of neurosteroids is their involvement in the control of mood disorders. Numerous behavioral investigations have shown that neurosteroids exert anxiolytic, anti-depressant, anti-aggressive, hypnotic, anti-convulsive, and anti-stress actions. (30)

In vivo studies indicate that progesterone, allopregnanolone (metabolite of progesterone), and DHEA exert neuroprotective effects in models of traumatic brain injury and in focal cerebral ischemia. (31*)

Neurosteroids play important functions in neurodevelopment and neuronal remodeling, including neurogenesis, axonal and dendritic growth, and synaptic connectivity. In addition to their protective effects on the brain, neurosteroids can regulate myelin formation and increase expression of myelin proteins in the sciatic nerve.

Neurosteroids can act at the transcriptional level through interaction with nuclear receptors, plasma membrane G-protein receptors, or act indirectly by modulation of neuropeptide (ligand) binding to their receptors. Therefore, neurosteroids modulate the action of the central nervous system (CNS), regulating synaptic transmission at different targets with rapid non-genomic effect on presynaptic receptors and long-term genomic actions. (32)

However, most of the actions of neurosteroids are mediated via allosteric modulation of neurotransmitter receptors: $GABA_A$/central-type benzodiazepine receptor (CBR) complex, N-methyl-D-aspartate, kainate, α-amino-3-hydroxy-5- methyl-4-isoxazole-propionic acid (AMPA), glycine, sigma, serotonergic, nicotinic, and muscarinic receptors. (33)

It appears that neuroactive steroids are the macro-hormones of bodily function, while neurosteroids are the micro-hormones that fine-tune the interactions amongst the neuro-circuitry of the brain. Neurotransmitters and their corresponding receptors are responsible for the inter-activity and reactivity of control and modulation systems within the brain. Failure of this system will lead to erratic transmissions which are perceived as major pathopsychiatric events. Depression and suicide, anxiety and panic attacks, and phobias and psychoses are all representative of this condition of unpredictable effects of neurosteroid dysfunction.

Cholesterol

As controversial as it is, Cholesterol is not the life threatening sterol that it has been portrayed as in the past 50 years of medical history. Our very existence is based upon the ability of the body to create and deliver cholesterol, which is required for viability and cell proliferation, and is the major sterol of mammalian cells. In fact, more than 90 percent of cellular cholesterol is located at the plasma membrane. (34)

Ingested cholesterol is either transported into the cell or retained in its bi-lipid outer membrane to regulate permeability to hydrophilic molecules. Upon entry into the cytoplasm, it is bound by carrier protein and transported to the different organelles within the cell. Some is converted to its esterified form and stored in lipid droplets and some is cleaved into its free form for use in production of either neuroactive steroids or neurosteroids based upon location.

Additionally, the endoplasmic reticulum serves as the major site of cholesterol synthesis. A class of lipid transport protein named caveolins bind and transport the de novo-synthesized cholesterol from the endoplasmic reticulum to the plasma membrane, as well as to other organelles within the cell. (35)

Steroidogenesis is the complex multi-enzyme process by which cholesterol is converted to biologically active steroid hormones. Under influence of luteinizing hormone (LH) cholesterol ester is inhibited and free cholesterol is enhanced for use in steroidogenesis. (36*)

Inhibition of steroidogenesis, by any means, can lead to a deficiency of neurosteroids and the stability of neuronal functioning and connectivity. The development of cognitive impairment and dementia can be accelerated by a lack of the important neurosteroid precursor; cholesterol. In a 2005 review of over 1,000 Framingham Heart Study cases, it was found that "Lower naturally occurring Total Cholesterol levels are associated with poorer performance on cognitive measures, which place high demands on abstract reasoning, attention/concentration, word fluency, and executive functioning." (37)

Luteinizing Hormone

Luteinizing hormone can cross the blood-brain barrier and has been found in cerebrospinal fluid, and is expressed by neuronal cells to initiate steroidogenesis with the production of neurosteroids from cholesterol.

Luteinizing hormone stimulates steroidogenesis by up-regulating the rate-limiting transport of cholesterol from the outer to the inner mitochondrial membrane by increasing the expression of the mitochondrial cholesterol transport protein — steroidogenic acute regulatory protein (StAR). Neurons and glial have been found to produce LH which regulates pregnenolone synthesis and secretion by modulating the expression of the LH receptor and the cholesterol transport protein StAR. (38)

Additionally, LH increases the expression of the P450 cholesterol side-chain cleavage enzyme (P450scc or CYP11A1) located on the inner membrane of mitochondria, which catalyzes the conversion of cholesterol to pregnenolone, the first product in steroid hormone biosynthesis. (39)

Pregnenolone

Commonly referred to as the "Mother of all hormones", pregnenolone sits at the pinnacle of two important hormone cascades. In one direction, it becomes progesterone (PROG) and in the other dehydroepiandrosterone (DHEA), both pathways have been found to influence neuronal functions and are likely to play an important role in the quality of aging in the central nervous system. (40)

The mechanisms underlying the memory promoting (promnesic) actions of Pregnenolone-sulfate (PREG-s) involve the modulation of neurotransmitter systems, including the N-Methyl-D-Aspartate (NMDA)-glutamatergic system ($GABA_A$), Sigma-1 receptors, and the central cholinergic system all resulting in enhanced acetylcholine (Ach) release within the cerebral cortex, amygdala and hippocampus.

The ability of the $GABA_A$ receptor to inhibit neurochemical transmission, in the form of an action potential, is based upon the conditions that modulate the receptor. Either directly or indirectly, neurodegenerative conditions (inflammation) can lead to the opening of the $GABA_A$ receptors with the influx of chloride ions (Cl^-). It is a sudden rise in the intracellular concentration of Cl^- that inhibits the action potential from firing. Loss of an action potential leads to a slowing of neurochemical transmissions that diminish the downstream release of ACh. This is a simplistic explanation of lost memories and learning. (41)

Pregnenolone-sulfate specifically inhibits the $GABA_A$ receptors from opening up to the influx of chloride ions with the net effect of continued neurotransmission and a potent steroidal enhancement for memory processes that are commonly lost in the aging process. (42)

Progesterone

Emerging data indicate that progesterone (progestins) has multiple non-reproductive functions in the central nervous system to regulate cognition, mood, inflammation, mitochondrial function, neurogenesis and regeneration, myelination, and recovery from traumatic brain injury. These effects in the brain are brought about through three principle mechanisms: regulation of gene expression, modulation of neurotransmitter systems, and activation of signaling cascades. (43)

Progestins regulate myelination in peripheral nerves via two distinct signaling mechanisms, involving either the intracellular PROG receptor

(PR) or membrane $GABA_A$ receptors, which are both expressed by Schwann cells. Progesterone and its metabolites have been found to stimulate myelination by oligodendrocytes in the central nervous system (CNS). (44) Progesterone and its 5alpha-reduced derivatives — dihydroprogesterone (DHP) and tetrahydroprogesterone (THP or allopregnanolone) — can promote Schwann cell proliferation and activation of the myelinating program of these cells through gene regulation. PROG is also a signaling molecule involved in the formation of new myelin sheaths, which are necessary for the efficient and rapid conduction of action potentials.

Neuroregenerative benefits of Allopregnanolone arise from its ability to influence the $GABA_A$ receptors to allow for the efflux of intracellular chloride ions (Cl-). As the concentration of intracellular Cl- drops, membrane depolarization occurs and activates voltage dependent L-type calcium channels. The intracellular calcium (Ca^{+2}) rise activates Ca^{+2} dependent kinases that ultimately lead to regulation of gene expression and protein synthesis of cell cycle proteins. (45)

Estradiol and progesterone simultaneously activate the MAPK/ERK pathway (46) as well as an alternate pro-survival pathway, the Akt pathway. Activation of Akt by estradiol and progesterone is associated with increase neuronal survival. (47)

In 2006, the ProTECT Study (Progesterone for Traumatic Brain Injury: Experimental Clinical Treatment) by Dr. Wright and colleagues, was able to show that the acute use of progesterone in individuals with moderate to severe traumatic brain injury had a significant decrease in mortality then the controls. The mechanisms behind progesterone's central nervous system effects are neuroprotection and decrease in cerebral ischemia. (48) Recently, the results of the ProTECT III study were sadly released showing that progesterone did not have the initial benefits as the original study in 2006 promoted. (49)

There are more than 4600 articles on pregnenolone and traumatic brain injury (50[L]) detailing the improved survival after an acute traumatic brain injury. (51)

DHEA

DHEA and DHEA sulfate (henceforth to be referred to as DHEA) are synthesized de novo in the adrenal glands and in the human brain, and central nervous system where levels of DHEA are six to eight times higher than blood levels. DHEA is found throughout the brain, with highest concentrations in the prefrontal lobe and hippocampus where DHEA incrementally increases glutamate, acetylcholine and norepinephrine release. DHEA acts as a $GABA_A$ receptor non-competitive antagonist and positive allosteric modulator at the NMDA receptor. DHEA has neuroprotective, antioxidant, antihypertensive, anti-inflammatory, and anti-glucocorticoid effects. (52*)

Pregnenolone, DHEA and their sulfate esters have been found to protect against beta-amyloid peptide-induced neurotoxicity and amnesia. Additionally, animal studies have documented beneficial effects of DHEA on obesity, diabetes, cancer, heart disease, immune, and nervous functions. With respect to the latter, the neurotrophic and neuroprotective effects of DHEA and its sulfate DHEA-s have been documented. Nanomolar concentrations of DHEA or DHEAS promote the survival and differentiation of cultured neurons. Both steroids also protected hippocampal neurons from the toxic effects of glutamate and stimulate neurite growth in cultures of cortical neurons isolated from embryonic rat brains by modulating the activity of NMDA receptors. When administered in vivo, DHEAS significantly attenuated learning impairments induced by the administration of the NMDA antagonist Dizocilpine. (53)

As a final comment on DHEA/DHEA-s, a 1999 study that was touted as the first double-blind, placebo-controlled trial of DHEA's antidepressant efficacy in major depression had data showing that DHEA had antidepressant effects in patients with major depression, and that antidepressant responses were directly correlated with treatment-induced increases in plasma DHEA and DHEA-S levels. They recorded a 50 percent improvement in symptom reduction. (54)

A Word about Alzheimer's disease

Science has shown us that there is a relationship between traumatic brain injury and the rapid onset of Alzheimer's disease. Common to both Alzheimer's and TBI is the appearance of elevated levels of Tau proteins leading to tangled fibrils, inflammation, and amyloid beta production. Most recently, UCLA published an article on their development of a PET scan technique that can pick up tau protein associated with acute TBI in NFL players. (55) A study funded by the NFL also found that players who had experienced a TBI while on the field were 19 times more at risk then the general population to develop Alzheimer's at a younger age. (56) So, the lines between trauma as a cause for Alzheimer's and genetic predisposition are being blurred to suggest that trauma is the trump card! (See Dr. Gordon's presentation on YouTube — Alzheimer's disease: A Hormonal Approach to Treatment.)

Testosterone

Testosterone has been found to provide an impressive modulating influence over the pro-inflammatory (TH1) and anti-inflammatory (TH2) systems in the body. Unfortunately, when there is overwhelming inflammation associated with oxidative stressor, many of the beneficial effects are lost (as with all the neurosteroids) or significantly diminished. (57*) Therefore, in a comprehensive approach to the treatment of inflammation and neurodegeneration, appropriate use of supplements and medications to alleviate a non-neuropermissive environment must be employed.

Testosterone influences neuroplasticity in different nuclei of the limbic system and also exerts neuroprotective effects, which can be mediated either directly or indirectly via its aromatization to estradiol. The administration of testosterone immediately after nerve injury promotes their survival and regeneration through actions mediated by the androgen receptor. (58)

A topic and concept that I have been trying to convey to my colleagues for more than ten years is the issue of dosing of testosterone and the risk of down-regulation of central neurosteroids. Studies have found that abusive doses of testosterone can lead to the negative feed-back and genomic decrease in the biosynthesis of neurosteroids. The full understanding of the mechanism involved is not clear, but when levels of allopregnenolone, pregnenolone, deoxycorticosterone, and others are reduced, there is a converse increase in agitation, aggression, and irritability. (59) Can this be the clear statement that these "minor" neurosteroids have a major beneficial effect on our emotional status? My experience says, "Yes!!"

In the past 20 years Dr. C.J. Pick of USC Keck School of Medicine, Department of Geriatrics, subdivision – Alzheimer's and Dementia Diseases has published innumerable studies and reviews on the benefits of androgens in Alzheimer's disease. (60[L])

Could it be that the evolution of Alzheimer's is just the overt expression of a more ubiquitous and surreptitious process brought on by both physical and environmental insults inclusive of medication and radiation? If so, we are all doomed unless we prepare for this inevitability by maintaining healthy, youthful levels of all our hormones — and not just when they fail us. Interventional endocrinology provides for preemptive assessments and treatments to avoid many of the anticipated attacks on our well-being, both physically and spiritually.

Estradiol

Studies that looked at gender and neurodegenerative diseases have found a pattern in both estrogen and progesterone levels. Gender differences exist in most disorders affecting the central nervous system (CNS), particularly the neurodegenerative conditions, with women typically having a later onset and greater severity of disease.

Due to the neurological damage that occurs with a stroke, these have been classified as a neurodegenerative disease. While men have a 33 percent higher incidence of stroke throughout most of their lifespan, women have significantly worse stroke outcome in terms of comorbidity and mortality. Furthermore, women who have had a stroke are four to twelve times more at risk of developing a dementia condition like Alzheimer's. Finally, women who used oral estrogens had a 29 to 44 percent reduced risk of Alzheimer's disease. (61)

Accumulated clinical evidence suggests that estradiol provides neuroprotection as has been shown in decrease risk and delayed onset and progression of Alzheimer's disease and schizophrenia, and enhanced recovery from traumatic neurological injury such as stroke and traumatic brain injury. Recent basic science studies show that not only does exogenous estradiol decrease the response to various insults, but the brain itself upregulates both estrogen synthesis and estrogen receptor expression preferentially at sites of injury and degeneration. (62)

The beneficial effects of estradiol on neuroprotection is brought about by a few well-defined mechanisms: genomic signaling, non-genomic signaling, antioxidant actions, and regulation of mitochondrial bioenergetics. (63)

The accepted concepts of hormonal regulation of biological functions centered on gene transcription and protein synthesis. This classic genomic model for steroid hormone action presumes that steroid hormones can freely cross the plasma membrane, enter the cytoplasm, and bind to and activate specific intracellular steroid receptor proteins. The bound steroid receptors act as transcription factors and bind to specific DNA response elements in target gene promoters, causing activation or repression of transcription and subsequently protein synthesis. (64,65)

As with other steroid hormones, estradiol also modulates gene expression by a second indirect mechanism that involves the interaction of endoplasmic reticulum with other transcription factors which, in turn, bind their DNA elements. In this case, endoplasmic reticulum modulates the activities of transcription factors to produce enhancements for cell survival. In addition, estradiol binding to endoplasmic reticulum may also exert rapid actions that start with the activation of a variety of signal transduction pathways. (66)

These estradiol-dependent alterations in cell survival, axonal sprouting, regenerative responses, enhanced synaptic transmission, and enhanced neurogenesis are regulated by mechanisms that are being defined at present. (67) Some of the mechanisms underlying these effects are independent of the classically defined nuclear estrogen receptors (non-genomic) and involve unidentified membrane receptors, direct modulation of neurotransmitter receptor function, or the known antioxidant activities of estrogen.

Supported by many in vivo and in vitro studies, treatment with estradiol enhances neuronal survival and recovery in animal models of TBI. In culture, estradiol protects neurons against excitatory amino acid and Beta-amyloid peptide toxicity, oxidative stress, and glucose deprivation. More recently, estradiol has also been shown to promote neurogenesis within the adult hippocampal formation, which is an area involved in recent and remote memory. An observation that may be particularly relevant for Alzheimer's disease is the decreased generation of beta-amyloid. Decreased levels of estrogen in post-menopausal women could thus contribute to the increased risk for the development of neurodegenerative diseases. (68)

Summary

Obviously, this was not a traditional approach to the science of Neuroendocrinology, but a step outside of the normal boundaries that have limited alternative approaches to the treatment of neurotrauma with subsequent neuropsychiatric complications. Over 20 years ago, Drs. Baulieu and Robel identified the presence of neurosteroids and their enzyme systems in specific areas of the brain — such as the cortex, hypothalamus, and amygdala. (69*)

On a macro scale, the hormones (neuroactive steroids) produced by the peripheral glands under the direction of pituitary trophic hormones, regulate many of the physical aspects of our existence, while the brain's neurosteroids control how we use it (the area below the neck). Neuroactive steroids are transported across the blood-brain barrier to influence genomic and non-genomic processes, while the neurosteroids have rapid effects on modulation of neurotransmissions, while influencing the slower genomic code. These delayed processes frequently relate to the up- or down-regulation of genes used to transcribe enzymes needed for neurosteroidogenesis.

During the aging process, the regulation of many of the neurosteroids and neuroactive steroids diminish due to illness, medication, X-ray irradiation, and probably more often than not, the accrued effect of lifetime traumas to the HP axis. This leads to increased inflammation with further loss of neurosteroids and disruption in neuro-connectivity. The end result may be expressed as an array of symptoms that are exemplified by anxiety, agitation, aggressiveness, depression, phobias, lethargy, and cognitive impairment.

The developing science behind the progesterone metabolite — allopregnanolone — is worthy of close attention and the addition to every treatment protocol. Over the past ten years, we at the Millennium have used moderate doses of pregnenolone to push the production of allopregnanolone from progesterone.

Allopregnanolone (Allo) is the most important neurosteroid, targeting both neurons and glial cells in central and periphery, primarily through rapid 'non-genomic' action via $GABA_A$ receptor (GABA-AR). Given these inherent properties, Allo is a promising drug for the development of novel neuroprotective and neuroregenerative strategies, as well as for the treatment of neuropsychiatric disorders. (70)

We feel so strongly about the science supporting allopregnanolone's benefits that we started a small pilot program using nightly doses of sublingual progesterone in veterans with blast trauma. Within a week, many experience better sleep, awaken with more energy, have clearer mentation (less foggy), less anxiety and depressive thoughts, and an improved outlook on life in general. (71)

The excitement here is in the potential that many of our traditional medications used for pathopsychiatric conditions will be replaced by neurosteroids like Ganaxolone. This is an Allo analogue that acts on the GABAergic system as a therapeutic alternative to the serotonin reuptake inhibitors. At present, it is the first neurosteroid analogue approved by the Food and Drug Administration for PTSD. (72)

The door is now open and soon more will follow.

Chapter 5: Neuroradiology in TBI

"You must understand that seeing believes, but also know that believing is seeing."

— Denis Waitley

Introduction

In addition to a physical examination, neurobehavioral evaluation, comprehensive neurosteroid and neuroactive steroid testing, another crucial role in the acute assessment and follow-up of a patient with a history of mild traumatic brain injury (mTBI) will be played by diagnostic imaging. Acutely, neuroimaging will help rule out the need for urgent surgical intervention. Post-injury, neuroimaging will address neuropsychiatric changes that are frequently being seen in patients with mild TBI months, and even years, after the insult. (1)

The neuroradiologic and neuropsychiatric worlds have conceptually merged in an effort to analyze the correlates between neuroimaging and the subsequent development of neurobehavioral changes. Unique to the population of mTBI patients, as opposed to moderate and severe cases, is the lack of clear anatomical alterations that are common to the other classifications. Therefore, functional imaging techniques will be needed to evaluate the impact of TBI on brain metabolism, neuron connectivity, regional blood flow, and expanding parenchymal deficits affecting recovery.

The majority of primary healthcare providers (MD, DO, ND, PA, and NP) will be exposed to the unique needs of mTBI survivors in the aftercare setting, and not in an emergency room. Aside from addressing their immediate and frequently demoralizing symptomatology, they will most likely be in need of functional neuroimaging (2) to assess the contributing factors leading to their cognitive and behavior deficits. (3*)

As I prepared for this chapter (2011), I was put into awe at the incredible technology that has been around for over a decade, if not longer. Reading research and clinical application papers one after another on each neuroradiologic procedure, I kept asking myself the same question over and over again, "Why hasn't this technology been put to use in all those TBI cases?" No one answered so, I kept on reading. (4)

There are ten radiologic procedures that will be reviewed here. Although not necessarily an all-inclusive list, but understanding that newer technologies are being worked out even at this very moment, the list will expand in time. It is logical that many of the newer technologies will be based on well-established procedures, like what has happened with the morphing of MRI to fMRI, MRI to DTI-MRI, MRI to H-MRS, and then the grand melding of a number of technologies into the Fusion Imaging MRI technique. (5) I have purposely not explained these abbreviations so that you are forced to read this chapter in its entirety. Live and learn.

Procedure	xRay	CTS	MRI	fMRI	PETS	SPECT	DTI	MRS	MEG	Fusion
Structural	X	X	X	X			X			X
Functional			X	X	X	X	X	X	X	X

Table 5.1: Over-view of neuroradiologic procedures and their assessments.

In the acute phase of assessment, the focus is on intracranial bleeding, as well as fractures of the calvarium. Once the patient is stabilized, advanced imaging technology can be used to further define the microscopic damage that is frequently associated with even mild TBI.

What follows is a walk-through of each radiologic procedure addressing their specific use as it pertains to an anatomical versus functional assessment of the patient with mTBI. Many of the functional studies will be obtained in the aftercare of the patients and not necessarily in the acute care setting for obvious reasons. The majority of the cases that we, as clinical physicians, will see are the mTBI cases that have developed new symptomatology months, years, or even decades after the initial insult. It is this temporal dissociation that frequently leads to our missing the TBI that set them on their course and into our care. Don't forget to ask!

Anatomic Imaging Techniques

Plain Film Radiography (X-Ray)

The best use of an X-ray is for:

Structural assessment of bones, as in looking for fractures…

…or foreign objects

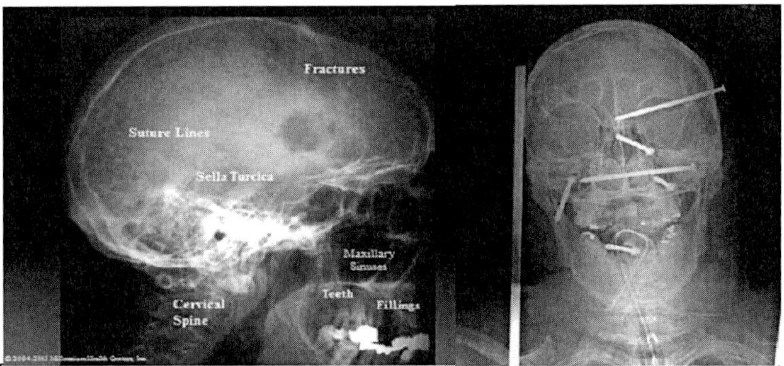

Figure 5.1: Plain x-rays of standard landmarks and foreign objects in a case of a contractor's angry wife. She nailed him for infidelity.

This is the oldest radiologic technique for looking past the skin and into the body. It is able to see calcified structures (bones) and any object with a high density, like bullets or nails. It cannot provide the needed visualization of internal structures of the skull (basilar fracture) or tell us whether there is disruption of any aspect of the vascular supply. Therefore, its use in closed head injury is inadequate, but may be used in assessing skull fractures or penetrating foreign objects.

X-rays are electromagnetic energy with a short wavelength. When directed at a target, X-rays can often pass through the substance uninterrupted, especially when it is of low density. Higher density targets like bone will reflect or absorb the X-rays. They do this because there is less space between the atoms for the short waves to pass through. Thus, an X-ray image shows dark areas where the rays traveled completely through the target (soft tissue or air) and shows light areas where the rays were blocked by dense material (such as bones, bullets, knives, and nails).

The taking of an X-ray is a simple procedure. The patient is positioned in front or on top of a photographic plate, while on the opposite side, the X-ray stream is released to pass through the patient and ends up exposing the film. Think of it as a human sandwich.

The use of this radiologic procedure in TBI is limited. Since its fundamental use is in the evaluation of dense objects, the information that can be supplied would be fracture of the skull. Unfortunately, due to the complexity at the base of the skull with overlapping structures, it is not uncommon to miss fractures of the basilar skull. Therefore, the plain radiogram has little evaluative value in TBI.

Computer Tomography Scan (CT-Scan)

The best use of the CT-Scan is for three-dimensional imaging of:

Bleeding, brain injury, and skull fractures in patients with head injuries.

Bleeding caused by a ruptured or leaking aneurysms in patients with a sudden severe headache.

A blood clot or bleeding within the brain shortly after a patient exhibits symptoms of a stroke.

Brain tumors.

Enlarged brain cavities (ventricles) in patients with hydrocephalus.

Diseases or malformations of the skull.

Diagnose diseases of the temporal bone on the side of the skull, which may be causing hearing problems.

Assess aneurysms or arteriovenous malformations through a technique called CT angiography.

Category	Definition
Diffuse Injury I (No Visible Pathology)	No visible intra-cranial pathology seen on CT scan.
Diffuse Injury II	Cisterns are present with midline shift < 5 mm and/or lesion densities present. No high- or mixed-density lesion > 25 ml, may include bone fragments and foreign bodies
Diffuse Injury III	Cisterns compressed or absent with mid-line shift 0–5 mm No high- or mixed-density lesion .25 ml
Diffuse Injury IV	Mid-line shift >5 mm. No high- or mixed-density lesion >25 ml
Evacuated mass lesion	Any lesion surgically evacuated
Non-evacuated mass lesion	High- or mixed-density lesion >25 ml, not surgically evacuated

Table 5.2: Marshall's CT Classification for Traumatic Brain Injury.

In many ways, CT scanning works like other X-ray examinations. In a conventional X-ray exam, a small burst of radiation is aimed at and passes through the body, recording an image on photographic film or a special image recording plate. Bones appear white on the X-ray, while soft tissue shows up in shades of gray, and air appears black. (6)

CT imaging is sometimes compared to looking into a loaf of bread by cutting the loaf into thin slices. When the image slices are reassembled by computer software, the result is a very detailed multidimensional view of the body's interior.

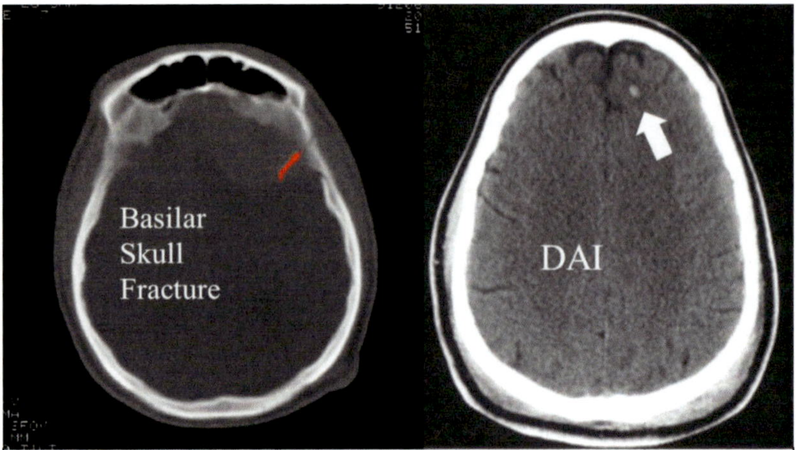

Figure 5.2: CT-Scan showing on left the Basilar skull fracture that can be missed on plain radiograms and to the right microhemorrhages associated with shearing of axons and blood vessels.

The use of this radiologic procedure in traumatic brain injury is the preferred imaging tool in the acute setting in the emergency room. It is fast and it can identify basilar skull fractures, as well as intracranial bleeding and clots, although it is limited in that the resolution is poor for lesions less than one to 1.5 cm.

Magnetic Resonance Imaging (MRI)

The best use of MRI in Neuroradiology is for:

Traumatic brain injury

Diffuse axonal injury (DAI)

Diagnosing multiple sclerosis (MS)

Diagnosing tumors of the pituitary gland and brain

Diagnosing infections in the brain, spine or joints

Diagnosing strokes in their earliest stages

In the beginning, it took almost five hours to produce one single image that were, by today's standards, quite ugly. Dr. Raymond Damadian, a physician and scientist, along with colleagues Drs. Larry Minkoff and Michael Goldsmith, labored tirelessly for seven long years to reach this point. They named their original machine "Indomitable" to capture the spirit of their struggle to do what many said could not be done. Their original machine is now in the Smithsonian Institution while thousands of modern MRI machines are in clinical use around the world. (7)

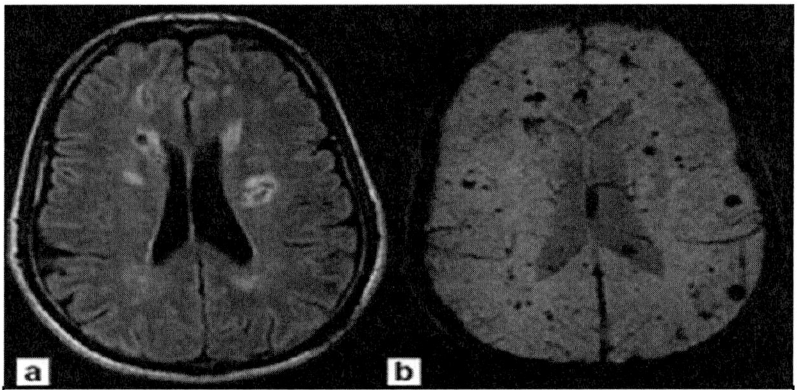

Figure 5.3: An MRI image showing the difference between (a) FLARE and (b) SWI. FLARE (fluid-attenuated inversion recovery) is a pulse sequence used in MRI which nulls fluids; for example, it can be used in brain imaging to suppress CSF effects on the image. SWI (susceptibility weighted imaging), originally called BOLD, uses a type of contrast in MRI different from traditional spin density, T1, or T2 imaging. This method exploits the susceptibility differences between tissues and uses the phase image to detect these differences. The susceptibility difference is the degree of magnetization of a material in response to an applied magnetic field.

The image above shows a comparison of a traditional MRI technique, FLARE (a), to an SWI image (b). Both images were taken of the same patient. Note the ‘voids’ in (b) that would have gone undiagnosed were a clinician to use only (a). The SWI image is possible through the use of algorithms that differentiate the densities of adjacent tissues. While signal density forms the basis of all MR scans, including (a), the SWI scan (b) is three to six times more sensitive as it accounts for the susceptibility of all brain elements, including hemorrhages — hence, the name Susceptibility Weighted Image. SWI is clinically appropriate in the diagnosis of: TBI, tumors, stroke, hemorrhage, MS, vascular dementia, and other brain disorders. (8)

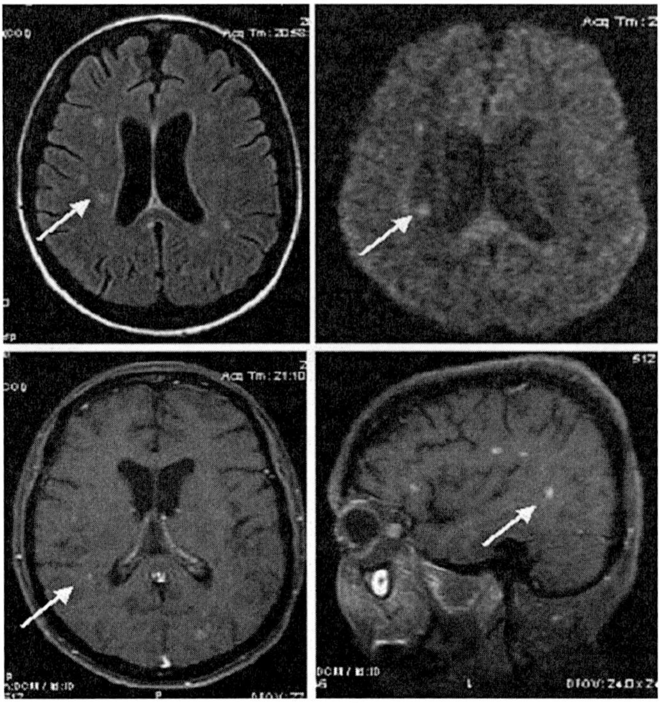

Image 5.4: MRI showing multiple traumatic calcifications with use of FLARE (except top right which is DTI).

Reductions in hippocampal volumes and lateral ventricular enlargement were significantly associated with impaired memory functions, memory complaints, and executive functions. Of the MRI parameters used, the best predictor for cognitive outcome was the volume of the lateral ventricle. There was only a modest relationship between severity of injury and cognitive performance. The results show that long-term memory impairments after TBI are associated with MRI volumetric measures. This suggests that the degree of diffuse injury leading to atrophic changes is prognostically more important than the initial severity of TBI. (9, 10)

Functional Imaging Techniques

Functional Magnetic Resonance Imaging (fMRI)

The best use of fMRI in neuroradiology is for:

The relationship between neuronal and psychological processes (11)

Functionality by proxy (12)

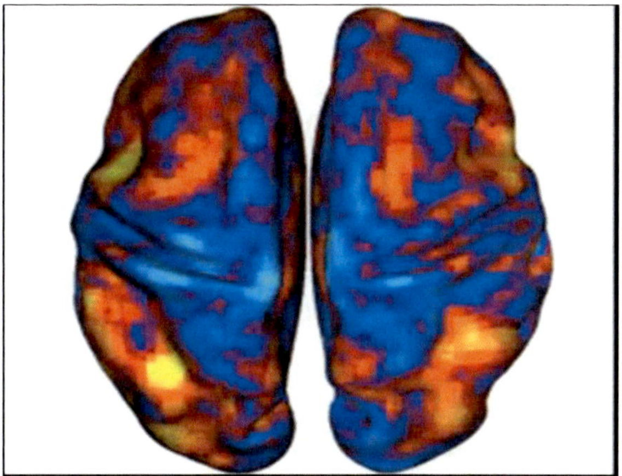

Image 5.5: Functional MRI studies look at how blood oxygen levels change, and assuming that this is connected to nerves firing and increased metabolism give a red color for high activity and blue for low.

Functional MRI makes use of a special signal called blood oxygen level dependent (BOLD) contrast. Blood flowing through the brain carries oxygen on hemoglobin molecules which also carry iron, and so they have a magnetic signal. It turns out that hemoglobin molecules have different magnetic properties when they are attached to oxygen than when they are not carrying oxygen, and this small difference can be detected with an MRI machine. (13)

Active areas of the brain tend to use more oxygen than those regions that are less active. As the oxygen gradient decreases in any active region, the brain compensates by inducing dilation of the local vasculature in order to restore the oxygen supply and gradient. The brain may even do this job a little too well, so that more oxygenated blood goes into the area than what was initially used. The MRI machine can detect the difference in signal that results from this increase in blood oxygen. (15)

So, functional MRI studies are not actually looking at neuronal activity directly, but are looking at how blood oxygen levels change and, assuming that this is connected to nerves firing, increased metabolism. Studies have shown that this assumption is usually correct, although sometimes you need to interpret the studies carefully if you think that the blood flow may not be as tightly coupled to nervous activity as usual. Diseases like vascular malformations, tumors, and even normal aging can change the relationship between neural activity and the local blood flow that results in BOLD signal. (16)

There are two main ways of looking at brain function using fMRI. One method focuses on finding specific areas of the brain that respond to some task or stimulus. For example, the person in the MRI scanner might be shown a flashing checkerboard at some points, and other times a blank screen. They may be asked to push a button whenever they see the flashing checkerboard. The signal during the task will then be compared to the signal when the task isn't being done, and the result will be a kind of picture of what brain regions were involved with seeing a flashing checkerboard and then pushing a button. (17)

The other way fMRI can be used is to evaluate neural networks. This involves figuring out what areas of the brain are talking to each other. If one area of the brain usually lights up at the same time as another, these two areas of the brain may be connected. No task may even be needed in order to do this kind of study. For this reason, these studies are sometimes called "resting state functional magnetic resonance imaging."

The information that comes from functional MRI studies is very complicated, and requires a lot of statistical analysis to become meaningful. This initially led many people to mistrust the results of functional MRI studies, as it seemed there were many possible opportunities for error in the analysis. However, as both researchers and reviewers have become more familiar with the new technology, results are becoming both more trusted, and trustworthy. (18)

Proton Emission Tomography Scan (PET scan)

The best use of a PET scan in neuroradiology is for:

Trauma to the brain

Alzheimer's disease

Stroke (restricted or reduced oxygen and blood in the brain that leads to cellular death)

Viral infections (viruses may cause inflammation and swelling in the brain's tissue)

Abnormal growths (tumors)

Changes in the brain's communication between neurons

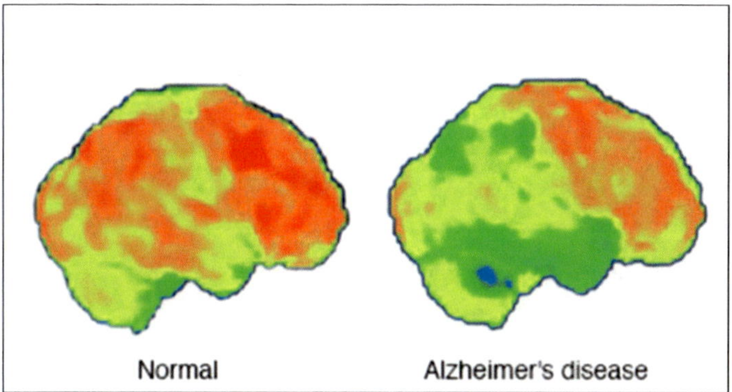

Image 5.6: A PET scan uses RED to indicate the highest level of activity while orange, green and blue represent progressively lower levels of brain activity.

PET neuroimaging is based on an assumption that areas of high radioactivity are associated with brain activity. What is actually measured indirectly is the flow of blood to different parts of the brain.

In mTBI, subtle changes occur in the normal pattern and regulation of blood flow, as well as glucose metabolism. Using standard FDG-PET (a radioactive glucose tracer) tracer, it was found that the greatest amount of disrupted glucose metabolism occurred at the site of contusion and continued outward for another 22mm. (19*)

In practice, since the brain is normally a rapid user of glucose, and since brain pathologies such as traumatic brain injury and Alzheimer's disease greatly decrease brain metabolism of both glucose and oxygen in tandem, standard FDG-PET of the brain, which measures regional glucose use, may also be successfully used to differentiate Alzheimer's disease from other dementing processes, and also to make early diagnosis of Alzheimer's disease, which is associated with traumatic brain injury. (20)

One of the main differences between PET scans and other imaging tests like CT scan or MRI is that the PET scan looks into the cellular level of metabolic changes in tissues. This is important because disease processes often begin with functional changes at the cellular level. A PET scan can often detect these very early changes, whereas a CT or MRI detect changes a little later as the disease begins to cause changes in the anatomical structure of the tissues. (21[1])

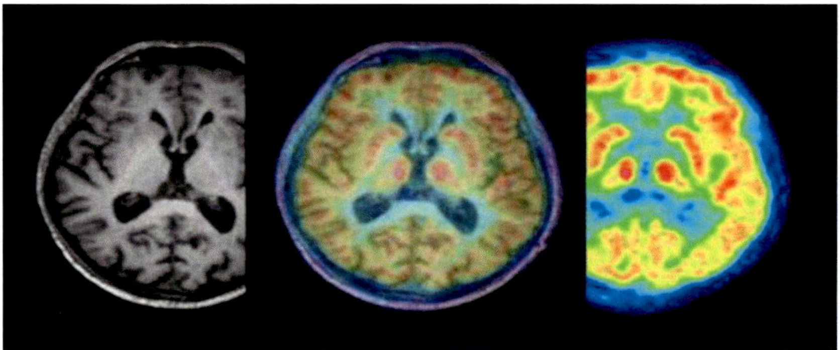

Image 5.7: An MRI/PET fusion scan showing on the left the morphology of an MRI scan and on the right the metabolic aspects of the PET scan. In the center is the image of the MRI/PET fusion scan disclosing morphologic areas of the brain with relative activity.

In 2008, the PET and MRI scan technologies were fused together resulting in the combination of molecular, morphological, and functional information that will allow for a better understanding of physiological and disease mechanisms in preclinical and clinical settings. (22)

Single Photon Emission Computer Tomography (SPECT Scan)

The best uses for a SPECT scan are:

Perfusion imaging (vascular flow)

Neurofunction (metabolism)

Receptor imaging (Parkinson's)

Refractory focal epileptogenic areas

Vasculitis

Neurolupus

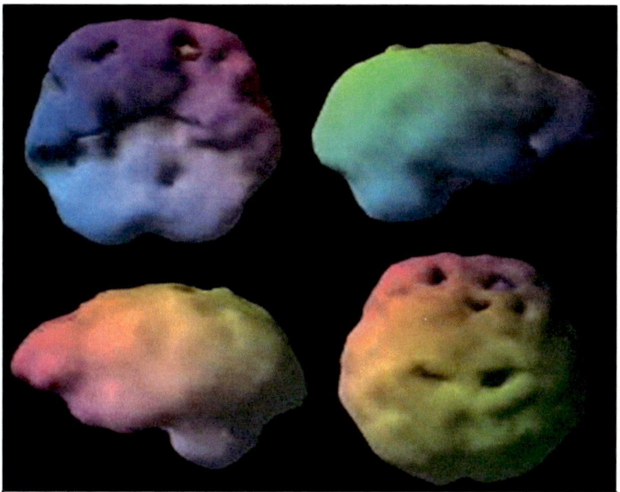

Image 5.8: This SPECT scan shows hypoperfusion in the Pre-frontal cortex that is associated with low dopamine.

This is a nuclear medicine technique that can be used in any organ system of the body, but its role in assessing perfusion or receptor imaging of the brain is primary. Using a radiopharmaceutical tracer, multiple 2-D images are obtained with a gamma camera that revolves around the imaging site in 360 degrees. The array of images captured is then computer processed to generate a 3-D construct. (23)

There are a number of tracers presently available, and more are under clinical investigation. The intravenous radiopharmaceutical 99mTc-HMPAO is used for cerebral perfusion imaging. HMPAO is a highly lipophilic compound, which crosses the blood brain barrier without resistance, and in proportion to cerebral blood flow. Once it has been taken up by neuronal tissue it binds to Glutathione, causing it to become both hydrophilic and trapped in the neuronal tissue, unable to be washed out. This process can take just a few minutes to complete and can give us a snapshot of brain activity. Unique to the brain is a process of perfusion auto-regulation: Those areas with the highest neuronal activity will utilize more nutrition, oxygen, and produce more metabolites then areas with less neuronal activity. In those areas of highest activity, there is a proportionate increase in perfusion and therefore, higher concentrations of HMPAO. An image of cerebral perfusion thus indirectly reflects cerebral metabolism. (24[1])

In patients that have sustained traumatic brain injury associated with subtle neuropsychological alterations, the SPECT scan can show anatomical abnormalities that were not seen on either CT or MRI scans. (25)

In a study looking at SPECT scans of 228 individuals, normal studies accounted for 52 (23 percent) and abnormal studies were present in 176 (77 percent). The specific findings were: basal ganglia hypoperfusion 338 lesions (55.2 percent); frontal lobe hypoperfusion 146 (23.8 percent); temporal lobes hypoperfusion 80 (13 percent); parietal lobes hypoperfusion 20 (3.7 percent); insular and or occipital lobes hypoperfusion 28 (4.6 percent). Patients' symptoms correlated with the SPECT brain perfusion findings. The SPECT were performed within three months of the date of the accident, and for the remainder, 106 (46 percent) over three months, and less than three years from the date of the injury. In early imaging, 382 lesions were detected in 92 patients, while imaging after three months detected 230 lesions in 84 patients. The study concluded that basal ganglia hypoperfusion is the most common abnormality, following mild or moderate traumatic brain injury, and is more common in patients complaining of memory problem and dizziness. Early imaging can detect more lesions than delayed imaging, and SPECT brain perfusion abnormalities can occur in the absence of LOC. (26[1])

Diffusion Tensor Imaging MRI (DTI MRI)

The best uses for a DTI-MRI scan are:

Traumatic brain injury.

Diffuse axonal injury.

Evaluation of central axotomy (severing of axons).

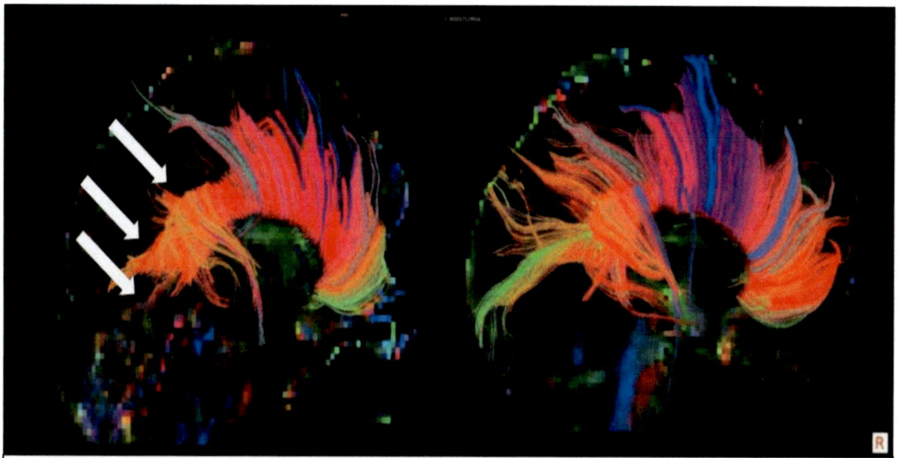

Image 5.9: DTI-MRI showing a deficit in the occipital lobe(left) and normal control (right).

Tractography is performed using data from diffusion tensor imaging (DTI) — a form of MRI. Water molecules diffuse more easily parallel to myelinated axons, when compared to the perpendicular direction. DTI uses this property to map the underlying axonal connections in the brain. One important measure is that of fractional anisotropy (FA), which represents the ratio of water molecules diffusing in parallel, as opposed to perpendicular directions, and thus reflects integrity of white matter bundles. Tears in these axon bundles from trauma may result in differential FA ratios because of the perpendicular flow of water out of these tears. (27*)

Conditions where the myelin or the structure of the axon is disrupted (such as trauma, tumors, and inflammation) reduce anisotropy as the barriers are affected by destruction or disorganization. Each anisotropy is linked to an orientation of the predominant axis (predominant direction of the diffusion). Post-processing programs are able to extract this directional information.

This additional information is difficult to represent on 2-D grayscale images. To overcome this problem, a color code is introduced. Basic colors can tell the observer how the fibers are oriented in a 3-D coordinate system. This is termed an "anisotropic map" where software can encode the colors (28) in this way:

> Red indicates directions on the X axis (right to left or left to right)
> Green indicates directions on the Y axis (posterior to anterior or from anterior to posterior)

Blue indicates directions on the Z axis (foot to head direction or vice versa)

In Figure 5.8, the tractography clearly shows interruption of long axons. It is these types of finding that can account for the changes in one's personality and cognition. Once treatment is started, the assessment of repair is best performed with the MEG scan, which can show the interconnectivity between different lobes of the brain.

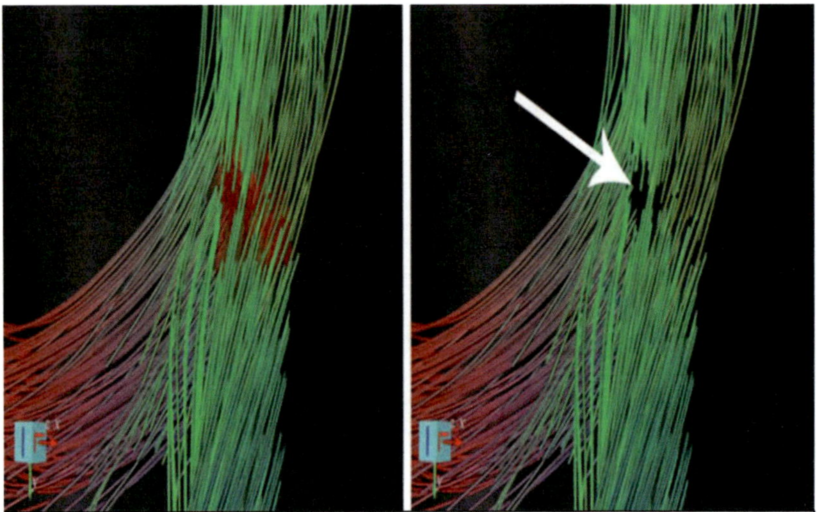

Figure 5.8: A high definition tractogram showing interruption of neurofibers (axons). This loss of interconnectivity can be followed using the MEG Scan discussed further in this chapter.

Proton Magnetic Resonance Spectroscopy (H-MRS)

The best uses for an H-MRS scan are:

Traumatic brain injury.

Diffuse axonal injury.

Evaluation of central axotomy (severing of axons).

Magnetic resonance spectroscopy (MRS) is an analytical technique that can be used to complement the more common magnetic resonance imaging (MRI) in the characterization of tissue. Magnetic resonance spectroscopy (MRS), also known as nuclear magnetic resonance (NMR) spectroscopy, is a non-invasive, ionizing radiation free analytical technique that has been used to study metabolic changes in traumatic brain injury, brain tumors, strokes, seizure disorders, Alzheimer's disease, depression and other diseases affecting the brain. (29)

Both techniques use signals from hydrogen protons (1H), but MRI uses the information to create 2-D images of the brain, while MRS uses 1H signals to determine the relative concentrations of target brain metabolites. Table 5.3 lists the common metabolites measured, and their relevancy in patients with TBI.

Proton MR Spectroscopy	
N-acetyl aspartate (NAA)	Is found almost exclusively in neurons at high concentration.
Choline (Cho)	Choline based chemistry is a vital constituent of the phospholipid metabolism of cell membranes. Increase levels of Choline is associated with conditions of myelin erosion.
Creatine (Cr)	Is present in both neural and glial cells.
Lactate (lac)	Is associated with anaerobic glycolysis, so the presence of Lip-Lac can reflect brain ischemia.

Table 5.3: Imaging markers located by H-MRS.

The main metabolites measured by H-MRS are: N-acetyl aspartate, which is a quantitative marker of neuronal health and is significantly decreased in demyelinated areas in multiple sclerosis; choline, which is a marker of inflammation and is elevated in cell proliferation; myo-inositol, which is a glial marker; lactate, which is an indirect indicator of ischemic and hypoxic conditions; and creatine and phosphocreatine, which are related to energy metabolism. Data from MRS studies are often expressed as changes in the ratio of N-acetyl aspartate to creatine or choline. (30*)

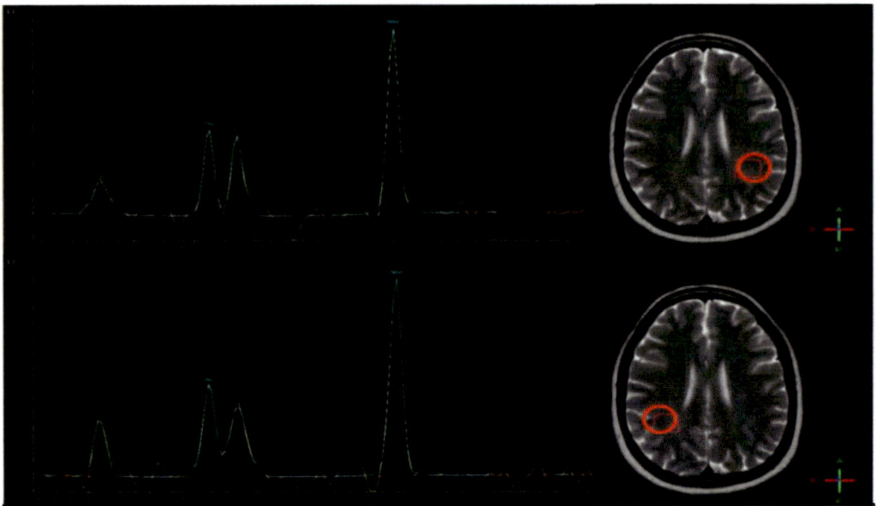

Figure 5.9: Proton MR Spectroscopy targets an area of cells and measures the presents of key metabolites. The quantities and the proportionate distribution of these markers can be interpreted to represent the health of the region under investigation.

When an area defect is seen on MRI (anatomical), the H-MRS is used to scan the same area for detection of the composition of metabolites, which is relative to the functioning of the cells in the target area. Based upon the analytical spectrum of each metabolite (NAA, Cho, Cr, and Lac), a definition of the status of the cells in the area under evaluation can be determined. The loss of NAA signal is associated with loss of cell membrane integrity, while elevation in lactate is relative to damage from ischemia and hypoxia. (31)

Magnetoencephalography (MEG)

The best uses for an MEG scan are:

Traumatic brain injury

Diffuse axonal injury

Functional neuronal disconnectivity

Functional neuronal reconnectivity

Neuroplasticity

Evaluation of central axotomy (severing of axons)

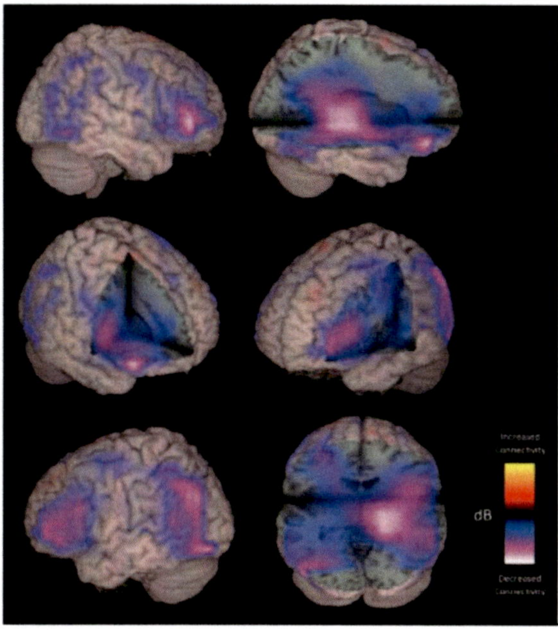

Figure 5.10: Using the MEG Scan to assess functional connectivity after TBI, as a means of quantifying a pathophysiological process that may otherwise only have clinical manifestations.

A pre- and post-study could be used to measure the return of neuronal functioning.

Magnetoencephalography (32) is an imaging technique used to measure the magnetic fields produced by electrical activity in the brain via extremely sensitive sensors called SQUIDs. (33)

One mechanism by which TBI is thought to affect cognition and behavior is through alteration of functional connectivity. That is, the brain's interconnectivity between different lobes can be disrupted by a single focal lesion having damaging effects not only locally, but also in remote connected sites.

Using the MEG scan to assess functional connectivity can offer a means of quantifying a pathophysiological process (disruption of connectivity) that may otherwise only have clinical manifestations. Magnetoencephalography has been used for studying functional connectivity in diverse diseases including brain tumors, schizophrenia, and stroke. (34)

In a key analysis of the MEG scan by a UCSF group, they collected one-minute resting-state MEG recordings of neuromagnetic activity in the alpha frequency band (eight to twelve Hz) in a group of patients and compared the results with cohort matched controls. The resting state alpha wave band has the greatest signal strength thereby making it the most accessible to be used to analyze interregional connectivity. (35)

It is postulated that disruption of long-interconnecting axonal tracts due to focal cortical and shearing injures will cause a reduction in the alpha-band MEG functional connectivity in TBI patients versus controls. The sensitivity of MEG scanning in TBI allows for the detection of injury, based upon decreases in functional connectivity that are absent in 3-T MRI studies. Frequently in TBI, there is an absence of focal lesions on conventional neuroimaging, but TBI can disrupt connectivity in widely disparate brain regions which MEG can detect. (36)

This same sensitivity can be used to monitor functional recovery based upon increases in alpha-band MEG functional connectivity. (37)

Magnetoencephalography also detects abnormally low functional connectivity in three out of five patients without radiographically evident traumatic lesions on 3-T MR imaging, suggesting a potentially high degree of sensitivity to brain injury. Furthermore, we observed in two cases that long-term recovery from the effects of TBI was accompanied by improvements in these areas of disrupted connectivity on follow-up MEG scans and, in one striking case, by the development of new areas of elevated functional connectivity compared with controls. (38) "Our results show that abnormal MEG functional connectivity can be localized to within one cm using short recording periods of one minute or less that can be easily performed in the clinical setting."

A regional compensatory response to brain injury called "over-connected" is detected in the recovering patients where the production of alpha-wave frequency is heightened. Study reports of reorganization in neural networks after brain injury (a phenomenon known as neuroplasticity) has been documented in young study participants supporting the premise that a greater capacity exists for neuroplasticity — in response to injury — in younger age groups. (39[1])

Summary

In the acute phase of TBI it is important to address all aspects of the primary injury, whether the etiology is penetrating or non-penetrating. Blunt head impact caused by a bat, slip and fall, or coming to a stop against the front windshield is also associated with a varying degree of rapid acceleration/deceleration. The cumulative results of these mechanical forces cause tissue distortion, compression, shearing, and swelling. Manifestations of these injuries include cerebral contusions, extra-axial hematomas (epidural, subdural, and subarachnoid hemorrhages), and diffuse axonal injury.

While contusions, epidural hematomas, subdural hematomas, and subarachnoid hemorrhage are commonly observed in moderate and severe non-penetrating TBI, the hallmark of penetrating TBI is cerebral laceration. (40) As a missile penetrates the brain, it tears the parenchyma, leaving a track with necrosis and hemorrhage (laceration). In the wake of the projectile, tissue is compressed, collapses and re-expands in a repeating wave-like pattern that further injures tissue.

Contusions are regions of hemorrhagic necrosis due to acceleration/deceleration. They most frequently occur in the orbitofrontal and anterior temporal regions and may be ipsilateral to the site of impact (coup) if the head is relatively immobilized when struck, or contralateral to the site of impact (contra-coup) if the head is not immobilized. While contusions may appear as multifocal areas of patchy hemorrhage, these hemorrhages may coalesce into a larger parenchymal hematoma. Roughly, one-third of contusion injures expand within the first 24 hours after injury. (41)

Epidural hematomas (EDH), observed in roughly five percent of patients with TBI, typically occur in the context of a skull fracture that involves the groove of the middle meningeal artery. (42) While laceration of the MMA is most commonly responsible for EDH, epidural bleeding may also occur from injury to the middle meningeal vein, the diploic veins, or the venous sinuses.

Subdural hematomas (SDH) are typically caused by rupture of the bridging veins and are often associated with severe underlying brain injury and high mortality. They usually occur over the cerebral convexities and are bilateral in roughly 15 percent; however, they may also occur along the tentorium or the falx. The mechanism of injury responsible for SDH differs by age group. Over 50 percent of SDH are caused by MVC in the 18 to 40 year age group, whereas falls comprise the vast majority of SDH in those over 65 years of age. (43*)

Subarachnoid hemorrhages result from tearing of small pial vessels. Blood is typically located over the cerebral convexities and is often confined to a few sulci or fissures. However, subarachnoid blood may distribute diffusely over the cortical surface, into the basal cisterns, or into the ventricles.

Diffuse axonal injury (DAI) is commonly observed after rapid acceleration and deceleration of the head, typically in the lateral plane. DAI is both a form of primary and a form of secondary injury. There may be immediate mechanical damage (primary injury) to structural elements of axons, such as microtubules, at the time of the trauma. This typically occurs in severe TBI that involves tearing of tissue. It has become evident, however, that axonal swelling, and ultimately axotomy (44), is the consequence of cellular cascades that are initiated by the physical trauma and continued by the secondary phase of injury.

Regions commonly affected include: the junction between cortex and white matter, white matter structures close to the midline (corpus callosum, internal capsule), the brainstem, cerebellum, and the corona radiata. Some have proposed the use of the term, “traumatic axonal injury (TAI)” or “diffuse traumatic axonal injury (dTAI)” to describe theses pathological and pathophysiological changes. (45)

The majority of patients that we see with TBI are those who have sustained a mild TBI (mTBI) and therefore, were never seen in an emergency room nor had a comprehensive evaluation until they developed symptoms that altered their functioning. These individuals, over the course of time, had developed changes in cognition and behavior with combinations of depression, anxiety, bursts of anger, lack of purpose, fatigue, loss of libido, phantom body aches and pains, and weight gain. A thoughtful history retrieving previous TBI or body injuries will open up the evaluation to include neuroradiologic evaluations looking at functionality of the brain.

The Millennium recommends using one or more of the following procedures to monitor treatment benefits based upon improvement in neurological functioning. The cost and availability of any of these procedures will probably be the bases for their selection. The order in which these neuroradiologic procedures are listed is based upon general availability. My personal favorites at the initiation of treatment are the DTI-MRI, SPECT scan, and the PET scan. The benefit of the MEG Scan, over time, can be as a treatment feedback tool to monitor neuronal regeneration and repair of connectivity provided by reestablishment of a Neuro-Permissive Environment (NPE).

Chapter 6: The Laboratory of TBI

"The mystery of life isn't a problem to solve, but a reality to experience."

— Frank Herbert, *Dune*

Introduction

The challenge to provide optimal treatment for patients with traumatic brain injury (TBI) is based upon a combination of two core issues: First, the selection of diagnostic laboratory testing that will allow for differentiation between central and peripheral hormonal disorders; and second, the critical interpretation of these results as they pertain to the concept of subclinical levels or insufficiency.

Our selection of laboratory testing for traumatic brain injury consists of those biochemical markers that will allow for a clear interpretation for both peripheral (neuroactive steroids) and central (neurosteroids) hormonal deficiencies and insufficiencies. The Millennium's TBI Panel 1 offers a robust assessment of the major and minor hormones allowing for correlation between central tropic hormones (1) and their peripheral target gland products: i.e., GH/IGF-1(liver), LH/testosterone/estrogens (testes/ovaries), TSH/T4 (thyroid), and ACTH/cortisol (adrenals). Additionally, carrier proteins (SHBG, ALS, thyroglobulin, and albumin) and metabolic markers are evaluated, along with cell counts and trace minerals. It is important to establish that each client's biochemistry is ideal and that there are no hidden conditions that will need to be addressed before instituting hormonal treatment. (2)

Once optimal laboratory assessment has been performed, it becomes the application of these results in the formulation of a treatment protocol; therefore, the interpretation of these results becomes the sine qua non (3) of the patient's improvement and quality of life.

Current conventional medical wisdom has offered us a foundation for the interpretation of laboratory results based upon a population study. However, in the words of Eugene K. Harris (4), "The conventional population-based normal (laboratory) range has been shown to be a generally defective reference criterion for assessing individual laboratory test results." It has been generally accepted that each assayed biochemical product has a range of acceptable "normal" or a "reference range" that is based upon two standard deviations. It has been the assumption that these ranges derived from a sampling group can be applied to all individuals. Instead, Harris proposed (in 1975 if not earlier), that the individual needs to be assessed based upon a series of laboratory results derived from their own blood, and not compared to the range of group results. His rationale behind this was based upon the individuality of the sampling and the dichotomy in the inherent ranges among people as being too variable to have any one range being called "normal" and used as a reference. (5)

This view has been substantiated by a growing number of published articles within the traditional endocrinology world, suggesting that we should start using the "median" of the range to optimize the health and/or recovery of a patient with traumatic brain injury. This concept of using the median of the range as a goal point for all hormones was introduced into my medical practice in 2001. Thereafter, having seen the added benefits to the patients' quality of life, the concept was included in many of the lectures that followed. The ideal or optimal range, for any hormone may be at the median of its range, as opposed to just being within the range. (6)

One of the challenges in interpreting laboratory results is the concept of a partial deficiency (insufficiency). This is where the measured hormone is within the lower aspect of the "reference range," but the patient has symptoms similar to someone with a complete deficiency. A recent NFL retiree came to us with neurobehavioral issues, along with pain in both knees, having had bilateral arthroscopic surgery. His testosterone levels (total, free, DHT, and DHEA-s) were already above the median. I called the patient to verify that he had never been on prescribed, over-the-counter, or illegally obtained hormones or steroid. He said, "No!" Upon his return to the office, we did a Provocative Testosterone Test (PTT) with 60mg of a blended testosterone. Five days later he sent us back our questionnaire, on which he had written, "I am 150 percent better." His knee pain was gone, and subsequently, his neurobehavioral issues improved.

As you continue in your reading of this chapter, as well as all those that follow, you will find that we use treatment protocols that raise hormone levels — slowly edging up toward the median number. In general, we find that many of the non-TBI patients do well at a number hovering around the median, while those with neurotrauma (TBI) and suffering from a number of common post-TBI symptoms, do well with levels above the median. The only way that you will discover an individual's perfect treatment range is to slowly increase the levels of hormones — and finally, treat the patient not the numbers.

Interpretation of Results

The concept to use reference values was introduced in 1969 by Gräsbeck and Saris (7) to describe fluctuations of blood analytes in well-characterized groups of individuals. It was intended to replace the more ambiguous concept of "normal values," and to ''establish a well-defined nomenclature and recommended procedures in the field.'' Their article promoted the concept that there is a clear distinction between healthy reference values measured in a healthy population (or individual) and patient reference values measured in those having various diseases. It is now commonly accepted that reference values describe fluctuations observed in healthy populations or individuals, which makes the definition of health, or characterization of health status, a perilous step.

The conceptualization of reference ranges goes beyond the traditional "normal" range to represent data from other groups of individuals besides the healthy. The object of studying biochemical analytes (8) in sick patients has not been to produce reference ranges, but to find specific values in the sick that allow for the optimal ability to discriminate between states of health and disease. The complexity of this correlation has failed to produce a reference range (RR) as such, so we are limited to using the reference ranges from apparently healthy individuals.

Statistical methods for analyzing reference values used to be restricted to the use of means (9), variances (10), and the well-known normal and lognormal (11) probability distributions. As problems involving reference values in clinical medicine deepened, statistical methods applied to them have necessarily become more extensive. The "reference range" is defined by a pair of numbers that represent the central 95 percent of a collection of values obtained from a specific group of individuals. On either side of this central core is another five percent, which represents 2.5 percent that lie below and 2.5 percent that lie above the central core.

Deficiency is that 2.5 percent below the range that is understood as that level of hormone or chemistry that is inadequate for optimal quality of life. My opposition to this, in general, is that they do not truly represent optimal functional ranges. How can I say that? Well, it is assumed that those individuals that are used to determine the ranges are healthy. That means no active diseases or taking medication that can adversely affect the testing modalities (RIA, ELISA, chemoluminescence, or LC/MS).

If the participant has had any previous injuries (TBI), medication, or exposure to radiation, it would impair the normal endogenous production of hormones, causing a shift in the statistical computations. Ideally, these individuals should have been eliminated from the sampling process in order to avoid sample bias. In effect, the post-injury hormonal levels could be decreased over the pre-injury levels; thereby, creating the impression that the levels are just part of the normal variance. Since the square root of the variance is the standard deviation (12), there would be either a shift up or down of the "normal range." And, if this is not enough, the standard deviation has the same dimension as the data, and hence is comparable with deviations of the mean. All of this is statistical jargon that means very little in the ultimate treatment of the patient.

Since 2004, the Millennium-TBI has evaluated thousands of laboratory results in patients with mild to moderate traumatic brain injury, and has clearly identified and supported the notion of the impact (no pun intended) causing an effect on normal hormone production. (13[L])

Insufficiency (partial deficiency) is that range of results within the lower 25 percent of the reference range, where the patient may have symptoms commonly associated in a patient with an absolute numerical deficiency. These are the patients that frequently do not receive the treatment they need, but are instead given a psychotropic medication and called "emotionally" impaired.

Case in point: A recent Graves' disease patient developed the usual post-operative hypothyroidism and was placed on L-thyroxine (0.10mg). She complained to her primary care physician of symptoms that are classically hypothyroid in nature, in light of an apparently "normal" TSH level. After a number of adverse interactions with her physician, she was told, "Patients who have normal TSH levels, and still have complaints of hypothyroidism, we place them on an anti-depressant."

Obviously, this patient refused the alternative treatment and subsequently appeared in our offices to receive a comprehensive thyroid panel (CTP3), which showed low-normal free-T4, low-normal free-T3, and a significantly elevated rT3. Adding 25mcg of triiodothyronine to her 0.10 mg L-thyroxine gave her symptomatic relief within 24 hours. (It also caused her to feel hyper, and so we reduced the T3 to 10mcg.)

Frequently, we see patients who have failed conventional treatment protocols (as is frequent with thyroid disease) because the treatment was based upon a limited laboratory assessment — usually just the TSH level, in lieu of a more robust approach. Nonetheless, conventional medicine looks at laboratory results in absolute black and white terms as either normal or abnormal, based upon a "reference range." If the range of a measured hormone is from ten to 90, and the patient's result comes in at 13, it is designated as being within the reference range without regard to any symptomatic complaints offered by the patient. It appears that we have lost our humanistic approach to medicine, and now treat the numbers — not the patient — while assuming that all lab results equate out to the same physiological responses across all different faces in the human race.

Since 1995, the Millennium has used a simplistic approach to the interpretation of laboratory results in all cases, and not just TBI. Our goal has been to bring the patient toward the median (the middle value) range for each hormone, and then to slowly increase toward the 75th percentile of that range — if indicated by their clinical response.

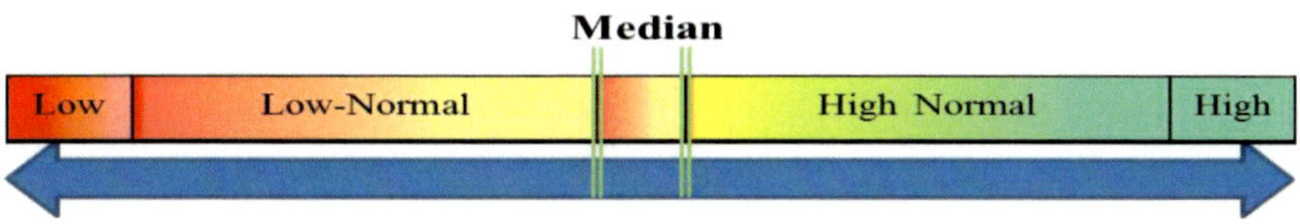

Figure 6.1 Optimal results with optimal treatment. Using treatment protocols to achieve a homeostatic balance so that each hormone hovers around its median range. Although this might be viewed as arbitrary, the concept of Homeostasis, a dynamic process, would place each hormone with points of its median if the net affect of both positive and negative feedback signaling was equal.

Using the above example: If the reference range of the hormone was between ten and 90, the median would be: [(10+90)/] = 50. Therefore, it would be our initial goal to raise the patient's level from their measured 13, toward 50. Frequently, as treatment ensues, the patient might notice improvement in some of their symptomatic complaints within days.

Upon subsequent laboratory testing, their level might be up from 13 to 27 and they note an improvement! What to do? Hold? There is no mandate to bring treatment levels to the median of the range if the patient is achieving beneficial results at a level that is higher than where they started, but lower than the median. This is the commonsense that we need to bring back into medicine, as well as acknowledging the uniqueness that each one of us possesses, and should be allowed to experience. Target levels do not address a patient's needs.

Hormone	Median M	Median F	Hormone	Median M	Median F
DHEA-s	200 ug/dL	277 ug/dL	Growth Hormone	5.0 ng/ml	5.0 ng/ml
T-Testosterone	690 ng/ml	44 ng/ml	IGF-1	>200 ng/ml	>200 ng/ml
F-Testosterone	14 pg/ml	2-4 pg/ml	IGFBP-3	4000 ng/ml	4000 ng/ml
DHT	< 52 ng/dl	< 30 ng/ml	TSH	2.5 mcu/ml	2.5 mcu/ml
SHBG	45 pg/ml	<75 ng/dl	fT4	1.5 ng/ml	1.5 ng/ml
Estrone	< 60 pg/ml	< 200 pg/ml	fT3	250 ng/dL	250ng/dL
Estradiol	<25 pg/ml	90 pg/ml	rT3	165 ng/dL	165 ng/dL
Progesterone	0.8 ng/ml	5-7 ng/ml	fT3/rT3 Ratio	> 1.06	> 1.06
Pregnenolone	210 ng/dl	210 ng/dl	TPO	< 35 IU/ml	< 35 IU/ml
Vitamin D3	> 60 ng/dl	> 60 ng/dl	ACTH (am)	< 35 pg/ml	< 35 pg/ml
LH	5.1 mIU/ml	22 mIU/ml	Cortisol (am)	< 15 ug/dl	< 15 ug/dl
FSH	7.0 mIU/ml	8.6 mIU/ml	Cortisol (pm)	7.3 Ug/dl	7.3 Ug/dl
Prolactin	11.25 ng/ml	13.75 ng/ml	Insulin	< 25 IU/L	< 25 IU/L

Table 6.1: These are the median "normal" blood result from Access Medical Laboratories of Florida that we use to guide our interpretations. Please note that female hormone results need to be correlated to the on-set of their menses if still cycling. Otherwise, the numbers used here are for peri- and post-menopausal women.

Table 6.1 represents the composition and median ranges for the 26 laboratory tests that are in the Millennium-TBI panel. The median ranges listed were the most current at the time of writing this book. It is important that you always double-check the lab ranges since they tend to change due to reagents, equipment, or overall technique.

The Millennium-TBI has been actively using the scale as depicted in Figure 6.1 (above) that includes the terms; Low, Low-Normal, Normal (median), High-Normal, and High. When the term "Low" is used, it tends to represent the clinical lab's interpretation of "low," which is a critical level for us. The use of "Low-Normal" implies that the results are below the median and "High-Normal" is above the median. The use of "High" therefore means that the level is above the laboratory's interpretation of "high." To confuse things more, when we receive a result of 100 and the median is 99 or 101, how do we interpret that? We tend to use a ten percent variance for the results; otherwise, 99 percent of the resulting levels would be either Low or High-Normal.

Throughout this chapter, we will be referencing lab results by name more than by any specific numerical reference point. We will assume that you "get it," and know how to look at your own laboratory's reference ranges and convert them into our discriminating language.

The TBI Testing Panels

The need for a comprehensive hormonal panel has become indisputable, based upon the scope of the literature clearly affirming how complex and convoluted the interactions between the diverse hormones are. Using the conventional approach of minimalism, the standard hormonal panels did not do much more than add to the confusion and failed to offer directions toward optimal treatment. Additionally, the impact of one's biochemical milieu can greatly affect hormonal production (i.e., B-12 deficiency can cause increased rT3). We were no longer just looking to identify the patterns suggestive of post-traumatic brain injury hormonal dysfunction, but were also looking for optimizing treatment. Frequently, we receive patients who have had outside laboratory work-ups and found to be hypogonadal. They were started on appropriate treatment, but failed to achieve optimal results due to labs having missed the concurrent DHEA-s deficiency or elevation in prolactin (PRO).

In the beginning, we had TBI laboratory panels that were based upon gender: a male and a female panel. As our knowledge increased, based upon the science behind the non-reproductive benefits of neurosteroids (NS) and neuroactive steroids (NAS), we found the gender gap between the differences in hormonal testing narrowed. So, we instituted a unified TBI testing panel that does not preference one gender over the other. As you continue your reading, the information will help support this approach, and help you to narrow this same informational gap with the science. As a preview, let me share that if a male's level of progesterone (PROG) is elevated, it can down-regulate luteinizing hormone (LH) via a central increase in prolactin (PRO), causing a reduction in testicular testosterone release. Henceforth, measuring this previously female only hormone in males might help pick up the cause for low LH and testosterone. (14[1])

Panel	Hormones	Abbreviation
✓	Growth Hormone	GH
✓	Insulin-like growth factor-1	IGF-1
✓	Insulin-like growth factor binding protein – 3	IGFBP-3
✓	Dehydroepiandrosterone-sulfate	DHEA-s
✓	Total Testosterone	T(T)
✓	Free Testosterone	F(T)
✓	Dihydrotestosterone	DHT
✓	Sex Hormone Binding Globulin	SHBG
✓	Estradiol	E2
✓	Estrone	E1
✓	Progesterone	PROG
✓	Pregnenolone	PREG
✓	Follicle Stimulating Hormone	FSH
✓	Luteinizing Hormone	LH
✓	Thyrotrophic Stimulating Hormone	TSH
✓	Tetraiodothyronine – Free	fT4
✓	Triiodothyronine – Free	fT3
✓	Reverse Triiodothyronine	rT3
✓	Triiodothyronine/ Reverse Triiodothyronine Ratio	T3/rT3 Ratio
✓	Cortisol	COR
✓	Adrenocorticotropic Hormone	ACTH
✓	Prolactin	Pro
✓	Vitamin D	Vit D
✓	Insulin	INS

Table 6.2: This is the panel that is being used by the Millennium Health Centers to assess both neurosteroids and neuroactive steroids.

Finally, a short comment about Access Medical Laboratories of Jupiter, Florida (15), which is a 25,000 square foot facility with all of the latest in laboratory technology, and where I am the Medical Director of Education, with the responsibility of sharing this impressive and cost-effective option (compared to the older laboratory practices of using RIA, ELISA, and chemoluminescence). The underlying mission of Access Medical Laboratories is to provide cutting edge analytical clinical medicine, with a reliability of nearly 100 percent. The majority of their hormonal and biochemical testing is performed on LC/MS/MS/MS, or Liquid Chromatography-Mass Spectroscopy[3]. I'm not sure I fully understand how it is done, but I do know that it does the job more accurately and consistently then any of the older technologies.

Anterior Pituitary Hormones

A number of meta-analyses have been performed to look at the effect of TBI on the anterior pituitary's production of hormones, and they have found chronic pituitary deficiencies (16) in 23 to 90 percent of the cases represented by mild TBI (80 percent), moderate TBI (15 percent), and severe TBI (five percent). The real issue is the elusive occurrence of pituitary insufficiency (17) (partial deficiency), where hormonal production (18) is not halted but is significantly reduced into the low-normal of the reference range. (19, 20)

A clear understanding of both the diurnal production and half-lives of each of the hormones will allow for a more accurate interpretation of the results, as well as a more effective design of your treatment protocols.

Using rational thinking; If GH levels are low to low-normal, and the BP-3 level is normal or even high-normal, GH was produced in adequate amounts during the normal nocturnal pulses. Furthermore, if IGF-1 and BP-3 are low-normal with a normal or low-normal GH, there might be something wrong with the liver. We see this pattern on occasion and send the patient out for a liver ultrasound — where fatty degeneration and cancer seem to play a role. So, remember to consider these!

The Growth Hormone System (GH/IGF-1 Axis)

The bulk of growth hormone production and release is between 8:00 p.m. and 4:00 a.m., with a half-life of about 20 minutes. Once GH enters the hypophyseal-portal blood supply (21), it takes about 30 minutes to arrive at its primary target organ — the liver — where it initiates the production of three groups of products: IGFs, BPs, and ALS. Knowing the characteristics of each of these three groups will allow for a more sound interpretation that will better support treatment.

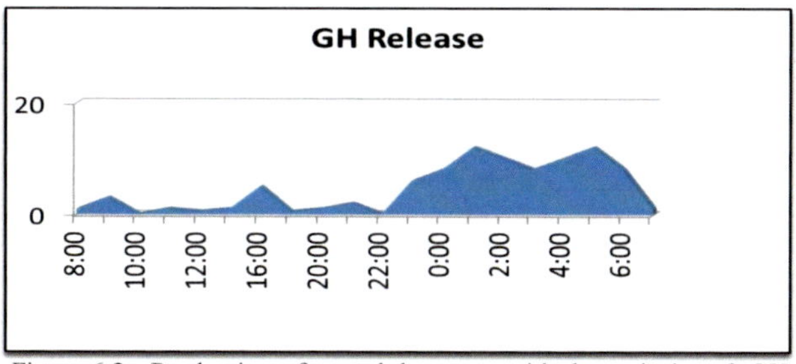

Figure 6.2: Production of growth hormone with the majority of GH released from 8pm to 4am with minor pulses throughout the day.

Free IGF-I has a serum half-life of approximately eight to ten minutes normally; however, when it is bound to insulin-like binding protein-3 (IGFBP-3 or BP-3), that half-life is extended to 20 to 24 hours (the half-life of IGFBP-3). As the circulating levels of IGFs rise, the negative feedback-loop down-regulates the expression of GH by decreasing both GHRH and its receptor.

Although there are six (and maybe even eight) major binding proteins (22) produced by the liver in response to growth hormone, IGFBP-3 (BP-3) is the one most referenced due to its high affinity for IGF-1 in both the serum and within the nuclear envelope. In the peripheral circulation, BP-3 carries IGF-1, extending its half-life from eight to ten minutes to between 20 to 24 hours, while within the nucleus it works with p53 to regulate mitosis and apoptosis. In the event that a cell's DNA mutates, posing a potential danger to the host, p53 levels rise, causing an increase in BP-3, which will bind most if not all of the IGF-1 within the nucleus. Recognizing the pro-mitotic (anti-apoptotic) characteristic of intranuclear IGF-1, and therefore its potential for propagation of an aberrant cell, we now appreciate the intranuclear presence of IGFBP-3 to down-regulate IGF-1 and assist the p53 apoptotic mechanisms (23) to protect the host from cancer (viruses too). (24) Therefore, the propaganda claiming GH causes cancer or increases the growth of cancer is not totally true, or even not true after reading the literature about IGFBP-3's ability to prevent cancer. (25) Unfortunately, the maximum benefit from p53 as "the most important anti-cancer mechanism in our cells" is lost, to some degree, due to its denigrated state of activity from the ubiquitous and world-wide zinc deficiency. (26) It appears that the activity of p53 is based upon the presence of zinc ions within its chemical structure — a metalloprotein. (27)

Acid labile subunit (ALS) is the third product induced by growth hormone's stimulation of the liver (another carrier protein specifically for the GH-system). (28) To recap, when IGF-1 is bound by IGFBP-3, it forms a binary molecule, which extends the half-life of IGF-1 from eight to ten minutes to 20 to 24 hours. When ALS binds to this complex (IGF-1 + IGFBP-3), it forms a ternary molecule that extends the serum half-life of IGF-1 to about 200 hours. Although ALS testing is available in some laboratories, it is not usually a part of a standard workup. The Millennium is presently looking at its use in research related to Secretropin® to evaluate how the laboratory results for IGF-1 might be influenced by the production of ALS.

No discussion of growth hormone can be complete without a few words about somatostatin (SS or SRIF) which is produced by neurons of the periventricular nucleus (PVN) within the hypothalamus. (29) These neurons project to the median eminence, where somatostatin is released from neurosecretory nerve endings into the hypothalamo-hypophyseal system through neuron axons. Somatostatin is then carried to the anterior pituitary gland, where it inhibits the secretion of growth hormone from somatotrope cells. The somatostatin neurons in the periventricular nucleus mediate negative feedback effects of growth hormone on its own release; and the somatostatin neurons respond to high circulating levels of growth hormone and IGFs by increasing the release of somatostatin, thereby completing the negative feedback loop reducing the rate of secretion of growth hormone. (30) As an aside, elevated levels of somatostatin can decrease the pituitary release of TSH (31), leading to a state of hypothyroidism.

Somatotropin (SRIF) has a direct inhibitory effect on growth hormone producing somatotropes of the anterior pituitary gland. Loss of the PVN within the hypothalamus will lead to the loss of inhibition and an elevation in the production of growth hormone. Again, the cause for the elevation in GH production and release must be assessed to determine if it is due to: (a) dysregulation of inhibition, (b) secondary to medication, and (c) pituitary adenoma. Once medication and pituitary adenoma have been excluded, the resulting elevation can be attributed to dysregulation of inhibition secondary to hypothalamic damage. At present, growth hormone deficiency in the majority of TBI patients is due to damage at the level of the anterior pituitary and not the hypothalamus. (32)

Laboratory Assessment

To minimize the influence of food and activities on their production, we normally perform a morning blood draw for GH, IGF-1, and IGFBP-3. The permutation for three items taken three different ways gives the table below with nine unique potential results (Table 6.3). By 9:00 a.m., the levels of GH and IGFs have gone through their natural decay curves, with low levels being anticipated. Since growth hormone does not have a binding protein like BPs for the IGFs, the levels are always significantly lower. So, having a morning level of GH of 0.03ng/ml might be considered low-normal or low, but if the IGFBP-3 is above 4000ng/ml (4.0pg/ml), nocturnal production of GH was normal. Otherwise, the level of BP-3 would be low-normal or low. Got it?

Laboratory Evaluation of (GH)-(IGF-1) Axis				
Serum Results	GH	IGF-1	BP-3	Comments
Optimal levels	▼M	M	M	No treatment indicated.
Optimal	▼M	M	▼	No treatment indicated. Check Liver if risks.
Evaluation needed	▼M	▼	▼	Ultrasound of liver. Steroid Abuse? Drugs?
Questionable	M	▼	M	Rapid Clearance. Check for IGF-1 antibodies
Laron's Syndrome	▲	▼	▼	GH Insensitivity. Give IGF-1.
Central Dysregulation	▼	▼	▼	Perform Glucagon Stimulant Test. TBI History
Positive	▼	▼	M	Perform GST. Quercetin?
Positive	▼	M	▼	Perform GST.
Questionable	▼	M	M	Rapid clearance. Check for GH antibodies.

Table 6.3: Assessment of the Growth Hormone System. The median (M), less than median (▼) and above the median (▲) are shown in this table to direct whether there is the need to treat. These results do not take into account supplementation with any growth factors or known products that alter the natural production of one or more of these results. d/or IGFBP-3 consider an ultrasound for liver and review any medication or supplements that might be affecting the livers ability to generate these hormones.

The median for GH is 5ng/ml, and the desirable quantity for IGF-1 is greater than 200ng/ml. A level of IGFBP-3 above the median of 4.0pg/ml (4000 ng/ml) is a good indicator of nocturnal GH production.

The likelihood that GH will be measured above the median or even close to the median, after a morning blood draw, is low. Therefore, the consideration of GH supplementation before a GH-pituitary adenoma must be assessed.

Another group of results that might need additional investigation is when GH is close to, but below, the median — and, the production of IGFBP-3 and/or IGF-1 are below the median. One must consider that there is a problem with the peripheral receptors, specifically within the liver. Questions to consider are: Is the patient consuming a medication or supplement that is interfering with the production of either IGF-I, BP-3, or both; or is there something going on with the liver? We have a GE VScan™ (33) in our office to help answer this question. Fatty degeneration, hepatoma, and Peliosis hepatis (excessive steroid use) are the most common findings in these cases. (34)

In a patient that has had disruptive head trauma, the most common pattern that we are seeing is one that has low to low-normal GH, IGF-1, and BP-3 levels — central dysregulation. If you find a young patient with normal to high-normal GH and low IGF-1 and BP-3 levels, you might consider a variation of Laron Syndrome or mosaicism of the GH receptors. (35)

Gonadotropic System (HPG Axis)

Just a quick comment about the hormones we typically refer to as "reproductive" or "sex" hormones like estrogen, progesterone, and testosterone. These are emerging as pleiotropic hormones, where the reproductive influence might be 40 percent and everything else they do amounts to 60 percent. I have peppered this document with a diverse array of readings that will support the concept that hormones are multifaceted and not to be ignored since they are just for sex! (36, 37, 38)

When assessing the impact of TBI on pituitary luteinizing hormone (LH) and follicle stimulating hormone (FSH) production in man, the natural inverse relationships do not exist where a low peripheral production of testosterone (free more than total testosterone) is met with a correspondingly high level of LH and/or FSH. In a TBI scenario, where hypothalamic-pituitary dysregulation has occurred, both the peripheral and central tropic hormones are low to low-normal. In order not to miss this relationship, we will spend some extra time with an in-depth discussion here, which can be extended to most other hormone pairs. (39)

First, in a perfect neuroendocrinologic world, if optimal homeostasis was achievable between the trophic hormone and its peripheral target gland, then there would be a balance between the forces of the positive and negative feedback loops, and the releasing hormone would be at the absolute median of its range… hypothetically. Unfortunately, you could not measure it since we are such a dynamic construct.

In our laboratory (Access Medical Laboratory), the median for LH, in a male is 5.1mIU/ml. When LH is high, it would imply that the peripheral production of testosterone/estradiol is low, thereby creating the positive feedback signal within the hypothalamus, leading to the release of gonadotropic releasing hormone (GnRH). The GnRH then stimulates the gonadotropic cells of the anterior pituitary to release LH. The increase in LH stimulates the Leydig cells of the testicles (if they are there) to produce more testosterone which, over time, becomes the negative feedback trigger to down-regulate LH production. When LH is below 5.1mIU/ml, it is assumed that the Leydig cells have produced a significant amount of testosterone to cause the negative feedback mechanism to be initiated. (40) This is the usual means by which all our hormones are regulated, save prolactin.

Therefore, when peripheral testosterone is low and LH is below the median, one can consider that there is an interruption in the hypothalamic-anterior pituitary-gonadal axis. This finding in either the male or female patient would translate to suggest that their TBI was significant enough to damage the regulatory mechanism for gonadotropic hormone production, and replenishment (supplementation) is indicated.

Gonadotrophic Releasing Hormone (GnRH)

Cells in the arcuate nucleus of the hypothalamus secrete gonadotropin-releasing hormone into the portal circulation ,and subsequently stimulate the release of both LH and FSH from the anterior pituitary. Gonadotropin-releasing hormone release is regulated by feedback from gonadal hormone levels, PRL levels, and other extra-hypothalamic structures in the brainstem and limbic system. (41)

Luteinizing Hormone

Luteinizing hormone (LH) is a hormone produced by gonadotroph cells in the anterior pituitary gland. In females, an acute rise of LH (LH surge) triggers ovulation and development of the corpus luteum. (42) In males, where LH had also been called interstitial cell-stimulating hormone (ICSH), it stimulates Leydig cell production of testosterone. In both genders, it acts synergistically with follicular stimulating hormone. (43)

When measuring the level of LH, one must keep in focus the purpose of LH on the testes or ovaries. The common hormonal pattern seen during primary ovarian or primary testicular failure is a low to low-normal amount of peripheral hormone production, corresponding to an elevating level of LH trying to induce a rise in the target hormone production. In primary failure, the target glands are incapable of responding to stimulation and cannot produce an adequate amount of the end-hormone to create a strong enough negative feedback signal to down-regulate the production of the signaling trophic hormone — LH, in this case. Thereby, in a dynamic setting, the level of LH continues to climb and will only drop when exogenous hormones are given to the patient. (44)

In central failure, due to trauma of the hypothalamus (hypothalamic amenorrhea) or pituitary gland (Sheehan's syndrome), the peripheral production of the target hormone(s) diminishes over time proportionate to the loss of the central trophic hormone production. A classical finding of central failure will be both a trophic and target hormone deficiency. (45, 46)

Interpretation of the results is important so that you do not miss an opportunity to improve upon the client's condition. Therefore, as a general conceptual approach: If the trophic hormone (i.e., LH, FSH, TSH, GH, and ACTH) is below the median and the patient is not on its corresponding hormone, then TBI induced central hormonal dysregulation must be considered. If the patient's trophic hormone (LH) is hovering at the median and they are not on hormone replenishment, and the peripheral hormone level is low to low-normal, then there is the suggestion of an incomplete central hormone dysregulation.

LH — Laboratory ranges (AML)

Male: Range = 1.7 to 8.6mIU/ML, median = 5.1mIU/ml.

Female: Range = 2.4 to 12.6 in follicular phase, 14 to 95.6 in ovulation phase, 1.0 to 11.4 in luteal phase, and 7.7 to 58.5 in post-menopausal phase. Ideal timing for female blood draw is day 21 or luteal phase. The median value must be established for each phase of the menstrual history, except we use the median of the luteal phase for menopausal patients (6.2mIU/ml).

Follicle Stimulating Hormone

In both males and females, FSH stimulates the maturation of germ cells. In males, FSH induces sertoli cells to secrete androgen-binding proteins (47), and its secretion is regulated by inhibin's negative feedback mechanism on the anterior pituitary gland. (48) In females, FSH initiates follicular growth, specifically affecting granulosa cells. With the concomitant rise in inhibin B, FSH levels then decline in the late follicular phase. This seems to be critical in selecting only the most advanced follicle to proceed to ovulation. At the end of the luteal phase, there is a slight rise in FSH that seems to be of importance to start the next ovulatory cycle.

Control of FSH release from the pituitary gland is unknown. Low frequency gonadotropin-releasing hormone (GnRH) pulses increase FSH mRNA levels in the rat; however, this doesn't directly correlate with an increase in circulating FSH. (49) GnRH has been shown to play an important role in the secretion of FSH, with hypothalamic-pituitary disconnection leading to a cessation of FSH. GnRH administration leads to a return of FSH secretion. FSH is subject to estrogen feed-back from the gonads via the hypothalamic pituitary gonadal axis. (50)

FSH — Laboratory Ranges

Male: 1.5 to 12.4mIU/ml, median = 7.0 (6.95) mIU/ml.

Female: The range can be 3.5 to 12.5mIU/ml during follicular phase, 4.7 to 21.5 in ovulation phase, 1.7 to 7.7 in luteal phase, and 25.8 to 134.8 in the post-menopausal phase. Again, the median value must be established for each phase of the menstrual history.

Pregnenolone

Under the regulatory influence of luteinizing hormone (LH), cholesterol is transported into the inner lining of the mitochondria where P450scc (CYP11A1) converts it to pregnenolone — the "mother of all hormones." (51) Thereafter, pregnenolone can go in three major directions to become (a) progesterone, cortisol, cortisone, aldosterone, (b) DHEA and DHEA-s, testosterone, dihydrotestosterone, estradiol, estrone, and (c) allopregnenolone .(52)

Pregnenolone is the first pro-hormone derived from cholesterol, and is both a neurosteroid and neuroactive steroid having significant benefits in the brain (see Chapter 4). Pregnenolone and its sulfated derivative, pregnenolone sulfate, enhance learning and memory in concentrations that are physiologically relevant. (53) In clinical application, pregnenolone was very well tolerated with minimal side effects, and did not affect weight, heart rate, blood pressure, menstrual cycle, or glucose levels. (54)

Pregnenolone — Laboratory Ranges

Males: Range 38 to 350ng/dl, median = 194 ng/dl.

Females: Range = 250 to 500ng/dl, median level = 205ng/dl.

Comment: The potential benefits from the use of pregnenolone justify achieving and maintaining a high-normal serum level, except in patients with a known history of seizure activity. (55)

Progesterone

Progesterone and its metabolites promote the viability of neurons in the brain and spinal cord. Their neuroprotective effects have been documented in different lesion models, including traumatic brain injury (TBI), experimentally induced ischemia, spinal cord lesions, and a genetic model of motor neuron disease. Progesterone plays an important role in developmental myelination and in myelin repair, and the aging nervous system appears to remain sensitive to some of progesterone's beneficial effects. (56) Thus, the hormone may promote neuroregeneration (57) by several different actions by reducing inflammation, swelling, and apoptosis; thereby increasing the survival of neurons, and by promoting the formation of new myelin sheaths.

In a 2006 study, 77 patients received progesterone, and 23 received placebo. The groups had similar demographic and clinical characteristics. Laboratory and physiologic characteristics were similar at enrollment and throughout treatment. No serious adverse events were attributed to progesterone. Adverse and serious adverse event rates were similar in both groups, except that patients randomized to progesterone had a lower 30-day mortality rate than controls (more than a 50 percent reduction in mortality). Thirty days post-injury, the majority of severe traumatic brain injury survivors in both groups had relatively poor Glasgow Outcome Scale–Extended and Disability Rating Scale scores. However, moderate traumatic brain injury survivors who received progesterone were more likely to have a moderate to good outcome than those randomized to placebo. This was the ProTECT study out of Georgia. (58)

Progesterone — Laboratory Ranges

Males: Range = 0.2 to 1.4ng/ml, median = 0.8ng/ml.

Females: Ranges = follicular phase 0.2 to 1.5ng/ml, ovulation phase 0.8 to 3.0, luteal phase 1.7 to 27.0, post-menopause 0.1 to 0.8. Median for postmenopausal patients is somewhat arbitrary, being based upon symptoms and the quotient from the estrogen-progesterone ratio (discussed later). Progesterone has so many important functions in the aging body that it is time to acknowledge these and to use it. (59)

Comments: In males, we use a small amount of progesterone (about 5mg a night), noting that there is the potential for down-regulation of LH with a loss of optimal production of endogenous testosterone. If the patient is on testosterone replacement therapy (TRT), then it is a moot point. Additionally, progesterone has been found to dose dependently inhibit the amount of 5-alpha reductase produced (5-AR), thereby decreasing the conversion of testosterone to dihydrotestosterone (DHT). This is a good thing because we want to maintain the levels of free testosterone and diminish the production of DHT in the serum.

The benefit of progesterone is in its conversion to allopregnanolone, a prototypic neurosteroid present in the brain and acting as a potent modulator of $GABA_A$ receptors; although, excessive amounts of progesterone can inhibit estrogen's ability to increase serum levels of 1, 25, dihydroxy-vitamin D. (60, 61)

DHEA and DHEA-s

Dehydroepiandrosterone (DHEA) is a metabolite of pregnenolone and is the precursor to down-stream hormones such as testosterone, dihydrotestosterone, androstenedione, estrone, estradiol, and DHEA-s. Both DHEA and DHEA-s have significant effects over psychological functioning and generation of myelin from oligodendrocytes. Additional biological actions of DHEA and DHEA-s include: neuroprotection, neurite growth, and antagonistic effects on oxidants and glucocorticoids. (62)

However, DHEA secretion decreases from the age of 30 years and is already decreased, on average, by 60 percent at time of menopause. Since there is no feedback mechanism controlling DHEA secretion within normal values, women with low DHEA will remain with such a deficit of sex steroids for their remaining lifetime. Without a replacement source of sex steroids after menopause, one can reasonably believe that low DHEA is involved, in association with the aging process, in a series of medical problems classically associated with post-menopause, namely osteoporosis, muscle loss, vaginal atrophy, fat accumulation, hot flashes, skin atrophy, type 2 diabetes, memory loss, cognition loss and possibly Alzheimer's disease. (63)

Since the literature is replete with articles about DHEA and DHEA-s having beneficial affects over the heart, immunity, inflammation, neuronal health, and cognition, we maintain their levels between the 75th to 95th percentiles of the range. (64) At these levels, women more often than men tend to experience oily skin and sometimes male pattern acne along the jaw line. This is due to the conversion of DHEA to DHT, which can be treated with saw palmetto with Pygeum africanum, or just by lowering the dose.

DHEA and DHEA-s — Laboratory Ranges

Male: Range = 88.9 to 487ug/dl, median = 287.9 ug/d.

Female: Range = 148 to 407ug/dl, median = 277 ug/dl.

Free and Total Testosterone

In a recent article by Dr. Ronald Swerdloff (UCLA Harbor General Hospital, Head of Endocrinology), he commented that maybe free testosterone should be given more significance in the assessment of hypogonadism over the total testosterone (TT) level. (65) When I read this I cheered! For as long as I can remember, the measurement of total testosterone has been the cornerstone for making the diagnosis of hypogonadism — regardless of the level of free testosterone. Serum total testosterone concentration represents the sum of unbound and protein-bound testosterone in circulation. But what did it really tell us and has it been the best test to evaluate not only the level of testosterone, but also bio-availability? It turns out that the total testosterone level has been used as the index for testosterone since the technology to measure direct free testosterone (FT) was lacking. What we have been measuring, according to an article in Clinical Chemistry was, "Total testosterone in blood bound to three plasma proteins: sex-hormone-binding globulin (SHBG), albumin, and corticosteroid-binding globulin." (66) We have found that the free testosterone is the form that binds to the cell wall androgen receptor to trigger the STAT (signaling transduction and translation) response. (67)

In TBI, the production of testosterone and estrogens are significantly affected.

In males, frequently LH and FSH are found in the low to low-normal ranges, with peripheral levels of testosterone being also low to low-normal. This is a characteristic finding in an individual who has central hypogonadism. On laboratory testing, free and total testosterone will frequently be low, as will both the LH and FSH levels. Corroborating this we frequently find levels of estrone and estradiol below the 25th percentile of the range for a male.

Total Testosterone — Laboratory Ranges

Male: Range = 280 to 1100ng/dl, median = 690ng/dl.

Female: Range = 6 to 82ng/dl, median = 44ng/dl.

Free Testosterone — Laboratory Ranges

Male: Range = 1.9 to 27ng/dl, median = 12 to 14ng/dl.*
*We have found this range to have the best clinical improvement to treatment.

Female: Range = 0.2 to 2.6ng/dl, median = 2 to 4ng/dl.*
*We have found this range to have the best clinical improvement to treatment.

Dihydrotestosterone

Dihydrotestosterone (DHT) is the 5-alpha-reductase (5-AR) by-product of testosterone, and is generally considered the active form of testosterone. When considering the form of testosterone supplementation to use, it is important to know where 5-AR is produced so that you can regulate the amount of DHT that is generated because of potential adverse side effects. There are three isoforms of 5-AR: steroid 5α-reductase 1, 2, and 3 (SRD5A1, SRD5A2 and SRD5A3). (68, 69, 70) Generally speaking, approximately five percent of produced testosterone converts to DHT in the serum. The skin has a significant amount of SRD5A1, so that topically applied testosterone can convert to DHT at a rate of 30 to 70 percent. (71) Since DHT comes from testosterone, elevated production of DHT comes at the expense of testosterone. Additionally, DHT derived from testosterone within the cell provides for optimal intracellular benefits that are attenuated when DHT is produced in the serum. Therefore, high levels of serum DHT and low levels of free testosterone are not the ideal balance. (72)

When evaluating the serum levels of DHT, it is best to keep it at the normal to low-normal range due to its documented side effects of thinning hair, oily skin, acne, testicular atrophy, and prostatic enlargement. It is within the cells that the beneficial effects of DHT hold precedence. Therefore, if the level of free testosterone hovers around the median range, the expectation is that there will be adequate amount of free testosterone to get into the cell for conversion to DHT. Once DHT is in the cell, there is some conversion to 3-alpha-androsteinedione, which up-regulates adenyl cyclase (AC) — a neurotransmitter.

Dihydrotestosterone — Laboratory Ranges

Male: Range = 11.2 to 95.5ng/dl, median = less than 54 ng/dl.

Female: Range = less than 30ng/dl, median = less than 15ng/dl.

Sex Hormone Binding Globulin

Sex hormone-binding globulin (SHBG) is a liver derived glycoprotein that binds to sex hormones — specifically: T, DHT and estradiol. The majority of serum T and DHT (approximately 60 percent) is complexed with SHBG, with the remainder bound to albumin. (74) In aging men, estrogen levels rise, resulting in an increase of SHBG and subsequently a global reduction of free testosterone. (75) After the age of 40 years, the capability for SHBG to bind to testosterone augments about 40 percent, which causes a decrease in libido, associated with the symptoms of aging and Andropause. (76)

Sex hormone binding globulin (SHBG) has for years been looked upon as a binding protein produced by the liver that forms an irreversible ligand with estrogens, or testosterone, as a means of regulating the availability of the free hormone compartment. The formation of this steroidal ligand complex alters the conformational ability of the hormone to bind to its cell wall receptor, thereby apparently inactivating it.

In the 2002 article, *Beyond Carrier Protein*, SHBG was also described to function as part of a novel steroid-signaling system that is independent of the classical intracellular steroid receptors. A steroid free (unbound to estrogen or testosterone) SHBG can bind to a cell membrane SHBG-receptor forming the SHBG–SHBG-r complex. In addition, a steroid bound SHBG can non-competitively inhibit the binding of SHBG to SHBG-r, and bind to its cell wall ligand the SHBG-r. Thereafter, exposing the SHBG–SHBG-r complex to a steroid leads to the formation of the steroid–SHBG–SHBG-r complex, which activates the STAT receptor, leading to the generation of the second messenger — cAMP – and a signal is born. (77)

Sex Hormone Binding Globulin — Laboratory Ranges

Male: Range = 10 to 80nmol/L, median = less than 45nmol/L.

Female: Range = 20 to 130nmol/L, median = less than 75nmol/L.

Estradiol

Estradiol is a pleiotropic hormone (78) that influences numerous non-reproductive functions such as bone and mineral metabolism, cardiac and vascular function, memory, cognition and mood, and the incidence and progression of age-related diseases. The discovery of three types of estrogen receptors (ERα, ERβ, and Membrane ER) has led to the expansion and reevaluation based upon potentially new targets and diverse mechanisms of estradiol's actions that have not been considered previously. (79)

Many lines of evidence suggest that estrogen has neurotrophic and neuroprotective properties. For many years, it has been known that 17β-estradiol promotes viability and survival of neurons in primary neuronal cultures increasing viability, survival and differentiation of primary neuronal cultures from different brain areas including: amygdala, hypothalamus, neocortex, and hippocampus. (80)

Neuroprotective effects of estradiol have also been described in basal forebrain cholinergic neurons and the nigrostriatal system (dopaminergic). (81) These laboratory research findings are in good agreement with the reported beneficial effects of estrogen replacement therapy on cognitive functions, regional cerebral blood flow, EEG activity, and severity of dementia in women diagnosed with Alzheimer's disease. (82) Clinical studies establish that estradiol influences aspects of memory, cognition, and mood in healthy young and postmenopausal women. In addition, it appears to delay the onset of, and slows the decline in cognitive function associated with neurodegenerative diseases such as Alzheimer's or Parkinson's disease, and may attenuate the extent of acute injury associated with stroke and traumatic brain trauma. (83)

Several lines of evidence suggest that females are less vulnerable to acute insults associated with cerebral ischemia, neurotrauma, hypoxia, and drug-induced toxicity. First, there are striking sex differences in the incidence, the pathophysiology, and the outcome of neurological injury. Pre-menopausal women suffer from cerebrovascular strokes less frequently than men, but this sex-related difference disappears in older postmenopausal women compared with age-matched men. (84)

Treating with estradiol in stroke-like, or traumatic brain injury, diminishes the extent of injury, and, in some studies, decreases mortality and behavioral dysfunction. Researchers have used several different treatment protocols looking at both physiological and pharmacological levels of hormones administered before, simultaneously with, or after brain injury. In general, it appears that pharmacological doses of estradiol or estrogen-like compounds protect even when given up to three hours following the onset of injury; whereas lower physiological concentrations of estradiol must be administered before the injury to exert protective actions. These researchers found that administration of low physiological levels of 17β estradiol for one week before permanent occlusion of the middle cerebral artery leads to a dramatic decrease in the extent of the infarct. (85)

Estradiol — Laboratory Ranges

Male: Range = 7.6 to 42.6pg/ml, median = less than 25.1pg/ml.

Female: Range = follicular phase 12.5 to 166pg/ml, ovulation phase 85.8 to 498pg/ml, luteal phase 43.8 to 211pg/ml, post-menopause is less than 5.0 to 54.7pg/ml.

Estrone

DHEA is metabolized to either androstenedione or testosterone, thereby giving rise to estrone (E1) or estradiol (E2), respectively. Depending upon which pathway dominates will dictate the amount of the specific estrogen produced. Studies have confirmed the finding that estrone-sulfate is an important plasma metabolite of estradiol, and have defined the production rate of E1-sulfate and its interconversions with estrone and estradiol. Monitoring the level of estrone is important due to the recent Framingham study showing an increased risk of diabetes in men with elevations in estrone. (86) The Millennium uses 25mg of 7-Keto-DHEA to diminish the levels of E1. The mechanism is unclear at this time.

Estrone — Laboratory Ranges

Male: Range = less than 60pg/ml, median = less than 30pg/ml.

Female: Range = less than 200pg/ml, median = less than 100pg/ml.

Estrogen-Progesterone Ratio (EP Ratio)

Since 2005, the Millennium has been working on what we have called the EP ratio, or estrogen-progesterone ratio. This is a simple mathematical ratio that produces a quotient that has been related to the probability of the patient developing symptoms associated with estrogen dominance, or confirms that they already have it.

Symptoms	< 250	250-1000	1000-5000	> 5000
Head Aches/Migraine	0-1	1	2	4
Sleep Issues	0-1	1	2	3
Sleep Deprivation	0	0-1	1	2
Anxiety	0	0-1	1	3
Depression	0	0-1	1	3
Panic Attacks	0	0-1	1	3
Mastalgia	0-1	1	3	4

Table 6.4: Using the calculation for Estrogen Dominance "(E1+E2)/P" produces the EP Ratio which has guided the Millennium Health Centers use of progesterone in the treatment of symptoms. Adjustments in estrogen dosing along with adequate amounts of progesterone have allowed for resolution of many of the patients symptoms. 0 = no symptoms and 4 = maximal symptoms

The computation is the sum of E1 and E2 divided by progesterone (the estrogen units are in ng/ml, while that of the progesterone is pg/ml). An example would be: E1 (40ng/ml) + E2 (90ng/ml) divided by progesterone (0.08) = an EP ratio of 1625. Most female patients have one or more symptoms of estrogen dominance when this number is above 1000.

Thyrotrophic System (HPT Axis)

Thyroid Stimulating Hormone

Sensing the circulating level of tetraiodothyronine (T4) and possible triiodothyronine (T3), the hypothalamus responds by either increasing or decreasing the release of thyrotrophic releasing hormone (TRH) based upon a state of deficiency or sufficiency. The thyrotropes of the anterior pituitary respond by releasing the thyroid stimulating hormone (TSH). TSH stimulates the iodination of thyroglobulin (tyrosine) and the formation of T4 (85 percent) and T3 (five percent) from coupling of two diiodotyrosince molecules (DIT) or one DIT and one monoiodotyrosine (MIT) molecules, respectively. (88*)

Measurement of TSH alone fails to provide adequate information to differentiate between suppression, dysfunction, or end gland failure. (89) Therefore, it is always necessary to perform a comprehensive thyroid assessment when the client is first seen, which will include: TSH, fT4, fT3, rT3, and sometimes TPO. Thereafter, the nature and extent of any follow-up thyroid testing will be based upon these initial findings. Many of our past clients' thyroid test results were within the median ranges, and therefore did not need supplementation. Some were found to have issues with elevated rT3, due to elevated cortisol, decreased B-12, or low iron and ferritin. A small amount of triiodothyronine (five to ten mcg) while correcting the underlying condition helped to improve common symptoms of mild hypothyroidism with and without cognitive and mood disorders. (90*)

Thyroid Stimulating Hormone — Laboratory Ranges

Male: Range = 0.27 to 4.2miu/ml, median = 2.235miu/ml.

Female: Range = 0.27 to 4.2miu/ml, median = 2.235miu/ml.

Tetraiodothyronine

Tetraiodothyronine (T4) is the main thyroid hormone produced in the follicular glands of the thyroid under the stimulation of TSH, which acts as catalyst for the intracellular process where organification occurs (91), and for the incorporation of iodine into thyroglobulin. Under this process, intracellular iodide is oxidized and conjugated onto tyrosine residues of the large glycoprotein thyroglobulin. (92) The ratio of T4 to T3 in the follicles is about 15:1, and when lysosomes release T4 and T3 into the serum it is about 11:1. The major binding protein in humans is thyroxine-binding globulin (TBG), which binds about 68 percent of circulating T4 and 80 percent of circulating T3, followed by albumin and transthyretin. (93) As with the majority of all hormones, T4 and T3 must exist in their free form in order to be an active ligand to their specific receptors. Only about 0.02 percent of serum T4 and 0.3 percent of serum T3 are normally free (unbound) and available to enter cells and signal thyroid hormone action. Tetraiodothyronine (T4) is the main hypothalamic regulating hormone that signals the "set point." (94)

Free T4 — Laboratory Ranges

Male: Range = 0.9 to 1.7ng/dl, median = 1.3ng/dl.

Female: Range = .9 to 1.7ng/dl, median = 1.3ng/dl.

Triiodothyronine (3, 5, 3' Triiodothyronine)

Triiodothyronine (T3) is produced from the deiodination of T4's outer ring 5'-iodide. Both active thyroid hormones, thyroxine (T4), and triiodothyronine (T3) exert negative feedback upon the hypothalamus and the pituitary with T4 being the primary. The laboratory testing for free T3 as opposed to total T3 is selectively that part of the T3 pool that is unbound. In conversation with Dr. Ronald Swerdloff (my guru) of the UCLA Department of Endocrinology, he confirmed that the free-T3 pool is theoretically a composite of both free-T3 and free-rT3.

Free T3 — Laboratory Ranges

Male: Range = 1.8 to 4.6pg/dl, median = 3.2pg/ml.

Female: Range = 1.8 to 4.6pg/dl, median = 3.2 pg/ml.

Reverse-T3 (3, 3', 5' Triiodothyronine)

Reverse-T3 (rT3) is produced from the deiodination of the inner ring of T4 (5), creating a non-functional stereoisomer. (96) In fact, studies have found that rT3 has the potential of blocking the T3-receptors (further decreasing the effectiveness of T3). Under conditions of stress, low B-12, low iron, low ferritin, and elevated cortisol, the rT3 production increases at the expense of T3. Recent articles show the sudden drop in T3 and the increase of rT3 within minutes of starting a surgical procedure (links to supportive documents: elective, surgical, surgical, surgical) and acute non-thyroidal illnesses. (97)

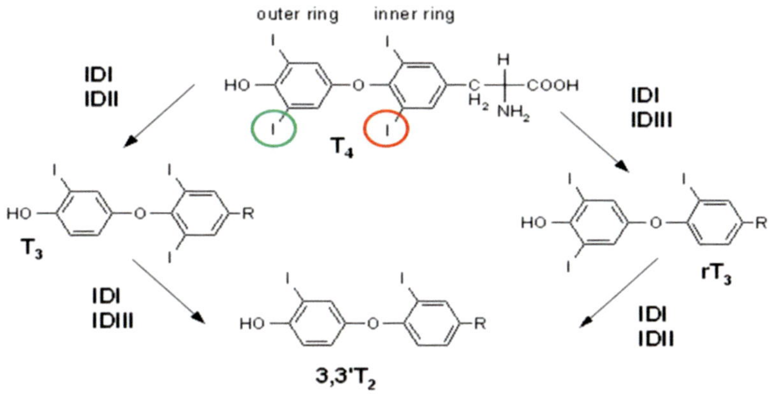

Figure 6.3: Triiodothyronine (T3) is produced by the deiodination of the outer ring at position 5′, while rT3 (reverse T3) is produced by the deiodination of the inner ring at 5.

Reverse T3 (rT3) — Laboratory Ranges

Male: Range = 80 to 250pg/dl, median = 165pg/ml.

Female: Range = 80 to 250pg/dl, median = 165pg/ml.

T3/rT3 Ratio

The importance of obtaining both T3 and rT3 values is so that you can see if the ratio favors the functional T3 or the non-functional rT3. When the level of rT3 is elevated and that of T3 decreased, the diagnosis of the low T3 syndrome [now the non-thyroidal illness syndrome (NTIS)] can be made. (98) This is determined by dividing the free T3 (pg/ml) by rT3 (ng/ml) and having a quotient greater than 1.06. Frequently, a patient with results below 1.00 has many of the symptoms associated with hypothyroidism, regardless of the apparent normalcy of the free-T4 or TSH levels. We occasionally see a low T3/rT3 Ratio (less than 1.00) with an elevation in the TSH level, normal free-T3, and low-normal T4. It appears that the conversion of T4 to both T3 and rT3 diminishes the presence of T4. Since T4 is the trigger for the hypothalamic set point for the HPT axis, TSH climbs.

In a patient with a centrally compromised production of TSH due to trauma, the peripheral production of thyroid hormones will decrease over time. Failure to maintain tonic stimulation of the thyroid gland will allow for a gradual drop in T4 due to normal peripheral conversion to T3. To further complicate things, growth hormone normally assists in the conversion of T4 to T3, but when GH is low there is a slowed conversion of T4 to T3, and when GH is elevated, there is an accelerated conversion. In a person starting on supplementation with GH, conversion of T4 to T3 is accelerated, thereby decreasing the amount of T4 and raising the amount of T3. (99) In a patient with TBI induced HPT axis disruption, a drop in T4 cannot mount a response from the HP axis and raise TSH production. The pattern of thyroid hormones that results is suggestive of a central thyroid deficiency.

Common Interpretation Error — TSH

The range of TSH is presently accepted as from 0.27 to 4.2uIU/ml, with the median at 2.2uIU/ml. Therefore, any level above the median indicates that the body is signaling the thyroid to produce more T4/T3. When there is HPT axis dysfunction (post-TBI), the low levels of T4 cannot be translated into a positive feedback response with an increase in TrH, and then subsequently TSH. Additionally, a normal or even decreased TSH in the face of low circulating T3 levels indicates a major change in HPT axis set-point. The mechanisms responsible for down-regulation of the central HPT axis are still uncertain, and most likely multifactorial. (100) Overtime, the TSH level falls or is maintained at a low level that is inconsistent with the peripheral low hormone levels. In medical practices where only the TSH is used for assessment, if the level is less than 1.0uIU/ml, or even 2.2uIU/ml, the patient is assumed to be making adequate amounts of thyroid hormones because it appears that the level of TSH is suppressed. Looking at it from our vantage point, the HPT axis is broken and cannot respond appropriately to the decreasing levels of peripheral thyroid hormones.

Common Interpretation Error — rT3

When one sees an rT3 level that is above 250pg/ml, this should make you stop and think about all the reasons why rT3 might be elevated. Yes, there have been many articles written in the past five years that acknowledge the influence of cortisol on the conversion of T4 to rT3. And, we know that cortisol goes up in situations that challenge us with stress (physiologic, surgical, nutritional, emotional, and chemical). We are also seeing the literature speaking of low B-12, ferritin and iron levels associated with elevated production of rT3. Look at your CBC results and if the MCV is elevated it can suggest a deficiency in B-12 or folic acid — and if low, the iron and ferritin levels need to be assessed as well. (101)

Corticotropin System (HPA Axis)

The HPA axis is a major part of the neuroendocrine system, and its main role is to subserve the body's response to a stressor (physical or emotional) that disrupts the homeostatic balance of the organism. Assessment of the HPA axis is important due to its potential deleterious effects on recovery (both centrally and peripherally) when regulation or production problems occur. Elevations in CRH and cortisol can interrupt the production of TSH and LH centrally, and preference the peripheral conversation of T4 to rT3 instead of T3. (102) In cases of hypothyroidism with elevation of cortisol, improvement in thyroid homeostasis can only occur once the hypercortisolemia condition is corrected.

Adrenocorticotrophic Hormone

Clinical studies in patients with different TBI severities — ranging from mild to severe — have described TBI induced HPA disruption resulting from pituitary dysfunction, alterations in adrenocorticotropic hormone (ACTH), and/or adrenal insufficiency. Plasma cortisol levels tend to increase after mild to moderate brain injury in the early post-injury period, whereas after a severe injury, cortisol levels are depressed. Activation of the hypothalamic-pituitary-adrenal (HPA) pathway begins with corticotropin releasing hormone, followed by ACTH, which stimulates the adrenal medulla to release corticoids (cortisol). This system is maintained in the majority of mTBI cases, but in some cases the sympathetic-adrenal-medullary (SAM) systems might over-ride the HPA. When this happens, there may be normal or depressed levels of ACTH with elevations in the production of cortisol. This adrenal dissociation seems to be based upon a hypothalamic mechanism, which excludes the normal feedback mechanism in favor of a direct one.

ACTH — Laboratory Range

a.m. Reference Range: 7:00 to10:00 a.m. is 7.2 to 63.3pg/ml, a.m. median is 35.25pg/ml.

Cortisol

Whenever the human brain senses a stressful event, the hypothalamic-pituitary-adrenal (HPA) axis is activated via the release of corticotropin-releasing hormone (CRH) from the hypothalamic paraventricular nucleus into the portal circulation, which stimulates the anterior pituitary corticotrophs to secrete adrenocorticotropic hormone (ACTH), in turn driving cortisol synthesis and secretion from the adrenal cortex. Feedback inhibition exerted by cortisol at the pituitary and the hypothalamic level controls its own release.

Cortisol — Laboratory Range

a.m. Reference Range: 7:00 to 10:00 a.m. is 6.2 to 19.4ug/dl, a.m. median is 12.8ug/dl.

p.m. Reference Range: 4:00 to 8:00 p.m. is 2.3 to 12.3ug/dl, p.m. median is 7.4 ug/dl.

Prolactin

Prolactin homeostasis is the result of a complex balance between positive and negative stimuli from both endogenous and exogenous stimulation. (103*) A number of mediators (of central, pituitary, and peripheral origin) are known to regulate the release and inhibition of prolactin, thereby making an accurate definition of normal prolactin serum levels difficult because of the high inter-individual variability. The hypothalamus secretes a prolactin-release-inhibiting factor (PIF) and a prolactin-releasing factor (PRF). Two important PIFs are dopamine and gamma-aminobutyric acid (GABA), while thyrotropin-releasing hormone (TRH) can act as a PRF.

When measuring prolactin in a patient who has sustained a TBI, we would like to see the results somewhere close to the median range for normal. If PRL is elevated, additional exclusionary assessment would be indicated to differentiate the cause of the PRL elevation as occurring from (a) dysregulation of inhibition, (b) secondary to medication, and (c) pituitary adenoma. Once medication and pituitary adenoma have been excluded, the resulting elevation can be attributed to dysregulation of inhibition secondary to hypothalamic damage.

Prolactinemia (hyper-) associated with traumatic brain injury is indicative of a significant trauma to the hypothalamus. Unlike the other anterior pituitary hormones, the hypothalamic control of prolactin release is predominantly of tonic inhibition. Therefore, patients usually present with galactorrhea, and due to the action of PRL to down-regulate LH-receptors, there is a decrease in the production of gonadal hormones.

Prolactin — Laboratory Range

Male = 4.1 to 18.4ng/ml, median = 11.25ng/ml.

Female = 3.4 to 24.1ng/ml, median = 13.75ng/ml.

Posterior Pituitary Hormones

The posterior pituitary, also called the neurohypophysis, differs from the anterior pituitary in that its primary hormones (ADH and oxytocin) are derived mainly from the long neuronal projections originating from the axons (104) of the magnocellular neurosecretory cells (105) extending from the supraoptic (106) and paraventricular nuclei (107) of the hypothalamus (108) into the posterior pituitary. Therefore, unlike the anterior pituitary that produces its hormones in situ, damage to the posterior pituitary (109) does not commonly lead to permanent deficiency in hormone production.

We generally do not test for these hormones since their deficiencies are usually detected and either resolve or are placed on treatment before they are seen in our office.

An Introductory Case: Putting It All Together

This is a 27-year-old male with a history of multiple TBIs from motocross at ages 16, 18, and 19 without loss of consciousness. The Glasgow coma scores were all 15, but his second accident at age 18, was associated with headaches and transient disorientation for 48 to 72 hours. He was seen by a number of physicians and placed on a combination of anti-depressants because he was considered to be treatment resistant. He continued with cognitive and neurobehavioral issues; bouts of anger, angry, mean, fatigue, and post-concussion type complaints. We performed only the Millennium-TBI panel, obtaining normal biochemistry from his physician.

Laboratory Results for Panel 1 (TBI Evaluation)

Example Case: Table 6.4 (Median = median of laboratory range).

Table 6.5: Example - Male (27) Multiple Concussions

	Marker	Result	Median
1	Growth Hormone	0.3 LN	5.0 ng/ml
2	IGF-1	101 LN	200 ng/ml
3	IGFBP-3	2600 LN	4000 ng/ml
4	DHEA-s	223 N	200 ug/dL
5	Total Testosterone	347 LN	690 pg/ml
6	Free Testosterone	7.39 LN	14 ng/ml
7	DHT	45.0 N	<52ng/dL
8	SHBG	23.0 N	<45 pg/ml
9	Estrone	9.0 N	<60 pg/ml
10	Estradiol	31.7 HN	<25 pg/ml
11	Pregnenolone	387 HN	210 ng/dl
12	Progesterone	1.40 HN	0.8 ng/ml
13	FSH	3.67 LN	7.0 mIU/ml
14	LH	1.34 LN	5.1 mIU/ml
15	Zinc	27.0 LN	95 mcg/dL
16	Prolactin	9.0 N	11.25 ng/ml
17	Insulin	11.0 N	12.5 miu/L
18	Vitamin D3	37.0 LN	60 ng/dL
19	TSH	2.7 N	2.5 mcu/ml
20	Free T4	1.28 LN	1.5 ng/ml
21	Free T3	3.6 HN	2.5 pg/dl
22	Reverse T3	280 HN	165 ng/dl
23	T3/rT3 ratio	1.28 N	> 1.06
24	Thyroperoxidase (TPO)	NA	< 35
25	ACTH	12.4 N	35 pg/ml
26	Cortisol	19.3 HN	15ug/dl_a m

Case Discussion

The majority of growth hormone is produced between 8:00 p.m. and 4:00 a.m., with small pulses of production throughout the day. The half-life of GH is about 20 minutes so by the time of the morning blood draw, the level will be naturally low. When it is elevated, I inquire as to the patient's use of either supplemental GH or Secretropin® (SRx). Therefore, we will initially accept this example patient's level of growth hormone (Line 1) as being normal in concept, but low-normal in quantity (LN).

Once GH enters the circulation, it can take about 30 minutes to start the stimulation of the liver to produce IGF-1 (IGFBPs and ALS too). Since IGF-1 has an eight to ten minute half-life, we would expect to see levels comparable to that of GH, however, because of IGFBP-3, which binds to IGF-1 and extends its half-life by 20 to 24 hours, we can have IGF-1 levels maintained at ideal levels (above 200 ng/ml). In this example scenario, the level of IGF-1 is low-normal (LN).

Binding protein-3 is the main carrier of IGF-1, and also has the longest half-life in this group of GH markers. Studies have identified the production of BP-3 as being logarithmically related (110) to the pulse production of GH. What this means is: As GH increases in the circulation, there is a paralleled production of BP-3 equivalent to the magnitude of the GH produced. This makes BP-3 the most reliable marker reflecting the effectiveness and magnitude of growth hormone's stimulation of the liver. Other stimulants that can increase BP-3 production, besides GH, are estrogen and quercetin. In this case's scenario, the level of IGFBP-3 is low-normal (LN).

In putting these three results together (Lines 1, 2, and 3), it appears that there was an inadequate amount of nocturnal growth hormone production to raise both the IGF-1 and IGFBP-3 to optimal levels. This is highly suggestive of a central GH deficiency caused by one or all of the patient's injures. Therefore, he will require a glucagon stimulation test (GST) to confirm hypothalamic-pituitary disruption as a cause.

Normally, the serum concentration of DHEA-s (Line 4) is 300 to 500 times higher than that of DHEA, and 20 times higher than that of any other steroid hormone. DHEA is derived from pregnenolone and is converted into several active metabolites, including: androstenedione, testosterone, estrone, estradiol, and estriol. The elimination half-life of DHEA is 15 to 38 minutes, whereas the half-life of DHEA-s is seven to 22 hours. Renal excretion accounts for 51 to 73 percent of the elimination of DHEA and its metabolites. (110.1) In this case, the level of DHEA-s is below the median, and therefore low-normal (LN), which appears to be inconsistent with the level of its precursor, pregnenolone (to be discussed).

The free testosterone (Line 6) result must be based upon a direct-measure methodology and not a calculated number. In a review of the derived results of free testosterone by calculation, there was up to a 34 percent variance between direct measurement techniques and calculation methods. (111) Access Medical Laboratory uses the LC/MS/MS/MS technology to measure free testosterone. In this patient, the level of free testosterone is below the median, and therefore low-normal (LN). It is important to base treatment not on the form of testosterone that circulates in the blood attached to carriers, but on that component that gets into the cell. (112)

Total testosterone (Line 5) represents an array of testosterones that are bound to carrier proteins, such as: SHBG, albumin, cortisol binding protein, and a number of minor and active metabolites. Therefore, it is important in general to monitor this component of testosterone to make sure that it is normal and not elevated, while the level of free testosterone is normal to high-normal for optimal response to treatment. In this case, the total testosterone is below the median, and therefore is low-normal (LN).

Dihydrotestosterone (Line 7) is considered the active form of testosterone (four times more anabolic than testosterone). This can imply that the natural quantity of 5-alpha reductase (5-AR) is high, or it was induced to be high by prior use of anabolic hormones. Elevated serum DHT can cause hair loss or thinning, testicular atrophy, prostatic hypertrophy, and oily skin (with or without acne). It is responsible for stimulation of the pilosebaceous organelle to produce sebum, which can improve the quality of skin (soft and lessening of wrinkles) or in excess cause oily skin with acne. Due to the structural difference between DHT and testosterone, DHT does not easily pass the blood brain barrier. Therefore, it is the free testosterone that passes the BBB and is converted by 5-AR to DHT, where it can influence the production of neurotransmitters. In this case, the level of DHT is above the median, and therefore is high-normal (HN).

The sex hormone binding globulin (Line 8) is the carrier protein for sex hormones (testosterone, DHT, and estrogens). The hepatic production of SHBG is influenced by circulating levels of estrogen and testosterone in a proportionate manner. When SHBG is elevated, it binds to free testosterone or free estrogen, decreasing their bioavailability. Therefore, keeping the levels of estrogens and testosterone within the normal physiologic range will prevent spiking of SHBG, DHT, and estradiol. In this case ,the SHBG is within the ideal range, and therefore is normal (N).

We started measuring estrone (Line 9) regularly when we noted the relationship between patients supplementing with DHEA and elevation. The natural hormonal cascade from DHEA allows for either androstenedione or testosterone to be formed. We found in patients supplementing on testosterone, or who had a naturally high endogenous level of testosterone, shunted their DHEA to androstenedione, which then metabolizes to E1. In this case, the estrone is normal (N).

Estradiol (Line 10) is derived directly from testosterone. Patients supplementing on testosterone, or who have a naturally high endogenous level of testosterone, can induce the enzyme estradiol synthetase (aromatase) and produce elevating levels of estradiol. Additionally, in male patients with a low zinc level, they tend to favor conversion of testosterone to estradiol. It appears that zinc is a natural aromatase inhibitor. (113) In this case, estradiol is above the medial, and therefore is high-normal (HN).

Progesterone (Line 11) is a metabolite of pregnenolone with the ability to decrease pituitary release of luteinizing hormone (LH), thereby reducing testicular production of testosterone from the Leydig cells. Additionally, progesterone is converted to allopregnanolone (ALLOP), an important neuroprotective neurosteroid and neuroactive steroid. (114) In the ProTECT study, where mortality was reduced by 50 percent in comatose TBI patients who received progesterone, it was the ALLOP metabolite that is perceived to have been the cause for the reduction in deaths. (115[1]) Allopregnanolone possesses a wide variety of effects, including: antidepressant, anxiolytic, stress-reducing, rewarding, prosocial, anti-aggressive, pro-sexual, sedative, pro-sleep, cognitive and memory-impairing, analgesic, anesthetic, anticonvulsant, neuroprotective, and neurogenic effects .(116) In this case, progesterone is above the medial, and therefore is high-normal (HN).

Pregnenolone (Line 12), the so called "mother of all hormones," is above the median, and therefore is high-normal (HN). Then we must ask why is PREG above the median and DHEA-s (and most likely DHEA) below the median? Take a look at the levels of progesterone and cortisol, which are both above the median. This pattern suggests the Pregnenolone Steal Syndrome, where the body redirects pregnenolone and DHEA, preferencing the production of cortisol due to the demand on this adaptogenic hormone. (117)

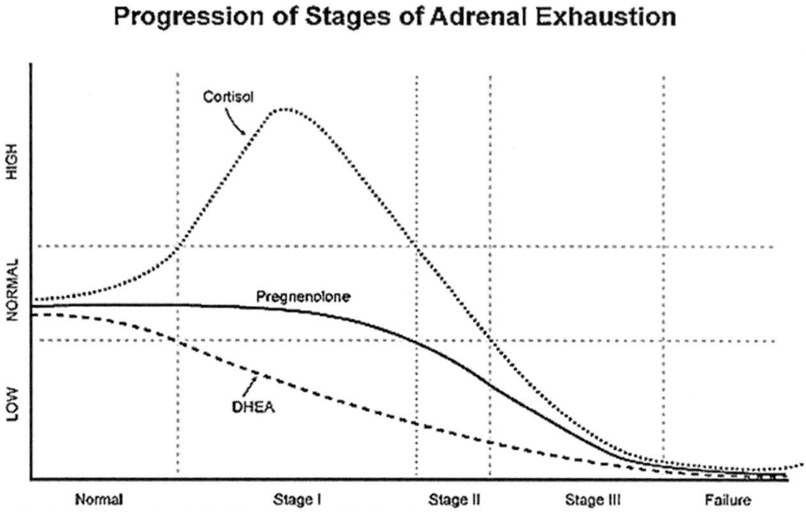

Graph 6.1: As the level of cortisol ascends there is a reciprocal drop in both Pregnenolone and DHEA (DHEA-s).

Follicle stimulating hormone (FSH) is low-normal (LN) not because of a high amount of circulating levels of sex hormones (testosterone, estrogen, progesterone), but because of the dysregulation of the HP axis from the TBIs. In patients on HRT, the FSH level can be used to monitor the adequacy of replacement treatment. When the level of FSH is below 1.0 to 5.0mIU/ml, it suggests suppression of the HP axis due to perceptively supraphysiological doses of hormones.

Luteinizing hormone (LH) is low-normal (LN), which would suggest that the testosterone level would be higher than what was found. Obviously, this patient has had injury to the HP axis, with interruption of the feedback mechanism, thereby being unable to sense the deficiency of testosterone and produce LH to increase testicular (Leydig cells) production of testosterone.

Prolactin (Prol) is normal (N), suggesting that there was no significant damage to the hypothalamus. When prolactin is low, consider the possibility that the patient is on a medication with dopaminergic activity (as in amantadine, L-dopa, and bupropion). This acts like prolactin inhibiting factors (PIF), causing down-regulation of the lactophors of the anterior pituitary gland. These patients tend to have symptoms of anxiety, panic, irritability, and insomnia. When prolactin is elevated, it can indicate the loss of hypothalamic PIF, suppression of prolactin release, or the presence of a prolactinoma. (118)

Zinc is an intracellular metal that is involved in over 300 biochemical pathways. (119*) We monitor it in regard to its natural aromatase ability, especially prior to starting any therapies with testosterone replacement. Additionally, low levels of zinc are associated with depression and poor protection of the brain from oxidative stressors due to diminished levels of superoxide dismutase. (120) Care should be taken when using more than 100mg a day, since it competes with both copper (Cu) and iron (Fe). In our basic nutritional supplements there is 4mg of copper, which is adequate enough to stop side effects relative to the immune system. (121)

Insulin is included as one of our surveillance markers for the metabolic syndrome, which is frequently seen in men and women over 50 years of age with low free testosterone. (122) This is a good pickup, since early detection can lead to total reversal. The insulin level here is normal and suggests a fasting level (less than 10mIU/L).

Vitamin D is no longer a vitamin — having been found to regulate gene expression as is the case with all hormones. What has been found is that vitamin D influences the ability of progesterone to function as a neuroprotective hormone, affects the production of testosterone, decreases autoimmune diseases, improves the immune system, decreases inflammation, enhances coronary functioning, decreases dementia and Alzheimer's disease, raises the pain threshold, improves bone metabolism, and increases hair growth. (123) This patient has a low-normal range of vitamin D3, which can negatively impact a multitude of systems that need to be improved upon. Vitamin D is low-normal in this case presentation (LN).

Thyroid stimulating hormone (TSH) has traditionally been the principal, if not sole, means by which physicians assess the functioning of the HPT axis. Alone, it is ambiguous at best; but, in conjunction with the full complement of thyroid related hormones, can tell an important story of function and biochemistry. What happens when TBI interrupts the hypothalamic regulation of the pituitary production of TSH? Most frequently, the level of TSH will progressively decrease, making us think that there is adequate or even an excessive amount of T4 circulating in the blood. TSH in this case is high-normal (HN).

The free T3 level (fT3) is actually a total free T3 measurement (TfT3) consisting of both the measured rT3 and T3. In this scenario, the free T3 appears normal at 3.6pg/ml, and will be accepted as optimal.

The free T4 level (fT4) is below the median ,with an above the median level of fT3 suggesting a few things: the conversion rate of T4 to T3 is rapid; the production of T4 has decreased while the conversion of T4 to T3 has increased, and GH levels are high. Healthy levels of GH have been shown to increase the rate of conversion of T4 to T3. In central hypothyroidism, the stimulation of the thyroid by elevation of TSH lags behind the conversion of T4 to T3; thereby disclosing a central thyroid issue.

Reverse T3 (rT3) is real. Yes, in normal individuals, it is made in small amounts and represents the deiodination of the inner ring 5'-iodine instead of the outer ring's 5-iodine. The effects of the inactive rT3 are to decrease the production of active T3, and also to block the T3 receptors. One could have a low-normal TSH, normal fT4, and normal to high-normal fT3, and a high-normal to high level of rT3, and have all the symptoms of hypothyroidism — the low T3 syndrome. (124) Reverse-T3 is high-normal (HN) in this case presentation.

Thyroperoxidase (TPO) is run in patients with hypothyroidism suspected of having Hashimoto's thyroiditis (increased occurrence of auto-immune diseases in those with vitamin D deficiency). (125)

Adrenocorticotropic hormone (ACTH) is an important marker of HPA axis communication, as well as a possible explanation for unexplained alterations in other hormones. Under stress (physical, emotional, nutritional, environmental, and chemical) ACTH can go up due to the production of CRH, which can down-regulate LH too. This is the connection between women with stress and alterations in their menstrual cycle. ACTH is normal in this case presentation (N).

Cortisol is the adaptogenic hormone that enables your body to function under an array of stressors. When the levels of cortisol are low, we experience adrenal fatigue, and when elevated, a Cushing's syndrome. Under prolonged stress, the adrenal gland's ability to produce functional amounts of cortisol fails, giving rise to adrenal fatigue syndrome (126), most likely the result of a combination of enzymatic deficiency, those used in the adrenal cortex to make not only cortisol, but also androgens (DHEA, DHEA-s, and androstenedione), mineralocorticoids, and glucocorticoids, and a deficiency of the precursors derived from pregnenolone. The presence of the Pregnenolone Steal Syndrome is an antecedent to the ultimate crash of the system, whereby pregnenolone and DHEA are shunted toward the production of cortisol (zona fasciculata produces cortisol and DHEA/DHEA-s is produced in the zona reticularis).

Elevation of cortisol has a direct route with central ACTH, and a peripheral one with the autonomic nervous system. This is how ACTH can be low, and there still be a significant elevation in cortisol. (127)

Case Summary

Based upon the GH axis, it appears that there is an incomplete or partial GH deficiency. This patient would be offered a glucagon stimulation test (GST) or a trial first of Secretropin® for up to three months. If the damage is at the hypothalamus, we might expect an elevation in the GH due to the loss of somatostatin inhibition. That does not seem to be the case here, and appears to be at the level of the pituitary, where a single pathway secretagogue might not work. Secretropin® has five different pathways that it addresses: somatostatin suppression, dopamine receptor 2 stimulation, ghrelin stimulation, GHRH receptor stimulation, and synthetic receptor stimulation. If Secretropin® fails to raise the level of GH, IGF-1 and IGFBP-3, we move to the GST and use rhGH.

The cascade from pregnenolone to DHEA/DHEA-s and then testosterone suggests that DHEA is being pulled into the Pregnenolone Steal Syndrome due to the low levels of DHEA/DHEA-s and testosterone, while there are high-normal levels of pregnenolone. Additionally, there is high-normal progesterone and an elevation in the a.m. cortisol level. The GST is a challenge test for both cortisol and growth hormone, and therefore can be used to "kill two birds with one stone."

The low level of luteinizing hormone, in light of low peripheral testosterone levels, can only support the diagnosis of a central hypogonadism.

Vitamin D3 is low, and increasing it to 80 to 100ng/dl might help with a number of the patient's issues: depression, sleep, anxiety, pain intolerance, reduced inflammation, improved immunity, and better production of testosterone. It is important that the level of calcium and consumption of calcium containing products be managed while treating the patient with 5,000 to 10,000 IU of vitamin D_3 a day.

The thyroid hormones are linked to the level of cortisol in that it is responsible for the increase in the conversion of T4 to rT3. Correcting adrenal stress with supplementation to stop the PSS can lead to an improvement in the high cortisol level. Iron, ferritin and B12 levels should be assessed since they too can affect the production of rT3 from T4.

ACTH is normal, with a high-normal amount of cortisol, which can be one of the causes for the increased production of rT3.

Treatment for this case will be addressed in Chapter 9; Treatment for TBI.

Conclusion

"Conclusions: To attain maximal improvement in mental and physical functioning, as well as in quality of life for victims of TBI, it is crucial that anterior pituitary hormonal function be assessed. Appropriate hormone replacement therapy for those patients with both TBI and TBI-induced pituitary function impairment could, for the first time, allow treatment and correction of underlying causes of TBI sequelae rather than merely symptomatic treatment." (128)

This concluding statement by Urban, Harris, and Masel in 2005 made it clear that neurotrauma, like traumatic brain injury, poses a substantial risk to pituitary function that is perhaps greater than previously appreciated. Patients with TBI should be screened prospectively for isolated, multiple, and panhypopituitarism at three month intervals during the initial year. It is well documented that patients with hypopituitarism (due to primary hypothalamic-pituitary pathologies) do benefit from hormonal replacement therapies. (129) We know this to be true firsthand with our treatment of patients since 2004.

The signs and symptoms of post-TBI hypopituitarism may be masked by what has been assumed to be merely a post-traumatic syndrome (PTSD). By increasing awareness among physicians of the risk of brain injury–induced endocrinopathies, and the need for appropriate endocrinological testing, may lead to improved quality of life with enhanced rehabilitation prospects. (130)

In severe and moderate TBI cases, the patient is seen and treated by trauma surgeons and neurosurgeons during hospitalization, and subsequently by rehabilitation physicians. The neuropsychologists and psychiatrists become involved and frequently place the patient on psychotropic medication, only to find that they frequently are resistant to monotherapy, a hallmark in TBI patients with testosterone dysfunction. The majority of these patients never have had a baseline hormonal survey, and fail to improve over years of traditional treatment and continue to suffer.

Nearly 80 percent of the injured have a mild form of TBI, and therefore never were evaluated in the ER or by their family physician. These individuals over the course of days, months, and years develop progressive symptoms associated with TBI. These are the people that must be targeted as being at risk of developing hypopituitarism. The Endocrinologists and Internists must be educated about TBI-induced hypopituitarism, and encouraged to actively share their expertise with other physicians ,and to document the presence or absence of clinical laboratory findings supportive of this condition.

Unfortunately, many of the patients who do have laboratory testing to assess hormonal dysfunction never receive treatment because of the two major flaws in the interpretation of laboratory results (a) the use of a fixed reference ranges that applies to everyone else, and (b), the failure to appreciate the integral relationships that exists between each central hormone and its peripheral product, as well as crossover relationships between the different hormones. Traditionally, we tend to look at each laboratory result as a single isolated number, and not in association with other results (e.g., cortisol and thyroid).

I believe I made it clear in the introduction that the statistical models that have been used for the “normal” and “reference” ranges are flawed in that they represent an artificial amalgamation of test results from an array of genetically different individuals. We need to treat each client as an individual, and collect results from them that represent their unique biochemical homeostasis — not using someone else’s.

The second issue of looking at lab results in relationship to other labs will not only help us to treat patients at much higher levels of interpretation, but we will be able to derive a better understanding of the interactions of each hormone with others. A classic example would be in both female and male patients who are receiving gender hormone replenishment (estrogen, progesterone, or testosterone) based upon low peripheral hormone levels and high LH and FSH levels. Once under treatment, a repeat lab shows that their hormone levels are increasing and their LH and FSH are decreasing. This would support an interpretation that they are receiving adequate amounts of hormone, which is returning them to a more homeostatic state.

Additionally, if the levels of LH and FSH fall below their median range, it would tell us that they are being over-treated. A similar situation occurs in hypothyroidism, with initial TSH levels being above 2.5ng/ml, and then with treatment, below 0.1ng/ml — obviously indicating that they are possibly receiving too high of a replenishment dose. Before I change anything in either of these cases, I always ask the patient how they are feeling — psychologically, physically, and physiologically — before changing anything. Otherwise, I would be treating the numbers instead of the patient. The optimal goal will always be to use the least amount of medication for the greatest and safest amount of benefits.

Chapter 7: The Neuropsychiatry of TBI

"My mission in life is not merely to survive, but to thrive; and to do so with some passion, some compassion, some humor, and some style."

— Maya Angelou

"It is not only for what we do that we are held responsible, but also for that which we do not do."

— Molière

Introduction

Antiquity shows that either the Egyptians or Mesopotamians developed the proto-psychological theory of the Four Temperaments (1), which is based upon the four fundamental personality types: sanguine (pleasure-seeking and sociable), choleric (ambitious and leader-like), melancholic (analytical and quiet), and phlegmatic (relaxed and peaceful).

However, it was the Greek physician Hippocrates who advanced this theory into a medical concept. He believed certain human moods, emotions, and behaviors were caused by the four bodily fluids called "humors," which were blood, yellow bile, black bile, and phlegm. Essentially, Hippocrates was not so far off, if we consider the four major hormones — somatotropin, gonadotropin, thyrotropin, and corticotrophin — as the "humors" that we now see as influencing our neuropsychology and physical well-being.

More recently, and with the further understanding of the impact of neurosteroids (2) on our psychological make-up, the diagnosis of neuropsychological conditions is no longer exclusively looked at as the sum total of one's life's experiences based upon nature and nurture, but as the interplay between external and internal factors that influence how we respond to the world around us.

Neurobehavioral Alterations

In traumatic brain injury (TBI), neurobehavioral alterations (3) have been seen as the primary factor attributing to long-term disability, which frequently include: difficulty remaining employed, maintaining social relationships, and participating in other social roles. In most cases of mild TBI, the cognitive sequelae are overshadowed by limitations caused by debilitating psychiatric problems such as: depression, suicidal ideation, anxiety, agitation, anger, paranoia, sexual dysfunction, and alcohol/drug abuse.

In 2002, Dr. Salla Koponen (4) reported results of a 30-year prospective study on neuropsychiatric sequelae involving Axis I (5) and II (6) psychiatric disorders after TBI. In this study on 60 patients, 48.3 percent experienced an Axis I disorder that began after TBI, and 61.7 percent experienced an Axis I disorder during their lifetimes. The most common disorders after TBI were: major depression (26.7 percent), alcohol abuse or dependence (11.7 percent), panic disorder (8.3 percent), specific phobia (8.3 percent), and psychotic disorders (6.7 percent). Fourteen patients (23.3 percent) had at least one personality disorder. The most prevalent individual disorders were: avoidant (15.0 percent), paranoid (8.3 percent), and schizoid (6.7 percent) personality disorders. Nine patients (15.0 percent) had DSM-III-R organic personality syndrome. Dr. Koponen concluded that, "Traumatic brain injury seems to make patients particularly susceptible to depressive episodes, delusional disorder, and personality disturbances. The high rate of psychiatric disorders found in this study emphasizes the importance of psychiatric follow-up after traumatic brain injury."

Although Dr. Koponen's study sample was relatively small, the results could easily apply to the over 410,000 Iraq and Afghanistan war veterans (7) who sought psychological help from the Veterans Administration in 2012. To further the significance of TBI, on January 3rd, 2013, NBC News reported that active service members committed suicide in 2012 at a record breaking pace: More than 349 took their own lives across the four branches — one every 25 hours — as a Department of Defense (8) spokesperson confirmed. The Army sustained the heaviest suicide toll at 182, a dark tally that marked another frightening first as soldier suicides last year outpaced the 176 Army members who were killed in combat while serving Operation Enduring Freedom, according to Pentagon officials.

Throughout the U.S. military, figures show that suicides increased by nearly 16 percent from 2011 to 2012. According to a Department of Defense spokeswoman, the DOD has been issuing annual reports that track suicides since 2008. More information can be obtained from the website: Suicide Prevention and Awareness. (9)

In another NBC News report, 28-year-old Army soldier, Spc. Brandon Barrett (10) presented at his parents' home in Tucson, Arizona on what was believed to be a leave following a brutal, year-long deployment in Afghanistan with the 5th Stryker Brigade. The family learned later that Brandon saw several of his buddies killed by bombs during his deployment. This deeply affected Brandon, leading to his alleged desertion from his unit. Brandon left his parents' home and drove to Salt Lake City where he donned his combat fatigues, boots, and helmet, then grabbed his AR-15 rifle, went to a hotel, and told an employee at the hotel to call the police.

A police officer arrived and Barrett shot him in the leg. The officer returned fire and killed Barrett with a bullet to the head. His family believes Barrett intended to commit "suicide by cop," as acknowledged by his brother Shane (a Tucson police detective). The Barrett family later learned that Brandon had confided to a chaplain within his unit, revealing that his year of combat in Afghanistan had left him depressed and anxious after witnessing the deaths of three teammates. This is not an uncommon neuropsychiatric condition that is being identified as post-traumatic stress disorder (PTSD), a condition that this physician believes is more frequently mild-TBI.

In addressing the psychological manifestations frequently seen in TBI patients, the question that is debated continues to be: Is this really a psychological process, or just the manifestations of an underlying illness? Is the depression, for example, as seen in hypothyroidism, really clinical depression, or just co-morbidity of the underlying insult to the brain? Therefore, which co-morbidity applies?

As a matter of reference, the original and more correct definition of co-morbidity — to indicate a medical condition existing simultaneously but independently with another condition in a patient — is indicated here. This is not to be confused with the non-standard definition of co-morbidity, which is: to indicate a medical condition in a patient that causes, is caused by, or is otherwise related to another condition in the same patient.

Emotions and Moods

Emotion has been defined as a reaction — psychological and physiological — which is subjectively experienced as strong feelings, many of which prepare the body for immediate action or reaction. (11) Certain emotions are considered primary emotions, and are thought to be innate. They include happiness, anger, sadness, fear, disgust, love, and surprise. Depression is considered a "mood state," and is generally more persistent than an emotion. Mood states are thought to function as moderators of emotional experiences. (12)

Emotions and moods are under the control of the brain. The limbic system (13[1]), located in the dorsolateral frontal and medial temporal lobes of the brain (Chapter 2), plays a major role in the production of emotions and moods. Included in the limbic system are: the hypothalamus (14) (which affects emotional responses through the control of the endocrine and autonomic system), the amygdala (15) (which is best known for its role in fear and aggression), the hippocampus (16) (which plays a critical role in memory formation and plasticity), and parts of the thalamus (17) (which receive sensory input and act as a way station for sending signals/messages to other parts of the brain).

Because the frontal lobes are actively monitoring and managing emotional input, there are major connections between the limbic system and the frontal lobes. Unfortunately, and due to their physical location in the skull, the frontal lobes are most susceptible to injury in acceleration-deceleration injuries — whether or not there is any external contact. Additionally, the hippocampus is highly susceptible to cellular changes that result in the production of neurotoxic agents, which are commonly seen in even mild traumatic brain injury (mTBI). As such, this chapter will address how TBI and alteration in neurobehavior frequently lead to emotions becoming volatile and unpredictable. Additionally, we will review major research studies relative to the impact of hormones on emotions and moods, understanding that the focus of this text is the impact of hormonal dysfunction on our global well-being.

The Challenge of this Chapter

I graduated from Swedish Covenant Hospital Medical Center (18) in 1985 after completing one year of rotating internship, followed by three years of a Family Practice residency program. I did not start out with flying colors, but ended up graduating with the highest awards and recognition by the residency staff and hospital nurses as someone who cared about the treatment of the patients, both physiologically and psychologically. During that program, I was introduced to endocrinology by Dr. Sidney Cruz, a large Filipino physician who was the antithesis of balanced hormones. He looked like a Buddha, and was a saint who enjoyed all the foods that he admonished his diabetic patients for eating. Nonetheless, even though I did not realize it at the time, he had set me in motion to arrive at this point in my life.

During my three years in the program, I saw many patients with thyroid disease who also experienced varying degrees of depression and mood disorders; that is, until their thyroid chemistry was corrected. Women with imbalances in estrogens and progesterone were perceived as evil until they were treated with appropriate hormonal supplementation (at that time, BCPs). Elderly men with dysthymia or frank depression (blue or melancholy) sat at home waiting for the big one (MI) since we never checked testosterone. (19) These men, as well as many of the women, were placed on tricyclic antidepressants and were forced into psychotherapy, never to have addressed the true underlying nature of their psychobehavioral transformation.

Thirty years later, the medical community, in light of tens (if not hundreds) of thousands of articles (20) linking hormonal deficiencies with psychological changes, refuses to draw a straight line connecting the dots. They acknowledge that TBI is associated with mood disorders, especially depression, and they also acknowledge the association of TBI with varying degrees of hormonal dysfunction; but, they fail to acknowledge that maybe treating the TBI associated hormonal deficiencies will improve the emotional-mood disorders.

The focus of this chapter is to present the evidence that hormone dysfunction, secondary to TBI, is directly associated with changes in personality and functionality that have led to the extensive use of antidepressants. Unfortunately, many of these patients experience treatment resistant depression (21) — a common denominator in those with TBI precipitated testosterone deficiency that goes unaddressed.

Once you are saturated with the information contained in this chapter, the association between laboratory-defined hormonal insufficiencies and well-defined premorbid neuropsychiatric symptoms will clearly become a treatment possibility with those hormones, rather than with psychotropic drugs.

The challenge will then be to institute these alternative pathways into your practice.

Depression

More than half of all individuals who experience TBI will become depressed in the year after their injury, and less than half of those who do become depressed are likely to receive adequate treatment. (22)

While depression is a relatively common diagnosis — affecting about 20 percent of the general population — individuals surviving TBI appear to be significantly more susceptible to varying degrees of depression, as evidenced by incidence rates ranging upwards to 77 percent. Additionally, the co-morbidity of TBI with anxiety, aggression, mood disorders, arousal, and sexual dysfunction is found to be about 44 percent. When the biochemical second-phase of TBI develops into a neuropsychiatric presentation, it tends to confound the ability of healthcare workers to assess the potential of a unified etiological theory; thereby, making the prescription of a psychotropic medication the quick and easy answer. (23)

Major depressive disorder (MDD) appears to be the most prevalent psychiatric disorder that develops after TBI, with a prevalence rate over 25 percent. The reported prevalence of MDD within the first year is 33 to 42 percent, and climbs to 61 percent within the first seven years. (24)

Data from a recent prospective study of 559 subjects hospitalized after TBI revealed the prevalence rate of 52 percent for probable MDD within the first year after injury. Notably, the increased risk of depression is not limited to those with moderate to severe TBI, as it is also present among those with mild TBI (mTBI). There is also an increased risk of suicide subsequent to TBI, with one study noting that ten percent reported suicidal ideation at one year post-TBI, and 15 percent attempted suicide by year five, post-injury. (25)

What to Treat?

The Diagnostic and Statistical Manual Text Revision (DSM-IV, 2000) (26), outlines the necessary symptoms which a patient must experience to be diagnosed with major depression. These include a depressed mood or loss of pleasure for two weeks, as well as the presence of four or more of the following symptoms: change in appetite or weight loss, insomnia or hypersomnia, fatigue or loss of energy, being restless or slowed down to a degree that is observable by others, feeling worthless, being unable to concentrate, having suicidal thoughts, planning or attempting suicide. (27[1])

However, patients suffering from various medical conditions — such as TBI — can have a prominent disturbance in their mood marked by many of the above characteristics, and yet not fulfill the criteria for major depression. Such a patient would be categorized as having a mood disorder secondary to a general medical condition (TBI). In these cases of mood disorder, and even frank depression arising from TBI, the question becomes what to treat: The cause or the symptoms? Unfortunately, we know the answer to this question: The symptoms are treated, and the underlying causation is never sought after. (28)

Depression following TBI is associated with worse global outcomes, worse social functioning during the first year post-injury, and lower health-related quality of life, even after controlling the medical, demographic, and neuropsychological factors. Those survivors of TBI with depression lasting more than six months experience deterioration in social functioning and quality of life. Depressed TBI patients also report more severe post-concussive symptoms (e.g., headache, blurred vision, dizziness, insomnia, memory and cognitive impairment, and progressive somatic complaints) when compared to non-depressed TBI patients. (29)

In non-depressed TBI patients, there is always the possibility that they may develop depressive symptoms when oxidative stress creates a sufficient amount of inflammation to disrupt neuro-connectivity and balanced biochemical functioning. This has been documented to take up to 17 years before symptoms of depression are exhibited, and is associated with the down-regulation of a number of neurosteroids. (30)

Several factors which have been suggested as being correlated with the development of depression after TBI include: lesion location (left dorsal lateral frontal lesions and/or left basal ganglia lesions, as well as possibly parietal-occipital and right hemispheric lesions), poor social functioning (less than high school education, unstable employment, and relationship difficulties) and previous psychiatric history (depression and substance abuse). (31)

A consistent finding in all types of neurotrauma has been the activation of proinflammatory chemistry derived from the immune system. Numerous studies have suggested that major depression is accompanied by immune dysregulation. Specifically, activation of the inflammatory response system (IRS) has been demonstrated by increased production of proinflammatory cytokines, such as: interleukin (IL)-1B, IL-2, IL-6, interferon (IFN)-G, tumor necrosis factor (TNF)-A, the soluble IL-6 receptor (IL-6R), and the IL-1 receptor antagonist (IL-1RA). These findings may be clinically important because proinflammatory cytokines can contribute directly to the development of depressive symptoms. Proinflammatory cytokines have been shown to induce stress-reactive neuroendocrine and central neurotransmitter changes reminiscent of those in depression, and it has been demonstrated that immunotherapy with IFN-G can precipitate depression. (32)

Additionally, a number of articles that asked the question, "Does TBI increase risk for substance abuse?" have found that there appeared to be an increased occurrence in those individuals with a prior history of abuse. Yet, confounding this perception is one of the concluding points by Bjork and Grant, which states that, "Behavioral evidence from 'clean' TBI survivors is mildly suggestive of decision-making deficits that may increase risk for drug abuse." The decision-making deficit is related to the executive functions of the frontal lobe, and therefore the proclivity toward substance abuse might be more akin to the area of trauma, and not the pre-morbid status of prior substance abuse. (33)

It is saddening when a popular celebrity (as well as anyone) commits suicide, and the media attributes it to a past/present alcohol or drug abuse scenario. Sensationalism does not allow for delving into the extenuating situations that might have fueled the negative outcome. Causative factors — such as open heart surgery causing neurotrauma — are not considered, even in light of the tens of thousands of articles addressing post-operative depression. It is always much easier to accept things at face value.

Robin Williams is a case in question. Although I do not have all the facts, I have some that are important enough to put down on paper. We know that Robin Williams had extensive open heart surgery in 2009 at the Cleveland Clinic to replace his aortic valve, fix his mitral valve, and correct an irregular heartbeat. This surgery could very well have taken six hours or more, barring any complications. During that time frame, the patient goes on a by-pass machine while the actual replacement is being performed. It is during this time frame that the potentials for damage to the hypothalamo-pituitary regulatory system might occur.

Contrasting prolonged surgical procedures with Sheehan's syndrome gives us a theoretical mechanism whereby patients might be at risk for developing hypopituitarism from interruption of blood flow through the hypophyseal portal system that supplies the pituitary gland. As in Sheehan's syndrome, it might take months for the diminution of anterior hormones to present as symptoms.

Additionally, intrasurgical monitoring of thyroid hormones has detected a transition from pre-surgery normal T3 to post surgery production of abnormal reverse T3 (rT3). This has been associated with increased symptoms of depression that can last for a year or more. (34, 35)

How to Treat Treatment-Resistant Depression?

Many of the patients seen by Millennium-TBI have presented with either atypical or treatment resistant depression. (36) Those with atypical depression are characterized as having less than the usual five of nine classic major depression symptoms to qualify as having a major depressive disorder (MDD), which are: (a) sadness or depressed mood most of the day or almost every day, (b) loss of enjoyment in things that were once pleasurable, (c) major change in weight (gain or loss of more than five percent of weight within a month) or appetite, (d) insomnia or excessive sleep almost every day, (e) physically restless or rundown that is noticeable by others, (f) fatigue or loss of energy almost every day, (g) feelings of hopelessness or worthlessness or excessive guilt almost every day, (h) problems with concentration or making decisions almost every day, and (i) recurring thoughts of death or suicide, suicide plan, or suicide attempt.

In patients characterized as treatment-resistant (37), they tend to fail monotherapy after a long period of rotating from one medication to another. Frequently, these individuals end up on two, three, or even four different medications without fully controlling their depression. Additionally, due to the cumulative adverse side effects of combination therapy, these patients frequently are placed on other medications to counter the side effects (methamphetamine, Adderall®). In a growing number of research articles, deficiencies of GH, thyroid, testosterone, and elevation in cortisol have been associated with TRD. (38)

That Ah-Ha Moment

Recently, I was involved in a discussion with a psychiatrist about hormones and their influence on depression and general neurobehavior. I was reciting a few of my favorite key articles when the question arose as to how many articles have been written on the subject of hormones and depression. So, that night I went home and posed the question to Google Scholar, and the resulting responses are what built Table 7.1, below.

Hormones and Depression	Results
Testosterone and Depression	70,400
Estrogen and Depression	99,300
Progesterone and Depression	53,600
Thyroid and Depression	235,000
DHEA and Depression	15,700
Growth Hormone and Depression	19,100

Table 7.1: A search on Google Scholar for published articles associating a specific hormone deficiency with the presence of depression yielded the following number of articles. The date range was between 2000-2012 and the articles were not screened for accuracy. MLG

With this table in hand, I started asking both patients and colleagues what they thought was the number of articles written between 2000 and 2012 that discussed a specific hormone and depression. Not having guessed any better, the common response was between two and 500 articles per hormone. When I shared the actual numbers, the typical response was, "Then why are we not testing for hormonal deficiencies before starting pharmaceuticals (drugs)?" Ah-ha!

A Brief Comment on Somatization

Regardless of what the clinical psychiatrists say about somatization (39) being a corporeal expression or manifestation of an overload of anxiety and depression, it can also be expressed as a breakdown in the energy management of the brain. Under "normal" conditions, the brain is capable of dealing with the production of electrochemical energy, which is used to run our bodies. Much of this energy (based upon the high utilization of glucose and production of ATP) is used to think, reason, analyze, and communicate. When there is a disruption in the normal production and use of energy, the excess leaks out and creates areas of hyperactivity. (40[1])

Under stressful situations, the brain increases the production of ATP, which has a lethal side effect in the concomitant production of free radicles. The radical group contains compounds such as: superoxide (O2) radicals, hydroxyl radicals, peroxyl radicals, alkoxyl radicals, nitric oxide (NO) radicals, and one form of singlet oxygen. The non-radicals group contains compounds such as: hydrogen peroxide, lipid hydroperoxide, singlet oxygen, peroxynitrite (ONOO), and hypochlorous acid. If these free radicles are allowed to accumulate they will cause cellular damage leading to either autophagy or apoptosis (Chapter 4). Depending upon the extent of the process, an expanding area(s) of the brain is involved, thereby increasing the potential for regulatory damage. The most probable mechanism is through the NMDA receptor, where excitotoxicity can cause a hyperactive state represented by: anxiety, panic attacks, insomnia, fibromyalgia, gastric symptoms, sleep deprivation, and non-specific, generalized, vague symptoms of pain. (41)

What helps to support this concept is that medications (such as benzodiazepines), minerals (such as magnesium and zinc), and hormones (pregnenolone and allopregnanolone) all block the activation of the NMDA channel — thereby inducing some degree of relaxation. Symptoms of irritable bowel, agitation, anxiety, and so forth will all diminish as well.

A recent study out of Turkey (42) looked at a group of men and women with somatization illness and found that the size of the pituitary gland was smaller than in the normal controls. Speculation as to the causative factor was not clear, but suggested that glucocorticoids played a role in the reduction in size of the gland.

In an article by Dr. Robert Dantzer (43), he believes that the presence of somatization and its construct of symptoms are derived from the activation of brain cytokines: "Proinflammatory cytokines produced by cells of the innate immune system in response to pathogen-associated molecular patterns and to endogenous danger signals act on the central nervous system via afferent and humoral pathways to trigger a brain cytokine system that organizes the sickness response in its subjective, behavioral, and metabolic components. There is evidence that prolonged activation of this system can precipitate the development of depressive disorders in vulnerable patients." Therefore, treatment might be best served by increasing the neurosteroids and diminishing the presence of oxidative reactants. (44)

Hormones and Depression

The following summaries will highlight a number of articles on the subject of hormones and depression, as well as a number of other clinical psychiatric presentations discussed in this chapter. Obviously, if you are in need of further support and justification for an initial hormonal work-up prior to the initiation of a psychotropic medication, you too, can always go to Google Scholar (scholar.google.com)

Another point of interest is that "partial" hormonal deficiencies, and not only frank deficiencies, can precipitate neurobehavioral disorders such as depression. (45) This concept of "partial" deficiency is what we refer to in the office as a "low-normal" result — commonly in the lower 25th percentile of the range. Articles supporting this concept address both testosterone (46) and growth hormone (47[1]) since they are significant in the realm of Neuropsychopharmacology. (48[L])

Growth Hormone and Depression

Traumatic brain injury has been recently recognized as a risk factor for cognitive impairment and hypopituitarism, presented most frequently with growth hormone deficiency (GHD). GHD is associated not only with changes in body composition, but also with impaired quality of life, cognitive dysfunctions, and some psychiatric sequelae, which are usually classified as "depression" or "atypical depression." (49) The impact of GH therapy on mental status in TBI patients is slowly being investigated as an important hormone to replace in order to regain optimal psychological and cognitive functioning. (50)

In this six-month, placebo-controlled study by Popovic-Doknic in 2010, patients with TBI precipitated growth hormone deficiency experienced improvement in both cognitive abilities (particularly verbal and non-verbal memory) and psychiatric functioning. The patients were treated with growth hormone for six months upon assessment, and then stopped on treatment until twelve months, when they were reassessed. In contrast, the severity of depression decreased, as well as intensity of: interpersonal sensitivity, hostility, paranoid ideation, anxiety, and psychoticism.

Somatization (51), obsessive-compulsive symptoms, and phobic anxiety decreased in all — except for one patient. (52)

In the Mahajan-Crown study in 2004, 61 percent of the patients with adult onset GHD, but none of the patients with childhood onset GHD, were found to have atypical depression at baseline. There were significant improvements in the depression rating scale scores after two months of GH therapy, with significant improvements in emotional reaction and social isolation scores from one month, and in energy levels and sleep disturbance from two and three months respectively. The authors concluded that: "A large proportion of GHDAs have unequivocal psychiatric morbidity, and suggest that a response to treatment can be seen after a short trial of GH therapy. We hypothesize that this rapid improvement of symptoms of atypical depression represents a direct central effect of GH therapy." (53)

Another interesting neuroendocrine assessment looked at a number of hormones and their effect on fatigue — specifically for: growth hormone (GH) reserve, thyroid, and cortisol and testosterone levels. Jeffrey Englander and his team found 53 percent reported fatigue on the Multidimensional Assessment of Fatigue (MAF) and 33 percent on the Fatigue Severity Scale (FSS), while 65 percent were found to have moderate to severe GH deficiency, 64 percent had adrenal insufficiency (low fasting cortisol), twelve percent had central hypothyroidism, and 15 percent of men had testosterone deficiency. (54) So, which comes first, hormonal deficiency or the change in neuroendocrine behavior — fatigue?

Testosterone and Depression

As unreported observations during the years 2001 to 2014, the Millennium Health Group has treated over 2,700 patients (males and females) with laboratory diagnosed suboptimal levels of free and total testosterone, associated with low dihydrotestosterone (DHT) and DHEA-s. Upon replenishing the hormones to optimal levels, both dysthymic and overt depressive symptoms improved — thereby allowing many of the patients to decrease or stop their antidepressant medication as directed by their treating psychiatrist. These patients were followed on a monthly basis with the Millennium Treatment Questionnaire©, that consists of 25 questions looking at psychological, physiological, and physical responses to treatment. The compilation of the results from these patients has supported our treatment protocols, and the development of newer and more robust treatments. Patient improvements were seen across the three areas of assessment within two to twelve weeks.

Based upon the results of these self-assessment questionnaires, the current medical literature was perused for evidence-based studies to provide support, and an understanding of the mechanisms by which benefits were gleaned. We wanted to understand why patients with low testosterone developed neurobehavioral symptoms, as well as why patients with traumatic brain injury fared better than their cohorts when testosterone was included in their treatment protocol.

The Rancho Bernardo study (55), the Health in Men Study (56), and the free testosterone study by Joshi (57) demonstrated that men with free testosterone levels in the lowest quartile had the higher occurrence of depression. Free testosterone levels below 170pmol/l (13.2ng/dL) are associated with depressive symptoms, while free testosterone levels below 220pmol/l (60.9ng/dL) (lowest quintile of our population) predict the onset of depressive symptoms.

Rubinow, Schmidt, and Ebinger (58), supported the findings that testosterone has many central nervous system effects, and can influence neuronal function: through binding to intracellular receptors, through modulation of ligand-gated ion channels (NMDA, Sigma1 and GABA), and through binding to neurotransmitter receptors. Furthermore, testosterone deficiency, as well as that of neurosteroids, have been found to be involved in the pathophysiology of mood disorders and suicidal behavior — again involving many of the receptors and neurotransmitters that are the target of traditional antidepressants. (59)

Hypogonadal men frequently show depressive symptoms, and testosterone replacement can improve these symptoms. (60) Testosterone and other androgens might have antidepressant properties. (61, 62) For example, it has been shown that testosterone gel may produce antidepressant effects in depressed men with low testosterone levels. (63)

In terms of traumatic brain injury, the greatest benefits from testosterone and the other neurosteroids are in their ability to attenuate the effects of the secondary phase of neurotrauma: the inflammatory cytokines. (64*) We have seen the destructive influence of a number of inflammatory processes set off by: mitochondrial dysfunction, oxidative stress, necrosis, as well as the non-inflammatory reduction in neurons by apoptosis, autophagy, and parthanatos. One of my mentors at USC Medical School is Dr. C.J. Pike, who has written extensively about androgens and Alzheimer's, as well as the anti-inflammatory benefits to testosterone. He discusses how testosterone and its metabolites have significant regulatory and neuroprotective roles in the central nervous system in which both inflammatory and non-inflammatory processes leading to loss of neurons is impeded. (65)

Protecting the natural metabolites of testosterone from DHT to androstanediol has been shown to be associated with improved seizure control and control of neuronal excitability and behavior. The use of any 5-AR blocker has been shown to impair the conversion of testosterone to down-stream androstanediol — a positive modulator of $GABA_A$ receptor causing a slowing of electrical impulses. (66)

Estrogen/Estrogen Dominance

Aside from estradiol's well-known function as one of the reproductive hormones, it has been found to be a pleiotropic hormone that influences numerous non-reproductive functions such as: bone and mineral metabolism, cardiac and vascular function (67), memory, cognition and mood, wound healing (68), and the incidence and progression of age-related diseases. (69)

Many of these functions are mediated through epigenetic and genomic modulation via estrogen receptors (ER-alpha, ER-beta, and recently recognized direct cell wall receptors) that initiate gene expression involved in the balance of apoptosis and cell survival (70*), mitochondrial function (71), the function of astrocytes (72), synthesis and secretion of neurotransmitters that modulate neuronal excitability or neuron/astrocyte interactions (73), expression of neurotrophins, growth factors and their receptors leading to enhanced neuronal viability (74), and expression of factors that influence dendritic or axonal elongation and synaptogenesis. (75) Overall, these are neuroprotective functions that can minimize the interruption of neuron-to-neuron communication that can cause both cognitive and affective dysfunctioning. (76)

When neurons are damaged, there is an increase in production of aromatase, an enzyme responsible for the conversion of androgens to estrogens. (77) The importance here is that under normal conditions, aromatase is restrictively produced in select regions of the brain. It is only after neurotrauma that there is induction of aromatase expression by reactive glia (astrocytes) in the hippocampus and in other brain areas. The regional increase in the formation of estradiol leads to the many beneficial effects already acknowledged. (78)

Estradiol has been found to significantly interact with the dopaminergic, serotonergic, and glutamatergic systems, giving it properties similar to those of atypical antipsychotic medications. (79[1]) Studies on schizophrenia show that the drop in estrogen levels from the follicular phase to the luteal phase can cause an exacerbation in symptoms. (80) This finding suggests that the initiation of cyclical hormone fluxes in women may serve as a protective function against the development of adolescent psychosis. This possibility is reinforced by the observation that, whereas men exhibit one main peak of schizophrenia onset in their late teens and early twenties, women show an additional onset peak at age 40 to 45 years, which is a time when estrogen levels are falling. (81)

Women are more vulnerable than men to develop anxiety or depression disorders (i.e., social anxiety, phobias, post-traumatic stress disorder, and general anxiety disorder). Changes in endogenous E2 levels may increase a women's susceptibility to anxiety and depression disorders, such as premenstrual dysphoric disorder and postpartum depression, which typically occurs concurrent with changes in endogenous E2 levels. (82)

The increased expression of aromatase in injured brain areas (83) suggests that this enzyme may be involved in the protection of nervous tissue by increasing local estrogen levels. Estrogen formed by astrocytes may be released as a trophic factor for damaged neurons, and be involved in the compensatory restructuring of injured brain tissue. Thus, estrogen released by astroglia may affect synaptic function, selective regeneration of neuronal processes, and local cerebral blood flow, which contributes to facilitation of neuronal recovery and reduction of neuronal death. (84)

Pregnenolone and TBI

Two powerful neurosteroids are pregnenolone and progesterone. Pregnenolone is the main precursor of various steroid hormones, including progesterone, and is referred to as the "mother of all hormones." Pregnenolone occurs as unconjugated steroid, and its fatty acid or sulfate esters. The CNS effects of pregnenolone and pregnenolone sulfate include: modulation of GABA-$_A$ receptors and effects on seizure susceptibility, anxiety, depression, and memory processes with some of these processes mediated through the hippocampus. (85) Pregnenolone sulfate is the source, and thereby the starting point for subsequent steroid synthesis pathways, and also an activating ion channel ligand. (86[1])

In a study by Morley (87), pregnenolone sulfate was effective over a wide-dose range. Alone or in conjunction with other treatments, pregnenolone might be more effective in treatment of memory deficits than substances having narrower therapeutic windows. Progesterone also affects a wide range of activities, including cognition and anxiety, with some of the effects being mediated through the hippocampus. (88)

The beneficial use of pregnenolone as a supplement is in its ability to provide substrate for progesterone and cortisol. In patients with adrenal fatigue, we have been able to increase the levels of cortisol within 30 days with the use of a combination of pregnenolone and DHEA — two important prohormones involved in the Pregnenolone Steal Syndrome (PSS). (89) Once the levels of these hormones are returned to normal, the patient has an improvement in memory, cognition, mood, and alertness.

Steroidogenesis Chart (Table 7.1)

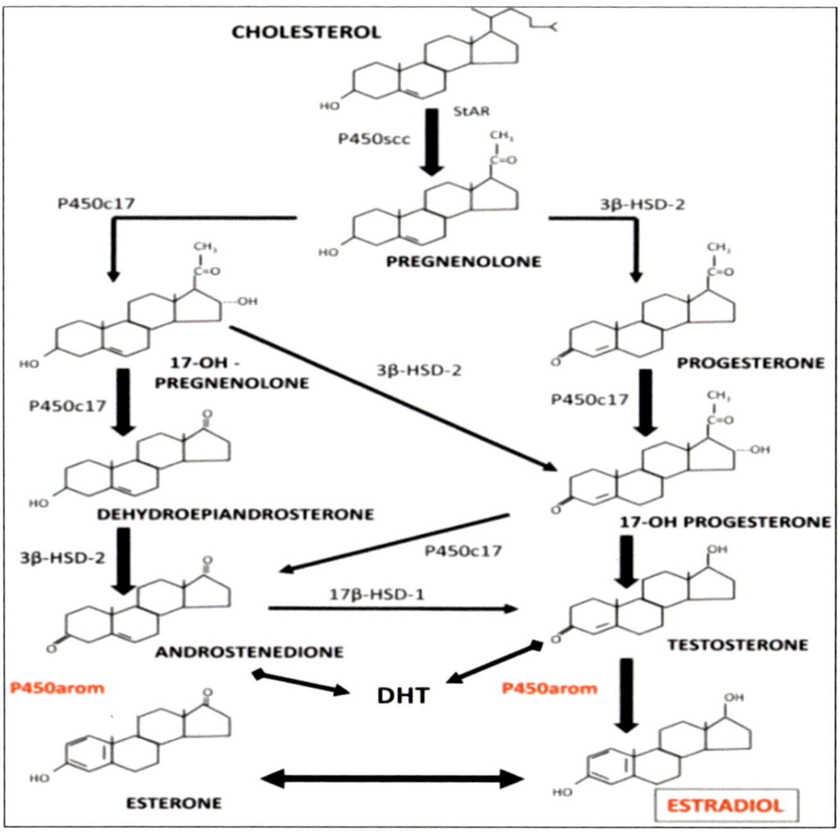

Progesterone and TBI

Progesterone (P4) is one of the two major active metabolites from pregnenolone (DHEA being the other). It is also an important neurosteroid being produced in the brain by Purkinje neurons. The importance of progesterone goes far beyond its participation in the menstrual cycle of women, and accounts for the protective edge that females possess in times of neurological challenge from TBI and vascular events. The genomic and non-genomic mechanisms behind progesterone's central nervous system effects are still being elucidated.

What we are seeing is that progesterone limits tissue damage and improves functional outcome after: blunt traumatic brain injury (TBI), stroke, spinal cord injury, diabetic neuropathies, and other types of acute neuro-injury. Progesterone appears to: protect or rebuild the blood-brain barrier (BBB), reduce cerebral edema, down-regulate the inflammatory cascade, and decrease apoptosis. (90*)

Progesterone regulation of mitosis of neural progenitors in the brain has a complex profile: A high level of Estradiol (E2) enhances hippocampal cell proliferation, whereas exposure to P4 resulted in blockade of the E2-induced enhancement of cell proliferation. In contrast to P4 regulation of E2-induced neurogenesis in vivo, P4 alone enhances cell proliferation in vitro. More recent results indicate that P4 induced a dose dependent significant increase in neural progenitor cells proliferation. The time course of P4-induced proliferation generated two important outcomes: First, P4-induced DNA synthesis occurred rapidly within the first one to four hours of P4 exposure, and second, it appears that P4-induced DNA synthesis does not persist beyond six hours — and that by eight hours, P4 no longer induces DNA synthesis. These data suggest that P4 is not driving a state of uncontrolled proliferation, but one that is limited. Lastly, a steroid specificity analysis indicated that P4 and its metabolite (allopregnanolone) were both proliferative agents. (91*)

The ProTECT (Progesterone for Traumatic Brain Injury: Experimental Clinical Treatment) study that is referenced throughout this text is notable because it was the first human study to look at the potential neuroprotective abilities of progesterone. The ProTECT study by, led by David Wright, was a phase II, randomized, double-blind, placebo-controlled trial conducted at a Level I trauma center. One hundred adult trauma patients who arrived within eleven hours of injury with a post-resuscitation Glasgow Coma Scale score of four to twelve were enrolled.

Subjects were randomized on a 4:1 basis to receive either intravenous progesterone or placebo. Neurologic outcome was assessed 30 days post-injury using the Glasgow Outcome Scale-Extended. Mortality in the progesterone group was reduced by approximately 50 percent as compared to the control group. Unfortunately, there was little comparative improvement in neurological functioning between the groups. In the patients noted as moderate TBI, their improvement was significant in terms of neurological functioning. (92)

In an animal model of traumatic brain injury, Deborah A. Shear (93) found that a single injection of progesterone can attenuate cerebral edema when administered during the first 24 hours after traumatic brain injury (TBI), but this regimen may not always produce functional benefits. In addition to its antiedemic effects, there is evidence that progesterone reduces both oxidative stress, due to lipid peroxidation, and excitotoxicity, by up-regulating ɣ-aminobuteric acid (GABA) and inhibiting glutamate release. (94)

Allopregnanolone (ALLO*) is a progesterone-derived neurosteroid with potent anxiolytic properties (95[1]) that acts as a positive allosteric modulator at the $GABA_A$ receptor. Allopregnanolone is a neurosteroid also produced peripherally in the ovaries and adrenal glands. In tissue culture, it acts on de novo in neurons and glia, in addition to synthesis in $GABA_A$ receptors with 20-fold higher potency than benzodiazepines and barbiturates, and modulates a broader range of $GABA_A$ receptors than either of these compounds. Due to its pronounced anxiolytic-like actions in rodent models and $GABA_A$ receptor activity, allopregnanolone shows promise as a mechanism for anxiolysis in psychiatric disorders. (96)

Thyroid Hormones and TBI

During the last 30 years, a plethora of scientific articles have appeared addressing the relationships between psychiatric disease and thyroid hormones. (97) These studies acknowledge the presence of changes in the hypothalamo–pituitary–thyroid (HPT) axis in patients with depression, but also in patients with other psychiatric diseases. The Millennium-TBI continues to see thyroid stimulating hormone (TSH) as the primary test used to determine the presence of a healthy thyroid, whilst a more robust and thorough evaluation consisting of fT4, fT3, and rT3 (review Chapter 6) is ignored.

The serum T4, both total and non-protein-bound (free), are consistently found as normal to increased in groups of depressed patients with approximately 25 percent of the patients having levels above the reference range. (98) These findings might be explained by the degree in severity of depression amongst the patients studied. This might be explained by an elevation in cortisol due to the frequent states of starvation, and thus may present changes in the HPT-axis similar to those seen in patients with non-thyroidal somatic illness with elevated serum T4 and rT3, and a reduced serum T3. One to four percent of patients with affective disorders are found to have overt hypothyroidism, while subclinical hypothyroidism occurs in four to 40 percent of these patients. (99)

Thyroid hormone receptors are widely distributed in the brain with highest concentrations in cerebral cortex, hippocampus, amygdala, choroid plexus, and olfactory bulb. The limbic structures, where thyroid hormone receptors are prevalent, have repeatedly been shown to be implicated in the pathogenesis of mood disorders. (100)

Thyroid hormones appear to have genomic, non-genomic, and structural influence in the mammalian brain. Genomic actions of T3 are mediated through the control and usually the increase of gene expression. Genes that are regulated by thyroid hormones are known to encode for proteins such as: myelin, neurotrophins, and proteins that are involved in intracellular signaling pathways. Non-genomic actions of thyroid hormones have been described in the brain and peripheral tissues. After binding to cytoplasmic thyroid hormone receptors, T3 appears to be able to rapidly activate the phosphatidylinositol-3-kinase protein pathway, and thereby achieves vasodilatory and neuroprotective effects. (101)

An important consideration in the recognition of thyroid related affective disorders, especially depression, is the change from pre-operative to post-operative levels of T3 and rT3. Considered to be precipitated by the increasing levels of cortisol during bodily stress (surgery), the levels of T3 decrease with an increase in the level of rT3. The normalization of these levels has been documented to take upwards of a year or more, and is related to the overall duration of the precipitating surgery. (102)

Finally, a heated debate exists in the medical literature assessing the benefits of a combination replacement therapy with both T4 and T3, as opposed to continuing with the standard monotherapy with T4. In a 1999 NEJM (103) article by Robertas Bunivicus, M.D., PhD, and others, "Patients with hypothyroidism, partial substitution of triiodothyronine for thyroxine may improve mood and neuropsychological function." This finding suggests a specific effect of the triiodothyronine normally secreted by the thyroid gland. The Millennium has used combination therapy for more than 20 years due to patients' perceived improvement in cognition and mental energy.

Desiccated Thyroid Extract (DTE) (104) was studied in patients on L-T4 therapy, which according to the authors, "Did not result in a significant improvement in quality of life; however, DTE caused modest weight loss and nearly half (48.6 percent) of the study patients expressed preference for DTE over L-T4." The preference was based upon an enhanced sense of well-being, cognition, and functionality. That is a significant improvement in quality of life!

DHEA and TBI

DHEA and DHEA-s have been found to influence the cerebral functioning in a number of ways. The structural neurological benefits of DHEA-s are in its ability to stimulate oligodendrocytes into making myelin, while DHEA appears to have a significant effect on the physical and mental well-being of 40 to 70 year-old individuals who were previously deficient, according to S.S. Yen. (105)

In the first randomized, controlled trial of DHEA in depression, Wolkowitz reported the beneficial effects of DHEA in a parallel-design study of 22 patients with major depression; however, only three of the subjects who received DHEA were not simultaneously receiving antidepressants. Nonetheless, the study reported a 50 percent reduction in depressive symptoms as per the Hamilton Depression Rating Scale (HDRS). (106)

A recent study by Peter Schmidt looked at the benefits of DHEA in midlife-onset minor and major depression in men and women aged 45 to 65 years. Using the HDRS after six weeks of administering DHEA (90mg/day for three weeks, followed by 450mg/day for three weeks) there was an associated improvement in the depression scale results by 50 percent or greater. Additionally, there was an improvement in Derogatis Interview for Sexual Functioning. Of note here is that the degree of benefit from DHEA administration on mood was directly correlated with the rise in DHEA-s. (107) Therefore, remember to include it in lab testing.

Cortisol

The Corticosteroids after Significant Head Injury (CRASH) trial, with more than 10,000 subjects in 40 countries, was halted because the treatment group had a significantly higher mortality rate than the control group. (108)

The question here is whether cortisol causes depression, or if the rise of cortisol is the response to depression and the stress that might have contributed to the depressive state. An answer to this was offered in 2009 by Dr. Clare (109), where the ratio of cortisol to DHEA (C/D) was assessed. In those patients with active depression, there was a high C/D ratio, which improved when patients were treated and their level of depression decreased.

Anxiety Disorders and TBI

Anxiety disorders are quite common after TBI to the extent that approximately 30 percent of injured patients have clinically significant anxiety. (110) Anxiety can have aspects of apprehension, uneasiness, or dread that occur in anticipation of either internal or external threats, which are perceived as unpredictable or uncontrollable. There are four subcategories of anxiety listed in the DSM-IV-TR that include: panic disorder (PD), obsessive-compulsive disorder (OCD), post-traumatic stress disorder (PTSD) and generalized anxiety disorder (GAD). (111*, 112)

TBI patients often experience generalized "free-floating" anxiety associated with persistent worry, tension, and fearfulness. (113) Increased activity of the aminergic system and decreased activity of the GABA inhibitory network is the proposed mechanism for the clinical manifestation of anxiety. (114) Right-hemispheric lesions are more often associated with anxiety disorder than left-sided lesions. (115)

Panic Disorder

Neuroanatomically speaking, the brain stem, limbic system, and prefrontal cortex have been implicated in the etiology of panic attacks (disorder). (116) Panic attacks are defined as discrete periods of intense fear, which develop abruptly and reach a peak within ten minutes with the presence of at least four of the following 13 symptoms: palpitations, sweating, trembling, shortness of breath, the sensation of choking, chest pain, abdominal discomfort, dizziness, de-realization, chills, paresthesia ,and fear of loss of control or death. (117[1]*)

Obsessive-Compulsive Disorder

OCD is characterized by recurrent obsessions or compulsions that are excessive or unreasonable. Obsessions manifest as persistent impulses, thoughts, or images that are intrusive, inappropriate, and time-consuming — while compulsions are repetitive behaviors (checking, ordering) or mental acts (praying, counting) that the patient feels driven to perform in order to reduce the distress of the obsession. Two recent epidemiologic studies have reported rates of OCD from as low as 4.7 percent to as high as 14 percent in patients who had sustained TBI. (118) Anatomically, the etiology of OCD has been linked to dysfunction of the orbital frontal cortex and subcortical circuits. (119, 120)

Post-Traumatic Stress Disorder

Post-traumatic stress disorder (PTSD) in relation to traumatic brain injury is an entity about which there has been much debate, since one of the essential criteria is that the patient who has been exposed to a threatening event must display re-experiencing symptoms: intrusive memories or distress when reminded about the particular trauma, recurrent dreams of the event, or the feeling that the trauma is recurring. (121) Additional diagnostic criteria for PTSD include: dissociative symptoms (de-realization, depersonalization and dissociative amnesia), marked avoidance of thoughts, feelings or reminders of the trauma, as well as marked arousal, which can be observed as insomnia, irritability, poor concentration, hypervigilance, or a heightened startle response. (122)

As I shared on the Joe Rogan Experience # 574 (123), PTSD in the pure sense, is a psychological event where the individual re-experiences the threatening event, provoking an array of symptoms as opposed to the physical trauma to the brain that occurs in a TBI. It is my belief that the two can co-exist, and that the injuries sustained by the TBI predisposed the individual to the susceptibility of the symptomatic complex associated with PTSD. We know that disruption of neurosteroids predispose the individual to mood disorders (124) by virtue of uncoupling of controlled neurological communication between the different emotional centers in the brain. (125)

Given that many TBI patients do not recall the event due to post-traumatic amnesia, which is a short interval after injury where the capacity to store and retrieve new information is lacking, one can argue that theoretically PTSD cannot occur in these patients. A study by Warden and colleagues reviewed 47 active-duty service members who had sustained moderate TBI with amnesia for the event. Using strict PTSD criteria, none of these patients qualified for the diagnosis, since no patient reported re-experiencing phenomena. However, when that part of the criteria was eliminated, then six patients (12.7 percent) received a diagnosis of PTSD. (126)

In a recent report of 100 patients involved in traffic accidents who sustained head injury with definite loss of consciousness, 48 percent reported PTSD at three months after the incident, and 33 percent suffered with this disorder one year later. (127) Some mechanisms to explain PTSD when there is a lack of recall of the traumatic event itself include: (a) recall of other distressing experiences associated with the event, which occurred either before or after the period of amnesia that then serves as the "trauma," (b) traumatic experiences may be processed by the limbic area of the brain at an implicit level outside awareness, and (c) learning of the traumatic event as told by others helps the patient to reconstruct the memory. (128[1])

Generalized Anxiety Disorder

A recently published epidemiologic study reported the rate of general anxiety disorder (GAD) in patients after TBI to be 1.7 percent (129), but this is in contrast to other research which has noted rates in the range of eight to 24 percent. This syndrome is marked by excessive worry and anxiety about a number of issues that occur almost daily for at least six months.

The patient is unable to control the worry, and experiences at least three of the six somatic symptoms, which include: restlessness, being easily fatigued, diminished concentration, irritability, muscle tension, or sleep disturbance. The symptoms of anxiety experienced by patients with TBI are usually attributed to the loss that patients feel in terms of their independence, as well as the relation to their prior level of high functioning. (130)

Anxiety and TBI — It Really Is "All In the Head"

The clinical case which follows is from Drs. Marc A. Cooper and Elspeth C. Ritchie of Washington, D.C., from the "To the Editor" section of American Journal of Psychiatry in Nov ember 2000. (131)

We report the case of a patient with previously undiagnosed hypogonadism whose anxiety symptoms improved after he received testosterone injections. Mr. A, a 34-year-old man, was diagnosed with generalized anxiety disorder (GAD). His symptoms included mental exhaustion, irritability, insomnia, poor concentration, and decreased libido. He unsuccessfully tried relaxation techniques and biofeedback before beginning treatment with buspirone, 30mg/day. After noticing improvement, he discontinued the medication after two months, but resumed taking it six months later, when his anxiety returned.

A review of his medical record indicated that he had undergone a right orchiectomy for an undescended testicle. Blood samples were taken for laboratory analysis: total testosterone was 185ng/dl (normal = 241 to 827), free testosterone was 8.9pg/ ml (normal = 18 to 39), LH was 18.7mIU/ml (normal = two to twelve) and FSH was 31.4mIU/ml (normal = one to eight).

The results of a physical examination and laboratory tests were within normal limits. Mr. A tapered his buspirone treatment and elected not to begin treatment with paroxetine. Mr. A was referred to an endocrinologist, who ruled out occult malignancy and prescribed testosterone enanthate, 200mg intramuscular, every two weeks. He reported resolution of his anxiety symptoms after one month. His concentration and libido increased, and he reported better orgasms. He tried to decrease the frequency of his injections, but remained on the bimonthly schedule after feeling his anxiety symptoms returning. He has been on the regimen for more than 18 months and has experienced no side effects.

Had this patient been on a short and intermediate acting combination of testosterones (propionate and cypionate), his response would have been more likely experienced within a few days to a week, based upon our experience at Millennium Health. The large single dose of enanthate is associated with elevation of estrogen and DHT, necessitating the use of an estrogen (anastrozole) and a DHT blocker (finasteride or durastride) since large doses of any testosterone are prone to producing these active metabolites of testosterone. The risk of both these forms of blockers have been discussed in detail in other portions of this book (Chapter 9), but they can block growth hormone production and release from the pituitary and stop the conversion in the brain of testosterone to DHT, which is a very important antidepressant and libido supporting hormone.

The literature supports a connection between hypogonadism and depression, as evidenced by untreated hypogonadal men scoring significantly higher in ratings of depression, anger, fatigue, and confusion than infertile and normal comparison men, and by the improvement of depressive symptoms after the administration of testosterone to hypogonadal men with depression refractory to selective serotonin reuptake inhibitors. Another study has shown that testosterone replacement therapy decreases anger, nervousness, and irritability in hypogonadal men. The temporal connection between the improvement of Mr. A's anxiety symptoms and replacement testosterone suggests an association between anxiety and hypogonadism. Based on this case report, it was suggested to include anxiety in the list of psychiatric manifestations of hypogonadism that improve with testosterone replacement therapy.

Agitation

Agitation after TBI is a frequently observed behavioral problem, and is a challenge to care providers. Nearly, one-third of the TBI patients exhibit agitation during the subacute stage of rehabilitation and in the post-traumatic amnesia (PTA) stage of recovery. (139)

The incidence of agitation has been reported to be from 35 to 96 percent (140) in the acute recovery period after TBI, and from 31 to 71 percent in patients who were followed one to 15 years after sustaining TBI. (141) A more current study of 158 subjects in an acute-care rehabilitation setting (most of whom had severe TBI) demonstrated that approximately 50 percent of these patients had post-traumatic agitation as measured by the ABS. This study noted that there were no statistically significant differences as regarding to gender in terms of the frequency, duration, or presentation and extent of the post-TBI agitation. (142)

Also, agitation has been a source of debate in the field due to the lack of agreement about a standardized clinical definition — the closest being personality change secondary to TBI (aggressive type), a proposal has been made to create a new diagnostic label (that of aggression), which could be subdivided into acute and chronic types. The former would be defined as lasting from a few weeks up to a few months and be essentially synonymous with delirium, while the latter would refer to the persistence of inappropriate verbal or physical behaviors beyond the two month time frame. From the physiatrist literature, an interdisciplinary definition has been suggested that would incorporate the elements of delirium, post-traumatic amnesia, and excesses of behavior that include some combination of aggression (verbal or physical), akinthesia, disinhibition, and emotional lability. (143)

In another recent study by Tateno and colleagues in 2003, it was found that 33.7 percent of 89 patients demonstrated significant aggressive behavior when measured with the Overt Agitation Severity Scale (OAS) (144) six months after their injury. The enormity of this problem is emphasized in a study by Bogner and colleagues, who reported that the presence of agitation in TBI patients receiving treatment in an acute rehabilitation center was predictive of a longer length of stay and a decrease in functional independence from a cognitive standpoint at discharge. (145)

Anatomically, agitation may be explained by damage to a number of different brain areas such as the hypothalamus, amygdala, medial temporal lobe, or orbito-frontal cortex — as these regions and their connections are involved in the regulation of emotion. (146)

Acute confusional state and acute agitated delirium are common syndromes after infarction of the right middle cerebral artery. Infarction in this territory, therefore, has an important clinical implication as a cause of these syndromes. Acute confusional state is a disorder in which cognitive and integrative functions become defective, reflecting disturbance of global attention, and is closely correlated with other right hemispheric global and directed attentional disorders. It is linked to damage to the right frontostriatal region and is associated with lesion volume. (147)

Aggressive Behavior

Aggression is a common neuropsychiatric sequela of traumatic brain injury (TBI), one which interferes with rehabilitation efforts, disrupts social support networks, and compromises optimal recovery. Aggressive behavior raises safety concerns, potentially placing patients and care providers in harm's way, although a study by Vani Rao in 2010 found that physical aggression to others is an uncommon event at three months post-TBI. (148) Beyond this period, aggression may be directed outwardly, manifesting as assaultive behavior, or directed inwardly, resulting in suicidal behavior. (149) Prior studies have shown that post-TBI aggression is correlated with depression, frontal lobe lesions, poor pre-TBI psychosocial functioning, and a history of alcohol and substance abuse. (150)

Aggression after traumatic brain injury is common, but not well defined. Sixty-seven participants with first-time TBI were seen within three months of injury and evaluated for aggression. The prevalence of aggression was found to be 28.4 percent, and to be predominantly verbal aggression. Post-TBI aggression was associated with new-onset major depression, poorer social functioning, and increased dependency on activities of daily living, but not with a history of substance abuse or adult/childhood behavioral problems. Implications of the study include early screening for aggression, evaluation for depression, and consideration of psychosocial support in aggressive patients. (151)

As published in The Journal of Neuropsychiatry and Clinical Neurosciences in 2003, Dr. Amane Tateno studied 89 consecutive patients with closed head injuries that were admitted to the University of Iowa Hospitals and Clinics. A diagnosis of TBI was substantiated by history of post-traumatic amnesia that lasted at least 30 minutes after the traumatic event. Dr. Tateno determined that in the first six months after an injury, aggressive behavior was found in 33.7 percent of TBI patients, while only 11.5 percent of patients without TBI exhibited aggressive behavior. (152)

The association of violent and impulsive behavior with abnormalities of the serotonergic system is one of the findings most consistently replicated in neuropsychiatric research. Furthermore, a specific subtype of major depressive disorder characterized by aggressive behavior and anger attacks has been reported to be associated with a dysfunctional serotonergic system.

Aggressive behaviors have also been related to the presence of brain lesions in specific locations — such as the hypothalamus, paralimbic areas of the temporal lobe, and the prefrontal cortex. On the other hand, an association between major depression and left prefrontal lesions during the early recovery period from TBI has been previously reported, making it conceivable that frontal lobe damage, including lesions of the ascending serotonergic pathways, contribute to the pathophysiology of both depression and aggressive behavior. (153)

Arousal and Attention

Impaired attention is a problem frequently observed in patients who have suffered traumatic brain injury. Its impact upon rehabilitation efforts is significant, since other cognitive processes such as learning, short- and long- term memory, problem-solving, and language skills are dependent upon one's ability to focus on various inputs. Often after TBI, the basic attention abilities recover, but studies performed years later reveal that TBI patients still struggle with cognitively challenging tasks, making it difficult for advancement and higher educational goals. (154)

Arousal and attention appear to be seamlessly related systems that are complex and widely distributed through the brain, and involve the ascending reticular formation of the brain stem (155*), which extends from the medulla to the midbrain (the hypothalamus, thalamus, basal forebrain, limbic system, anterior cingulate and parietal, temporal, and prefrontal cortical areas). Damage to any of these regions via mechanical injury or diffuse axonal impairment can disrupt the various neurotransmitter pathways (noradrenergic, dopaminergic, and cholinergic), which play key roles in the modulation of arousal and attention. (156) Evidence for the latter neurotransmitter's role in this cognitive domain was highlighted in a recent study of TBI patients whose neuropsychological profile demonstrated decreases in sustained attention and reaction times, while the morphometric analysis of their brain imaging revealed reduced gray matter density in the regions of all the major cholinergic pathways. (157*)

When a patient sustains TBI, the physiologic state known as arousal, which is defined by the level of wakefulness and the intensity of stimulation needed to elicit a meaningful response by the individual, can be altered by varying degrees. Whereas in normal consciousness, the person is fully awake and able to respond cognitively and emotionally to both internal needs, as well as to external stimuli, the drowsy patient sustains wakefulness only with the application of some form of external stimuli. These patients are often inattentive, glary-eyed, spaced, and confused.

Selective loss of the hypocretin-producing neurons causes sleepiness and cataplexy in over 90 percent of patients with narcolepsy. Injury to the hypothalamus is common in patients with TBI, but its clinical impact remains unclear. It was recently found that TBI patients have a marked reduction in cerebral spinal fluid (CSF) hypocretin-1 levels in the first days after injury. Even after six months of recovery, many TBI patients with excessive daytime sleepiness (EDS) have persistently low hypocretin-1 levels. Thus, it was hypothesized that post-traumatic sleepiness is caused, at least in part, by injury to the wake-promoting hypocretin neurons. (158*)

Coma and obtundation are common during the acute period post-TBI, but even after six months of recovery, 43 percent of patients continue to have symptoms of sleep disorders. The recent findings suggest a key role for the neuropeptides hypocretin-1 and -2 (orexin-A and -B). Hypocretins are made by a small cluster of neurons in the lateral hypothalamus that play an essential role in promoting wakefulness. (159) This is the foundation for the use of medication such as modafinil, dextroamphetamine, methamphetamine, and methylphenidate. Frequently, the daytime fatigue is really caused by the side effects of over-medication of the patient with pain medication and psychotropic drugs.

Sexual Dysfunction

Neuroanatomically, decreased libido has been related to lesions of the medial orbital gyrus of the frontal lobe, hippocampus, anterior thalamus, and hypothalamus. Specifically, damage to the hypothalamus can lead to a diminished release of GnRH, thereby decreasing LH release from the pituitary and ultimately failure of the testicular Leydig cells from producing testosterone. (160) Additionally, and as support for performing a comprehensive laboratory work up, elevation in prolactin secondary to damage to hypothalamic prolactin inhibiting factor neurons (also dopamine), can cause down-regulation of LH release leading loss of optimal testosterone production.

After TBI, a patient's sexuality can be altered in a variety of ways, and he or she can experience difficulties not only with libido and the physical sexual act, but also develop problems with self-esteem and relationship skills. In TBI patients, the rate of sexual dysfunction has been reported to be in the range of four to 71 percent. (161)

Individuals after TBI report frequent physiological, physical, and body image difficulties, which negatively impact sexual activity and interest. For men, post TBI predictors of sexual difficulties included: age at interview, age at injury, and having milder injuries — however, depression was the most sensitive predictor of sexual dysfunctions. For women post TBI, predictors of their sexual difficulties included age at injury and having milder injuries; however, depression and an endocrine disorder combined were the most sensitive predictors of their sexual dysfunction. (162)

What you have just read above has been the clinical dogma by the psychiatric world. Looking critically at the age-related development of sexual dysfunction in elderly males, you see the lack of sexual confidence, loss of libido, lack of full erection, weak ejaculation, pre-mature ejaculation, and loss of assertiveness all layered on a platform of dysthymia or depression. When taking a (sexuality) history in a young male who has sustained a traumatic brain injury, their complaints parallel the elderly male's complaints (163[L]) — not due to depression, but due to the loss of hormones such as testosterone, estrogen, hypocretin (orexin), and dopamine.

There is no doubt that in both genders, replenishment of the free testosterone levels helps to improve this condition in more than 80 percent of the cases. The question is which of these came first — sexual dysfunction, depression, or testosterone deficiency?

Estrogen Dominance Syndrome

I have added this section on EDS so that we don't miss it as an important causative factor for many psychological maladies that interrupt the potential of quality of life for many females. In this condition, regardless of TBI, a woman can have a disproportionate elevation in estrogens, or a naturally low level of progesterone generating a hormonal environment where the estrogen-progesterone ratio is estrogen dominant. Dr. John Lee (164) started promoting this concept of estrogen dominance decades ago, although it fell onto deaf ears. Today, many of those to whom I have presented the estrogen-dominance lecture quickly realize that there is a need to address this ratio in order to maximize a woman's health.

Estrogen Dominance symptoms and conditions	
Acceleration of the aging process	Breast cancer Breast tenderness
Allergies	Fibrocystic breasts
Cervical dysplasia	Endometrial (uterine) cancer
Cold hands and feet as a symptom of thyroid dysfunction	Decreased sex drive
Depression, anxiety, agitation	Early onset of menstruation
Dry eyes	Copper excess
Autoimmune disorders; lupus erythematosus, thyroiditis, Sjogren's disease.	Fat gain, especially around the abdomen, hips and thighs

Table 7.2: Estrogen dominance is a frequently undiagnosed condition that can be simply corrected by performing adequate labs and replenishing progesterone.

Looking at the lists of symptoms associated with EDS, it is no wonder that once this process begins, and there is no enjoyment of life. Many of these women suffer from additional issues associated with sleep-deprivation syndrome, as a sequela to EDS. Elevation in estrogens does not allow for the beneficial effects of progesterone, its sulfated form, or any of its important metabolites like allopregnanolone (ALLO). As discussed above, ALLO is an important neurosteroid that has influence over many neuropsychopharmacological processes that lead to calmness and clarity. Therefore, it is important to assess the EP ratio in every woman pretreatment and thereafter, while on treatment.

In women who present to your practice with headaches (migraines or not) associated with PMS and peri- or post-menopausal symptoms, it is imperative that you assess estradiol (E2), estrone (E1), and progesterone (P) to determine if there is an issue of estrogen dominance. This is based upon the equation (E1+E2)/P with a quotient less than 250 being most favorable. In the event that the resulting quotient is greater than 250, progesterone therapy will help immensely (Chapter 9).

Conclusion

Not only are the neuropsychiatric complications of TBI numerous and complex, but the standard approach to the treatment of neurobehavioral symptoms associated with post-traumatic brain injury are non-functional. It does not work because we have, in our ignorance, decided to substitute an array of synthetic medication for the missing biochemistry that is encumbered by neurotrauma. Where is the Celexa® or Lamictal® gland in our bodies? Isn't it more logical that if we are deficient in hormones [neurosteroid (NS) and neuroactive steroid (NAS)] that have been shown to be associated with precipitating psychobehavioral dysfunctioning, that these should be replaced first, before a symptom-masking drug is tried? You think (AV)?

Obviously, and in light of the overwhelming amount of literature addressing both the clinical application and research, the impact of hormonal deficiencies and replenishment on the emotional and cognitive status of the individual are being ignored. The articles cited here are but the proverbial tip of the iceberg in terms of how much supporting documentation shows that each hormone has an impact on the quality of one's neuropsychology.

It is therefore the position taken, that TBI is associated with the development of some degree and extent of hormonal deficiencies (relative or absolute), and that these deficiencies are what precipitate the bio-hormonal environment associated with alterations in neurobehavior.

A great gap that exists, and hence the main hindrance in a more successful treatment protocol for our veterans as well as civilians with neurotrauma, is the conceptual terminology of post-concussion stress syndrome (PTSD) and traumatic brain injury (TBI). PTSD is a near 100 percent psychoneurobiological condition that is devoid of a physical component found to exist in nearly 100 percent of the traumatic brain injury patients. Yes, these two can appear to overlap, but the question that needs to be answered is: By treating the patient's underlying hormonal disruption with appropriate replenishment and not masking drugs, does the patient improve? If the patient improves with application of both NS and NAS, then there is no need for other forms of medication. If there are residual conditions that mandate protecting the patient from harm, then it makes sense to use them cautiously, and with the goal of tapering them off in the near future.

I was reading an article on PTSD where the author offered an example of a woman involved in a MVA some 18 months prior to her visiting with him due to classical PTSD symptoms (reliving the event which is triggered by entering a car). He also described the slow progression of the patient with issues of mood, attention, concentration, and sleep disturbance. He indicated that the patient was the driver in the car, and that she sustained minor injuries without focal involvement of her head. This is not PTSD —

it is a primary TBI with a secondary co-morbid component that we will call PTSD. It is my belief that the TBI-precipitated cerebral dysfunctioning of the NS/NAS creates the appearance of PTSD. Fix that hormonal milieu and then take another look!

In conclusion, it stands to reason that the most rational approach to these individuals would be to assess their hormonal status, and then to appropriately replenish those deficient or insufficient to physiologically optimal levels to obtain an optimal response. Anything less, would fail to treat.

Chapter 8: Supplementation in TBI

"We will continue to do all we can to protect the public health against these dietary supplements that have been found to cause serious illness and injury."

— Andrew von Eschenbach, former FDA director, 2005 to 2009

Introduction

As you have learned in previous chapters, traumatic brain injury has an overt phase of damage (primary) that might be represented histologically by ''focal'' anatomical lesions; such as laceration, contusion, intracranial hemorrhage (1), diffuse axonal injury (2), and cavitation (3) — all of which produce cerebral edema. (4) The secondary damage (biochemical, delayed), which is produced by complex processes, is initiated at the moment of injury and with the death of the first brain cell — be it an astrocyte (5), neuron (6), microglia (7) or oligodendrocyte. (8) Additionally, the peripheral damage to the limbs, abdomen or thorax creates additional sources of inflammatory molecules (IL-6, specifically) that pass through a disrupted blood brain barrier (BBB) to cause additive damage and biochemical havoc. (9) All these processes are subversive to the ability of the brain to recover, generating that non-neuropermissive environment. The net effect is the onset of subclinical pathologies that can take minutes, hours, days, weeks, months or even years to appear. The "silent epidemic" or "stealth syndrome" does exist. (10)

In response to the typically short-lasting primary injury mechanism, there is a second wave of long-lasting pathological changes called the secondary injury mechanism. (11) These pathologies include metabolic changes (acidosis), neuroinflammation, axonal injury, vascular abnormalities, and neuronal and glial cell death. Metabolic changes include abnormal levels of oxygenation (increasing free radicals ROS), altered cell metabolism, disrupted energy production (mitochondrial damage), diminished systemic hormonal secretion, and an upregulation of inflammatory activity. (12)

Inflammation occurs in response to damaging stimuli, triggering the release and activation of cytokines and chemokines, and the activation and proliferation of microglia and astroglia in the central nervous system. (13, 14) Vascular abnormalities are marked by aberrations in the water content of the brain parenchyma, dysregulation of water channels, and a compromised blood-brain barrier (BBB). These primary and secondary injury processes may lead to a range of neuropsychiatric symptoms, including various forms of memory and learning deficits, anxiety, and depression. (15[1])

The first stages of cerebral injury after TBI are characterized by direct tissue damage and impaired regulation of cerebral blood flow (CBF) and metabolism. This ''ischemia-like'' pattern leads to accumulation of lactic acid (16) due to anaerobic glycolysis (17), increased membrane permeability, and consecutive edema formation. The second stage of the pathophysiological cascade is characterized by terminal membrane depolarization along with excessive release of excitatory neurotransmitters, activation of NMDA, AMPA, and voltage-dependent Ca^{2+} and Na^{+}-channels. Ca^{2+} activates lipid peroxidases, proteases and phospholipases, which in turn increase the intracellular concentration of free radicals. (18) The end result is a damaged system (brain) being overwhelmed by mounting sources of free radicals that are being generated by expanding mechanisms of inflammation.

It has been proposed that neurons regulate their energy supply by releasing glutamate to be taken up by astrocytes, thereby turning on glycolysis. This process and the subsequent conversion of glutamate to glutamine are proposed to use glycolytically-derived ATP, thus producing lactate which is exported to neurons as a substrate for mitochondrial oxidative phosphorylation. Under anaerobic conditions, more and more glutamate is released to provide ATP for neuronal activities. Unfortunately, under these conditions the demand for energy rises and the potential for excitotoxicity grows, which can lead to further neurodegeneration and loss of function. (19)

Redox Terminology

Substances that have the ability to reduce other substances (cause them to gain electrons) are said to be reductive or reducing and are known as reducing agents, reductants, or reducers. (20) The reductant (reducing agent) transfers electrons to another substance, and is thus itself oxidized.

And, because it "donates" electrons, the reducing agent is also called an electron donor. (21) Electron donors can also form charge transfer complexes with electron acceptors. (22) Reduction is the *gain* of electrons or a *decrease* in oxidation state.

Substances that have the ability to oxidize other substances (cause them to lose electrons) are said to be oxidative or oxidizing and are known as oxidizing agents, oxidants, or oxidizers. (23) That is, the oxidant (oxidizing agent) removes electrons from another substance, and is thus itself reduced. And, because it "accepts" electrons, the oxidizing agent is also called an electron acceptor, hence the name. (24) Oxygen is the quintessential oxidizer. Oxidation is the loss of electrons or an increase in oxidation state. (Don't worry, I wrote this and I still can't remember which one is which.)

Addressing Oxidative Stress in TBI

The cell's energy supply is protected from conditions that damage mitochondria by an inducible transcriptional program of mitochondrial biogenesis, which operates in large part through redox signals involving the nitric oxide synthase and the heme oxygenase-1/CO systems. These redox events stimulate the coordinated activities of several multifunctional transcription factors and co-activators also involved in the elimination of defective mitochondria (Autophagy) and the expression of counter-inflammatory and antioxidant genes, such as IL-10 and SOD-2, as part of a unified damage-control network. (25*)

Free radical-induced oxidative damage reactions and membrane lipid peroxidation (LP) have clearly been shown to represent the secondary phase injury mechanisms in traumatic brain injury. (26) In addition to the disruption of the cell-membrane phospholipid architecture, as well as subcellular membranes (*organelles*), LP results in the formation of cytotoxic aldehyde-containing products that bind to cellular proteins impairing their normal functions. The use of specific antioxidant agents to prevent and remove the causes of oxidative cytotoxicity precipitated by TBI (non-permissive environment) will be a key factor for optimizing the potential for long-term recovery. A number of pharmaceutical and natural alternative agents have been recognized as providing protection and recovery from free radical damage.

Free radicals are highly reactive compounds which are mostly generated during cellular respiration and normal metabolism. Their possession of unpaired electrons in their outer shell causes them to be more reactive than their corresponding non-radicals. This is because they act as electron acceptors, and essentially "steal" electrons from other molecules and thereby modify their chemical structures — an action which is referred to as oxidation. (27)

Free radicals are liberated from a variety of sources, including inflammatory cells, dysfunctional mitochondria and excitotoxic mechanisms, which are stimulated by increased glutamate and aspartate concentrations. Superoxide radical is the most commonly occurring cellular free radical and it is produced when an oxygen molecule gains one electron from another compound.

There is a vast amount of evidence implicating oxygen-derived free radicals, as well as other high-energy oxidants, as playing mediatory roles in diverse pathological conditions. They have also been shown to be key contributors in the secondary events following brain injury; including the formation of the oxygen radical, superoxide anion, which is believed to be one of the final events of several metabolic pathways in the cascade that leads to delayed neuronal death after traumatic or ischemic brain injury. Cellular injury caused by reactive oxygen species (including free radicals, peroxides and oxygen ions), is believed to occur as a result of oxidation of poly-desaturated fatty acids in lipids, oxidation of amino acids in proteins, damage of the DNA, and inactivation of specific enzymes by oxidation of co-factors. (28)

Oxygen free radicals are produced continuously in tissues, and even though they are considered to be destructive agents, they can sometimes be useful. It is believed that they act as secondary messengers in intracellular signaling cascades, which are responsible for the induction and maintenance of the oncogenic phenotype of cancer cells. They may also function as anti-tumorigenic species.

Normally, a state of equilibrium exists between tissue oxidants and antioxidant activities. This balance can, however, be upset as a result of excessive free radical generation, depletion of endogenous antioxidants or failure to repair oxidative injury induced by reactive oxygen species. The resultant condition is referred to as oxidative stress (OS). Enhanced oxidative stress associated with increased production of free radicals has been implicated in the disruption of neuronal homeostasis induced by traumatic brain injury. (29[1])

Traumatic brain injury (TBI) leads to massive production of reactive oxygen species (ROS), which in turn mediate further damage via various cellular molecular pathways, including damage to cellular components like lipids, proteins and nucleic acids, with neuronal death occurring as a result of impairment of cellular calcium homeostasis, tissue acidosis and oxidative stress. OS is also thought to, at least in part, initiate or influence autophagy — a process whereby cellular components are digested by enzymes within the same cell. Experimental data indicate that the destructive oxidative events following TBI reach their peak within the first 24 hours of injury, and that the brain damage that occurs as a result of the impact can be the cause of death or irreversible permanent disabilities in affected patients. The degree of oxidative injury in clinical TBI is, however, not yet completely understood. (30)

Antioxidants are compounds whose actions include: inhibition of the formation of reactive oxygen species and binding of metal ions needed for catalysis of their generation, and scavenging of reactive oxygen species or their precursors. (31) They inhibit other oxidation reactions by being oxidized themselves. Endogenous antioxidant scavenger mechanisms help to defend cells against oxidative injury. Two major groups of these compounds are recognized as: antioxidant enzymes (such as superoxide dismutase [SOD], catalase and glutathione peroxidase), and low molecular weight antioxidants (LMWA). (32) The latter group contains directly acting agents (such as ascorbic acid, glutathione, lipoic acid, uric acid, α-Tocopherol, ubiquinol, and carotenoids) and indirectly acting antioxidants (e.g., chelating agents). The above mentioned low molecular weight antioxidants are also capable of chelating metal ions, thereby reducing their catalytic activity to form ROS and also scavenge them.

Lipid Peroxidation

Cellular membranes are composed of phosphatidylcholine (PC), phosphatidylethanolamine (PE), phosphatidylserine (PS) and phosphatidylinositol (PI), sphingomyelin (SM), ceramide and gangliosides, cholesterol and cholesterol esters, acylglycerols, and fatty acids. (33) The membrane's phospholipid bilayer provides a selectively permeable barrier while also being a platform that is essential for the proper functioning of membrane-bound proteins. "Cholesterol is one of the most important regulators of lipid organization as its structure allows it to fill interstitial spaces between hydrophobic fatty acid chains of phospholipids." The neutral lipids such as PC and SM reside on the outer layer, whereas PS, PE, and PI reside on the inner layer of the membrane. The distribution of cholesterol between the layers determines membrane fluidity and can alter the membrane function. (34)

In addition to their role as structural components of the cell membrane, phospholipids serve as precursors for various second messengers such as arachidonic acid (ArAc), docosahexaenoic acid (DHA), ceramide, 1,2-diacylglycerol, phosphatidic acid, and lyso-phosphatidic acid. Lipids comprise a large number of chemically distinct molecules arising from combinations of fatty acids with various backbone structures. Overall, mammalian cells may contain 1,000 to 2,000 lipid species. Lipid metabolism may be of particular importance for the CNS, as this organ has the highest concentration of lipids next to adipose tissue. (35)

Within a rising environment of oxidative stress there is production of ROS, NO, peroxyl, and nitryls along with blood byproducts such as heme. (36) These free radical generating agents all create damage to the cell membrane's composition of lipids, generating an increased concentration of end products of lipid peroxidation. However, it is likely that increased oxidative damage occurs in most human diseases and plays a significant pathological role in only some of them. Peroxidation appears to be important in atherosclerosis, and in worsening the initial tissue injury caused by ischemic or traumatic brain injury. Oxidative stress can damage many biological molecules such as proteins and DNA, and are often more significant targets of injury than are lipids.

Therefore, it is imperative, as a proactive approach to any individual with TBI, that these secondary reactive and indolent destructive processes be curtailed if not halted. This chapter will introduce you to a number of treatment options that are supported by evidence-based science to support their use. When to start their use will always be "now."

About Our Recommendations

TBI involves primary and secondary injury cascades that underlie delayed neuronal dysfunction and death. Oxidative stress is one of the most notorious secondary injury mechanisms at the foundation of global inflammation. A close relationship exists between levels of oxidative stress and the pathophysiology of TBI. However, other cascades, such as an increase in proinflammatory cytokines, also play important roles in the overall response to the trauma. Pharmacologic intervention, in order to be successful, requires a multifaceted approach. Naturally occurring flavonoids (37) are unique in possessing not only tremendous free radical scavenging properties, but also the ability to modulate cellular homeostasis leading to a reduction in inflammation and cell toxicity. (38)

The recommendations listed here are based upon stand-alone dosing where one product or supplement is used at a time. When more than one supplement is added to the regimen, consideration to the benefits of synergistic interactions needs to be considered. It is impossible to categorically state what the dosing is for any product that is combined with another or even with four or five other supplements. Therefore, if using a single component product, we start with it for about four weeks before adding another product or products. Some of the supplements we use do have multiple components, but we have used and monitored their effects for many years and are comfortable with the outcome and low side effects.

The new line of synergistic products under the brand name, *Perfect Protocol*, have been developed and tested in our offices, or are embellished forms of products from other longtime manufacturers of excellent products. A point of concern here is that there are so many supplements with notable "evidence-based" support that we tend to overload in excess in search of the Holy Grail. Don't do this. Work to systematically and methodically find the best combination of products for health and well-being.

Nutraceuticals for Oxidative Stress

Melatonin

N-Acetyl-5-methoxytryptamine (melatonin) is produced in the pineal gland and readily crosses the blood brain barrier (BBB) to enter neurons and glial cells. (39) It is a potent scavenger of peroxyl and hydroxyl radicals, shown to prevent both initiation and propagation of lipid peroxidation and stimulate brain glutathione peroxidase. (40) Melatonin acts as an antioxidant in both lipophilic and hydrophilic environments because of its solubility properties. Recently, it was shown that melatonin inhibits nitric oxide synthase (41), thus preventing the toxic effect obtained after its interaction with superoxide radicals. (42)

It was 2010, the exact month I don't remember, but I was in Mexico City getting ready to participate in a medical program sponsored by the Instituto Mexicano Del Seguro Social (IMSS). I was sitting in the front row when a healthy sized gentleman walked onto the stage and began his lecture on melatonin. During the 47.5 minutes of his presentation, I learned more about melatonin then I had ever known to even exist. That evening, while shooting back tequila shots at dinner, we had a chance to introduce ourselves. This was Dr. Russell J. Reiter of Texas and, in my estimation, one of three, if not the most, noted researchers on melatonin. He and his colleagues published a 25-page paper: Melatonin: A Multitasking Molecule (43*), which is by far my favorite of his recent works, and one you might want to read in its entirety. (The point here is you can still be professional and have fun too.)

Recommendation: We begin treatment with 0.5mg a night, increasing by 0.5mg each week until tolerance is achieved. At that point, we back down by 0.5mg looking for resolution of morning the morning symptoms. Optimal treat with melatonin should start as soon as possible, with the dosage being titrated from 0.5mg up to tolerance. Tolerance is reached when the patient complains of increased morning fogginess, lethargy, or headache.

L-Carnosine

Carnosine (beta-alanyl-L-histidine) is a naturally-occurring, pluripotent, homeostatic agent which is found with its family members — homocarnosine, and anserine — in both the muscles and brain of humans. Carnosine can chelate zinc ions, suppress amyloid-beta peptide toxicity, inhibit production of oxygen free radicals, scavenge hydroxyl radicals and reactive aldehydes, and suppresses protein glycation. (44)

Glycated protein accumulates in the cerebrospinal fluid (CSF) of Alzheimer's disease (AD) patients. Homocarnosine levels in human CSF dramatically decline with age. Cerebrospinal fluid composition and turnover is controlled by the choroid plexus, which possesses a specific transporter for carnosine and homocarnosine. Carnosine reacts with protein carbonyls and suppress the reactivity of glycated proteins. Carbonic anhydrase (CA) activity is diminished in AD patient brains. Carnosine is a CA activator. Protein cross-links are present in neurofibrillary tangles in AD brain. Carnosine stimulates proteolysis thereby helping to dissociate the cross-linkage and inflammatory damage. (45)

The antioxidant activity of carnosine compounds has been examined by testing their peroxyl radical-trapping ability at physiological concentrations. Reactive oxygen species, reactive nitrogen species, copper and zinc ions, glycating agents and reactive aldehydes, protein cross-linking and proteolytic dysfunction may all contribute to Alzheimer's disease. (46, 47) Carnosine has been found to catalyze their removal from the brain and muscles. (48)

Recommendation: As a single product we recommend 1000mg a day; however, when in combination with other brain protective supplements (pregnenolone, DHEA, Quercetin), only 250mg a day to start.

Vitamin C

Ascorbic acid is considered a powerful hydrophilic scavenger in biological fluids and tissues. Humans and other primates have lost the ability to synthesize ascorbic acid and rely on dietary sources of this compound. Vitamin C is distributed throughout the brain, and its concentration in the cerebrospinal fluid is about tenfold higher than in the plasma. The vitamin serves as a strong reducing agent by donating electron(s), thus directly neutralizing reactive oxygen species (ROS). In addition, it also acts to recycle the tocopherol radical to its active reduced form. However, ascorbate may also acquire a strong pro-oxidant activity by reacting with iron ions in the so-called Udenfriend reaction to produce highly toxic hydroxyl radicals (XX). This reaction might occur in the brain after injury following mobilization of iron ions and their interaction with ascorbic acid. (49,50)

Recommendation: We like the fat soluble ascorbyl palmitate (AP) due to its enhanced absorption into the brain, as opposed to the hydrophilic form of vitamin C. (51) Dosage: 500 to 1000mg twice a day.

IV Bar Consideration: Check that the client is not Glucose-6-phosphate dehydrogenase deficiency (G6PD) prior to using high doses of vitamin C. (52) Otherwise, mix 15grams of vitamin C into 250 ml D5W or normal saline (0.9 percent) and give it over 30 minutes. This may be repeated weekly if indicated.

Vitamin B-12

Is it possible to prevent atrophy of key brain regions related to cognitive decline and Alzheimer's disease (AD)? One approach is to modify non-genetic risk factors, for instance by lowering elevated plasma homocysteine using B vitamins. In an initial, randomized controlled study on elderly subjects with increased dementia risk, they showed that high-dose B-vitamin treatment (folic acid 0.8 mg, vitamin B6 20 mg, vitamin B12 0.5 mg) slowed shrinkage of the whole brain volume over two years. They also demonstrating that B-vitamin treatment reduces, by as much as seven-fold (7x reductions), the cerebral atrophy in those gray matter (GM) regions specifically vulnerable to the AD process, including the medial temporal lobe. In the placebo group, higher homocysteine levels at baseline are associated with faster GM atrophy, but this deleterious effect is largely prevented by B-vitamin treatment. (53)

Recommendation: Orally, we use Nano-B12 from QSM Scientific which delivers 250mcg per pump, which is placed under the tongue and held for 60 seconds. A starting dose of two pumps (500mcg) every other day or daily as needed up to four pumps Monday-Wednesday-Friday. For injectable, we use Hydroxycobalamin 0.5mg three times a week to daily.

IV Bar Consideration: Use Myer's Cocktail with Hydroxycobalamin (1mg) once a week for four to twelve weeks.

Nicotinamide

Nicotinamide (niacinamide; NAM; vitamin B-3) is the amide form of nicotinic acid (niacin) and is currently used in the treatment of pellagra, a vitamin deficiency. (54) It has been identified as a neuroprotective agent and has been shown to increase growth factors in a mouse model of Huntington's disease, reduce excitotoxicity in vitro, prevent cell death from oxidative damage both in vitro and in vivo, and improve behavioral and histopathological outcomes following experimental TBI and stroke. The potential for nicotinamide as a therapeutic agent for disorders such as stroke and TBI was first recognized when it was shown to be successful at reducing damage seen in models of oxidative stress, in addition to preventing damage associated with neurotoxic lesions. (55)

Research has shown that early use of NAM limited the area of cavitation at the point of maximal contusion and improved upon the overall level of neurobehavioral recovery. (56)

Recommendation: The results from a number of studies indicated that the long term use of 50mg/kg dose resulted in strong behavioral and histological neuroprotective effects following TBI.

IV Bar Consideration: Use Myer's Cocktail once a week for four to twelve weeks.

N-Acetyl Cysteine

N-acetyl cysteine (NAC) has been commercially available for about 40 years as Mucomyst, being used for pulmonary issues and also as the antidote for acute acetaminophen toxicity in the emergency room. An impressive group of recent articles (17,500 in all) found that NAC has both antioxidant and anti-inflammatory benefits in TBI. In 2013, Michael Hoffer used NAC in an active theater of war (Iraq and Afghanistan) study on mild and moderate TBI cases produced by blast injury. The studies clearly showed that initiation of treatment with NAC within 24 hours of injury led to better outcome in terms of headache, confusion, memory loss, and sleep issues. (57)

Recommendation: Acute injury dosing: four grams a day divided into two grams in the morning and two grams at night for four days. The dose is lowered to three grams in divided doses of 1.5 grams morning and evening. Post injury dosing: If the initial injury was more than one week old, we start our patients on 500mg twice a day because we are using a number of other nutraceuticals products as are listed here.

Diindolylmethane

Diindolylmethane (DIM) is one of the active phytochemicals found in cruciferous vegetables along with Indole-3-carbinol (I3C). (58) In fact, it takes two molecules of I3C hitting your stomach acid (HCl) to produce one molecule of DIM. The list of benefits for either or both DIM/IC3 has been growing from decreasing the production of carcinogenic estrogen metabolites (4(OH) & 16(OH)), to being adjunctive to Taxol (59) to enhance induction of apoptosis in a number of cancers. (60)

Another benefit found in DIM/IC3 is their influence on inflammatory cytokines. DIM significantly decreased the release of nitric oxide (NO), prostaglandin (PGE_2), tumor necrosis factor α, interleukin (IL)-6, and IL-1β cells treated with Lipopolysaccharides (LPS). DIM inhibited LPS-induced increases in protein levels of inducible NO synthase (iNOS) (61), which were accompanied by decreased iNOS mRNA levels and transcriptional activity. The mRNA levels of phospholipase A_2 decreased (62), whereas neither cyclooxygenases-2 protein (63) nor transcript was altered by DIM. In addition, DIM suppressed LPS-induced nuclear factor-κB (NF-κB) transcriptional activity, NF-κB DNA-binding activity, translocation of p65 to the nucleus, and degradation of inhibitor of κBα. (64)

Recommendation: A dose of 200 to 300mg a day in divided doses.

Quercetin

Quercetin is one of a broad group of natural polyphenolic flavonoid substances (similar in effect to resveratrol) (65) that are being investigated for their widespread health benefits. (66*) Among flavonoids, quercetin is the most common flavonoid in nature, and it is mainly present as its glycosylated forms — such as quercitrin (3-rhamnosyl quercetin) or rutoside (3-rhamnosy-glucosyl quercetin). Flavonoids exert several biological activities, which are mainly related to their ability to inhibit enzymes and/or to their antioxidant properties, and are able to regulate the immune response. These activities may explain the beneficial effects that flavonoid intake exerts in different human pathologies — including hypertension, inflammatory conditions, and cancer. (67)

Quercetin has been found to increase mitochondrial biogenesis in muscle and brain as indicated by increases in gene expression of PGC-1 (68), SIRT1 (69), mitochondrial DNA (XX), and cytochrome c enzyme concentration. All of these reflect an increase in mitochondrial function with increased fat utilization over carbohydrates. The net effect is an improvement in energy production that projects out to be an improvement in muscle endurance. (70)

Recommendation: Quercetin 500mg twice a day.

Coenzyme Q10

Coenzyme Q10 (CQ10) is the only lipid antioxidant that is synthesized in mammals by all cells, and its biosynthesis is a very complex process which involves the participation of at least nine gene products in all the species studied. The redox functions of CQ10 are due to its ability to exchange two electrons in a redox cycle between the oxidized (ubiquinone, CQ10) and the reduced form (ubiquinol, CQ10-H_2). This redox reaction can be driven either by the simultaneous transfer of two electrons in a single step, or by two sequential steps of one electron transfer through a partially reduced semiquinone intermediate. These redox forms allow CoQ10 to act as antioxidant. (71*)

Coenzyme Q10 is an essential cofactor of the electron transport chain, as well as a potent free radical scavenger in lipid and mitochondrial membranes. Supplementation with CQ10 increased cerebral cortex concentrations which resulted in a significant increase in cerebral cortex mitochondrial concentrations of CQ10. These results show that oral administration of CQ10 increases both brain and brain mitochondrial concentrations. They provide further evidence that CQ10 can exert neuroprotective effects that might be useful in the treatment of neurodegenerative diseases and the sequelae associated with TBI. (72)

Note: Statins lead to dose-dependent reductions in coenzyme Q10, a key mitochondrial antioxidant and electron transport carrier that serve to help bypass existing mitochondrial respiratory chain defects. (73)

Recommendation: Depending on what else is being taken, the amount of Co-Q 10 can range from 60 to 250mg a day. Therefore, we start with 60mg once a day if not on a statin and 100mg if on a statin.

Pyrroloquinoline Quinone

Pyrroloquinoline Quinone (PQQ) is a micronutrient that is naturally found in foods such as soybeans, parsley, and green pepper. Recent clinical research suggests that as an antioxidant it may influence nerves and neurological health, as well as cognitive function, by supporting several signal transduction pathways that are important in maintaining mitochondrial homeostasis and oxidative metabolism. (74, 75*)

PQQ also promotes healthy levels of nerve growth factor and supports synaptic and intracellular neuronal responses by maintaining healthy N-methyl D-aspartate (NMDA) receptor activity. The NMDA receptor is the primary conduit for excitatory glutamate neurotransmission and is regarded as an important target for maintaining neuronal health. Several studies suggest that PQQ may promote learning ability and memory. In a double-blind, placebo-controlled clinical trial conducted in 71 middle-aged individuals, PQQ supplementation over a twelve-week period supported healthy cognitive performance, and a combination of PQQ and CoQ10 provided greater support than PQQ alone. (76)

PQQ is analogous to combining some of the best chemical features of ascorbic acid (reducing potential), riboflavin (redox reactions), and pyridoxal (carbonyl reactivity) cofactors into one molecule and is more efficient than those substances correspondingly. (77)

Recommendation: Our dosing of PQQ is always with Co-Q10, dosing 20mg and 60mg respectively.

Ribose

Aside from being the sugar moiety in DNA (Deoxy-ribose-Nucleic Acid) and RNA (Ribose Nucleic Acid), ribose is also the backbone of every energy molecule produced in our body from ATP, ADP, AMP to all the others (such as cAMP and cGMP).

In order to provide the optimal potential for the body to manufacture ATP, and therefore provide for energy, all the substrates for producing ATP, and for the regeneration of ATP from ADP, must be available. Researchers have demonstrated that oxidative phosphorylation (OP) is the main mechanism initially providing energy to power neuronal activity, and that the main subcellular mechanisms underlying information processing (i.e., presynaptic action potentials, neurotransmitter release, postsynaptic currents and postsynaptic action potentials) all consume oxygen, and that an astrocyte-neuron lactate shuttle is not needed for oxidative phosphorylation to occur. (78) Therefore, supporting all aspects of OP with an ample amount of substrates will ensure that the neuronal production of ATP, as well as NADH+, will be present to provide the needed energy to maintain function.

Recommendation: When indicated, we start on five grams of ribose powder in a bottle of water (16 oz.), one to three times a day.

Glutathione

Glutathione is a tripeptide (glutamate-cysteine-glycine) molecule, and is the most abundant non-protein thiol found in the brain. Glutathione acts as an antioxidant via its capacity to serve as a substrate for the enzyme glutathione peroxidase and seems to mainly be found in astrocytes. Nitric Oxide (NO) can react with superoxide O^{2-} to form peroxynitrite and its reactive intermediates, which can react indiscriminately with proteins, DNA, thiol, and other cell components. Under this scenario, neurons in culture with glutathione-depleted astrocytes exhibited a two-fold increase in cell death over a range of NO donor concentrations. These findings suggest that astrocytes protect neurons from NO toxicity by a glutathione-dependent mechanism. (79)

Optimizing benefits obtainable with glutathione can be achieved with a nanoliposomal based product that has a high absorptive capacity and delivery to the brain. We start our patients on 50mg of a liposomal glutathione twice a day (two pumps in the morning and two pumps at bed time).

Recommendation: 50 to 100mg once or twice a day.

IV Bar consideration: As a stand-alone IV solution, we suggest 800 to 1000mg per infusion, once a week for ten to twelve weeks. Note: Do not place glutathione into any solution with vitamin C as it will cause reduction of the glutathione.

Alpha Lipoic Acid

The lipid-soluble dithiol a-lipoate (ALA) is absorbed from the diet, crosses the BBB, and is taken up by cells. It possesses a wide spectrum of activities as a metabolic antioxidant, and its reduced form (dihydrolipoate) exits the cells to act as an extracellular antioxidant. Alpha-Lipoate scavenges a large variety of species including hydroxyl radicals, hypochlorous acid, NO, peroxynitrite, hydrogen peroxide, and singlet oxygen. It is also an effective chelator of transition metals and may regenerate various antioxidants (such as ubisemiquinone, dehydroascorbate radical, and glutathione disulfide) to their active form. Thus, α-lipoate and its reduced product act as potent antioxidants in both intra and extracellular environments, and were recently reported to show neuroprotective properties in traumatic brain injury induced pathology. (80)

Lipoic acid may also have lipid peroxyl radical (LOO•) scavenging effects, but it is more likely to be indirect via the regeneration (i.e., re-reduction) of other endogenous electron-donating antioxidants including vitamin E, glutathione and vitamin C.

Recommendation: A starting dose of 400mg a day up to 800mg as a single agent.

PEG-SOD

The earliest studies of free radical scavenging compounds in TBI models were carried out with Super Oxide Dismutase (Cu/Zn SOD) (81) based upon the work of Kontos and colleagues who showed that post-traumatic microvascular dysfunction was initiated by ROS generated as a by-product of the arachidonic acid cascade(82), which is massively activated during the first minutes and hours after TBI.

The work of Kontos showed that administration of SOD prevented the post-traumatic microvascular dysfunction. This led to clinical trials in which the more metabolically stable polyethylene glycol (PEG) conjugated SOD was examined in moderate and severe TBI patients when administered within the first eight hours after injury. Their work showed that administration of SOD prevented the post-traumatic microvascular dysfunction. Although an initial small phase II study (83) showed a positive trend, subsequent multi-center phase III studies failed to show a significant benefit in terms of increased survival or improved neurological outcomes. (84)

The benefit of using PEG (polyethylene glycol) conjugation to other compounds or medications is to enhance their delivery to the system. In the work by Kontos and colleagues showed that the administration of SOD prevented post-traumatic microvascular dysfunction. This led to a small clinical trial in which polyethylene glycol (PEG) conjugated SOD was used in moderate and severe TBI patients within the first eight hours after injury. (85) Noted was some improvement; but, when repeated in a phase III study, the benefits were not significant.

Recommendation: Although the phase III studies in moderate to severe cases of TBI failed to show significant benefits, we use PEG-SOD in our mild TBI (mTBI) cases in a sublingual delivery system. The response has been a reduction in the "fogginess" within a few days to a week.

Curcumin

Curcumin's immunomodulating and antioxidant activities suggest that it might be a useful adjunct in the treatment of neurodegenerative illnesses characterized by inflammation and inflammatory processes — Alzheimer's disease, hemorrhage, anoxia, ischemia, and traumatic brain injury. (86) Curcumin's potential therapeutic benefit in neuroinflammatory syndromes is based upon its effect on chemokine production. As has been discussed elsewhere, chemokines, as well as cytokines, have been demonstrated in the pathogenesis of a variety of central nervous system disorders accompanied by inflammation, which supports a non-neuropermissive environment. (87)

As is true of other naturally occurring polyphenolic compounds (such as caffeic acid phenyl ester, rosmaric acid and resveratrol), curcumin possesses antioxidant properties that may reduce the production of free radicals and improve cell viability under conditions of enhanced oxidative stress, as is found in stroke and TBI. In neuropathological processes associated with neutrophilic infiltrates (such as encephalitis and traumatic brain injury), chemokine, macrophage inflammatory protein-2 (MIP-2) appears to play a pivotal role in the induction and perpetuation of inflammation in the brain. (88)

Reports have also promoted curcumin's ability to influence a list of diseases by its immunomodulating abilities: anti-carcinogenic, anti-mutagenic, anticoagulant, antifertility, anti-diabetic, antibacterial, antifungal, antiprotozoal, antiviral, anti-fibrotic, anti-venom, anti-ulcer, and hypotensive activities. Its anticancer effect is mainly mediated through induction of apoptosis. Clinically, curcumin has already been used to reduce post-operative inflammation. Safety evaluation studies indicate that both turmeric and curcumin are well tolerated at a very high dose without any toxic effects. (89)

Recommendation: Standardized powder (curcumin): 400 to 600mg, three times per day.

Pregnenolone

Pregnenolone has been referred to as the "mother of all hormones" for being the first steroid generated by the mitochondrial metabolism of cholesterol and representing the key substrate at the head of two important pathways (cortisol/aldosterone on one side and testosterone/estrogen on the other). This critical step in steroidogenesis is rate limiting and essential in needing sufficient amounts of cholesterol, which is converted within the oligodendrocytic mitochondria to pregnenolone. (90) Failure to supply ample amounts of cholesterol to be converted by oligodendrocytes can equate out to a deficiency in myelin production.

Diethylstilbestrol, tamoxifen, cocaine, and other drugs have been described to interfere with steroidogenesis by down-regulation of cytochrome P450 side-chain cleavage enzyme. Without adequate amounts of cholesterol, there cannot be significant amounts of pregnenolone to generate all the steroidal hormones. When there is a deficiency of cortisol, the conversion of pregnenolone to DHEA is down-regulated in favor of the life-saving benefits of cortisol — the Pregnenolone Steal Syndrome. (91)

Pregnenolone is also a neurosteroid being found throughout the brain tissue, but in highest concentration in the hippocampus. It appears that its central benefits are derived when it becomes pregnenolone-sulfate (PS). PS allosterically inhibited $GABA_A$ receptor currents and enhanced N-methyl-D-aspartate (NMDA) receptor function. PS has been found to regulate learning and memory in extremely low concentrations.

Recommendation: 50 to 100mg of pregnenolone a night with DHEA.

Warning: Care should be taken in those individuals with a history of seizure activity since PS has been associated with precipitating activity. (92)

Dehydroepiandrosterone

Dehydroepiandrosterone (DHEA) and its sulfinated active metabolite (DHEA-s) are both neurosteroids (NS) and neuroactive steroids (NAS) with significant functions — both in the peripheral organ systems and centrally in the brain. They have been discussed extensively elsewhere in this book and therefore, at this point, we will focus on their use for modulation of phase II damage by inflammatory mechanisms that curtail a neuropermissive environment. (93)

There is abundant evidence that inflammatory mechanisms within the CNS contribute to cognitive impairment via cytokine-mediated interactions between neurons and glial cells. Cytokines facilitate cellular mechanisms that modulate neuronal and glial cell function to facilitate neuronal regeneration or neurodegeneration affecting cognition. According to the article by Caleb E. Finch (my guru at USC, who has authored a number of articles and books on the Neuroendocrine Theory of Aging) has proposed that cytokines (like IL-6) that are actively transported through the BBB affect neuron-to-neuron communications causing a diminution in cognition. (94*)

Dr. Finch summarizes that, "The cause of this age-related cytokine dysregulation is unclear and could include normal homeostatic responses and disease processes. One possible mechanism is suggested by findings that DHEA inhibits IL-6 secretion from human mononuclear cells in vitro. Thus, an age-related increase in IL-6 could be due to a loss of tonic inhibition by DHEA as levels of this adrenal hormone decrease with advancing age. Advanced glycation end products (AGEs), reactive derivatives of non-enzymatic glucose macromolecule products that accumulate in human tissues with age, are implicated by way of induction of pro-inflammatory cytokine expression through nuclear factor- kβ (95) transcription factor-dependent pathways."

Recommendation: A starting dose of 25 to 50mg at bedtime so that the morning blood level of DHEA-s is within the 75th to 99th percentile of the range (400 to 500ng/ml).

Furthermore, some organizations that teach HRT (hormone replacement therapy) promote the practice of giving DHEA in the morning. I have been unable to substantiate this recommendation, as there is prominent information promoting nighttime use to get the benefit of a 20 percent increase in the production of GH. (96)

Vitamin D3

If any "vitamin" has gone through a rebirth, it has to be vitamin D. Vitamin D is no longer recognized as just a vitamin, but rather as a secosteroid hormone (97) with the same cholesterol backbone as other steroids (including PROG) and with its own class of nuclear steroid receptors and signaling mechanisms. (98, 99) In general, vitamins act as co-factors in chemical reactions while hormones influence our genomic expression by regulating gene activation and transcription. In its biologically active form (1,25 dihydroxyvitamin D3) is a hormone with sites of action throughout the CNS. Additionally, vitamin D can be considered a neuroactive steroid having met the same criteria as others in this classification. (100)

Vitamin D deficiency has been associated with many systemic disorders, including infectious (101), inflammatory and autoimmune conditions (102), cardiovascular disease (103) hypertension and atherosclerosis, neuromuscular function, cancer, neurodegenerative diseases, and neuropsychological and functional outcomes in the elderly population. (104) In fact, vitamin D deficiency appears to be correlated with many, if not most, of the problems associated with advanced age — especially those with an inflammatory component. (105) There is also evidence that the level of serum vitamin D is a key marker of frailty (106), and that it is associated with elevated levels of IL-6. (107)

Of all the endocrine and nutritional disruptions that affect the elderly population, vitamin D deficiency has recently received considerable attention, partly because an estimated one billion people worldwide exhibit vitamin D deficiency, or insufficiency. (108) In the northeastern United States, studies show a prevalence from 32 percent in healthy adults (109) to approximately 50 percent for adolescents and preadolescents. (110) The most dramatic statistics for vitamin D deficiency, however, come from studies in the elderly population, which show that 40 to 100 percent of community-dwelling American and European older men and women are vitamin D deficient. Even higher averages are seen in the ill and institutionalized. (111)

Vitamin D is structurally similar to many sterol hormones and is obtained through both dietary intake and endogenous biosynthesis from cholesterol in the skin. Following intake or biosynthesis, vitamin D undergoes enzyme catalyzed sequential hydroxylation to yield its active form (1,25 dihydroxyvitamin D, or calcitriol). Despite being established to play a vital role in calcium homeostasis peripherally, the functional role of vitamin D in the CNS has remained elusive. Recent research has suggested that the cells in the brain not only possess the hydroxlase responsible for vitamin D activation, but that multiple regions in the brain abundantly express the nuclear vitamin D receptor. (112) Binding of vitamin D to its nuclear receptor, in turn, leads to its association with other transcription factors, such as retinoic acid receptor. Subsequently, this complex binds to vitamin D response elements in genomic DNA, thus augmenting gene transcription. Vitamin D induced alterations in gene transcription are now believed to modulate a myriad of neuronal properties including: proliferation, differentiation and maintenance of calcium homeostasis. (113)

More recent research has suggested that vitamin D supplementation and the prevention of vitamin D deficiency may serve valuable roles in the treatment of TBI, and may represent an important and necessary neuroprotective adjuvant for post-TBI progesterone therapy. (114*) Progesterone is one of the few agents to demonstrate significant reductions in mortality following TBI in human patients in preliminary trials and phase III multi-center trials currently in progress. Similarly, in vitro and in vivo studies have suggested that vitamin D supplementation with progesterone administration may significantly enhance neuroprotection. (115) Vitamin D deficiency may increase inflammatory damage and behavioral impairment following experimental injury and attenuate the protective effects of post-traumatic progesterone treatment. (116)

Recently, we have added thyroperoxidase (TPO) to all patients with a history of hypothyroidism, or in those that we suspect of having an autoimmune hypothyroid condition. This is because of recent articles emphasizing the immunomodulating abilities of vitamin D (117) and the close relationship of vitamin D deficiency and Hashimoto's thyroiditis (118), as well as Graves' disease (119, 120) and polyarthritis. (121) These newfound associations of vitamin D open up another avenue of approach for medical intervention of a deficiency state by the replenishment of the missing compound, and not by masking or suppressing the symptoms.

Recommendation: After testing the levels of all the vitamin D (D3, 25OH, and 1,25-OH) we start the patients on 5,000 IU a day and increase to 10,000 IU a day. We monitor calcium levels as an indicator of excessive vitamin D. The goal is to get the vitamin D level to 60 to 100ng/ml.

Nanoliposomal vitamin D: A number of nanoliposomal products for TBI and BHRT are in the dietary and compounding pipeline. The convenience of the delivery system allows for a significant reduction in overall dosage of a product, as well as enhanced delivery to the circulatory system and therefore, the brain.

Green Tea

One of the most abundant compounds in green tea extract is the potent antioxidant Epigallocatechin-3-gallate (EGCG) (122), which is capable of crossing the blood-nerve and blood-brain barrier and exerting neuroprotective benefits in peripheral nerve injury, spinal cord trauma, and ischemic stroke.

Epigallocatechin-3-gallate also displays neuroprotective properties in animal models of chronic neurodegenerative diseases, including: amyotrophic lateral sclerosis, Parkinson's disease, and Alzheimer's disease. Epigallocatechin-3-gallate's neuroprotection has largely been attributed to its potent antioxidant and anti-inflammatory properties. Theanine (123), another important component of green tea extract, exerts a multitude of neuroprotective benefits in experimental models of ischemic stroke, Alzheimer's disease, and Parkinson's disease. (124) Theanine, like EGCG, contains multiple mechanisms of neuroprotective action including protection from excitotoxic injury and inhibition of inflammation.

As with most other natural compounds, no human trials have been conducted to investigate the effects of EGCG and/or theanine on reducing or treating brain injury following TBI; however, preliminary evidence has suggested that green tea-derived compounds may indeed modulate neuronal function in human subjects. For example, a randomized, placebo-controlled trial demonstrated that administration of green tea extract and L-theanine, over 16 weeks of treatment, improved indices of memory and brain theta wave activity on electroencephalography, suggesting greater cognitive alertness. (125, 126)

Additional studies have also suggested that green tea extract may decrease cognitive decline in the elderly, and that L-theanine and theogallin-enriched green tea or caffeine may increase brain theta wave activity and performance on tasks requiring attention, respectively. Collectively, these studies suggest that green tea consumption or supplementation with its derivatives may bolster cognitive function acutely and may slow cognitive decline. (127)

Recommendation: A cup of well brewed green tea can deliver about 300 to 400mg of EGCG. Green tea extract supplements are accessible over the counter in various forms. Standardized green tea extract is 90 percent total polyphenols, and one capsule equals five cups of tea. For a green tea extract standardized for 80 percent polyphenols and 55 percent EGCG, a daily dose of 400 to 1,000mg green tea extract is recommended.

Phosphatidylcholine

Neuronal membranes contain different types of lipids present in varied amounts: glycerolipids (60 percent), sterols (20 percent), glycosphingolipids (15 percent), and sphingomyelin (five percent). Phosphatidylcholine (PC) represents about 58 percent of the membrane phospholipids, thereby being the principal and essential component for mammalian neuronal membranes. (128)

When neuronal damage occurs, it will be regenerative processes that will help to repair the damage. The process is started with neuronal differentiation, which is characterized by neuritogenesis, neurite outgrowth, polarization, pathfinding, and synaptogenesis — each being critically dependent on membrane biosynthesis consisting of phosphatidylcholine and growth factors. The word "neurite" pertains to any projection from the cell body of a neuron such as an axon or a dendrite. A feature of neurites is that they undergo dramatic changes in length and shape during development in which the outgrowth is tipped by the growth cone, or axon elongation following the body growth. (129) In a non-neuropermissive environment, attempts at regeneration of the growth cone are inhibited by an oligodendritic cell product called NOGO-A, which is an axonal growth inhibitor. (130) NOGO-A is also responsible for blocking attempts to regenerate the microvasculature lost during TBI and other forms of intracerebral hemorrhages. (131)

Recommendation: We use an oral product starting with 400mg twice a day, increasing to 400mg three times a day after a month.

IV Bar Consideration: We use 1,000mg of PC in 50cc of sterile water or D5W infused over 30 minutes on a weekly basis for ten to twelve weeks.

Phosphatidylserine

Phosphatidylserine (PS) is a naturally occurring phospholipid, and represents a major component of cell membranes. While PS is important for the basic maintenance of all cell membranes, it is found in a relatively higher concentration in brain cells. The predominance of PS in brain cell membranes points to its role in an assortment of nerve cell functions — most importantly, neurotransmitter release and synaptic activity. Clinical studies strongly suggest its ability to support and improve brain functions such as mental concentration and memory retention, which typically begins to decline with age. (132)

In two double-blind, randomized, placebo-controlled trials of PS (coordinated by T.H. Crook, PhD), the first group of subjects were selected on the basis of their degree of measurable losses in memory, judgment, and abstract thought, as well as changes in personality and behavior. The treatment group received 300mg of phosphatidylserine per day, and showed significant improvement in name-face acquisition (learning names and faces), name-face delayed recall (recall of names and faces) and delayed non-matching (facial recognition). (133)

Recommendation: As a stand-alone product, 100mg of PS three times a day is the starting dose.

DL-Phenylalanine

DL-Phenylalanine is a combination of the well-tolerated essential amino acids: d-phenylalanine and l-phenylalanine. (134) Together, these compounds promote mental functioning, support a positive outlook, and relax the musculoskeletal system. L-phenylalanine is a precursor to tyrosine, which converts to the neurotransmitters norepinephrine, epinephrine, dopamine, and 5-hydoxytryptophan (5-HTP). By maintaining healthy tyrosine and endorphin levels, dl-phenylalanine nutritionally supports mental acuity and emotional well-being, while relaxing stressed muscles and joints. (135)

Recommendation: Starting at 500mg on an empty stomach prior to each meal, and increasing to 1000mg after two weeks, seems to allow for a consistent response without any gastric reactions. I used this product for about five weeks and lost 14 pounds due to the reduction in my sugar craving. (As a hypoglycemic, I cannot stay away from carbohydrates.)

Tocopherols and Tocotrienols

The human body has an antioxidant defense system with two lines of antioxidant defense within the cell. The first line is found in the fat-soluble cellular membrane consisting of vitamin E, beta-carotene and coenzyme Q. Of these, alpha-tocopherol is the most potent vitamin E member as an antioxidant that acts upon the cell membrane to protect from free radical generation of lipid peroxidation with disruption of membrane stability. The second line is found inside the cell. The water-soluble antioxidant scavengers include vitamin C, glutathione peroxidase, and superoxide dismutase. (136)

Of the numerous vitamins commercially available, vitamin E has been at the forefront of many studies investigating its potential neuroprotective benefits. (137) Vitamin E is a collective term for eight naturally occurring compounds, four tocopherols (alpha-, beta-, gamma-, and delta-) and four tocotrienols (alpha-, beta-, gamma-, and delta-). (138) Vitamin E is a potent, lipid-soluble, antioxidant that is present in high concentrations in the mammalian brain.

In several animal models of brain injury such as ischemic stroke, subarachnoid hemorrhage and Alzheimer's disease, administration of alpha-tocopherol or its potent derivative alpha-tocotrienol has been shown to lessen oxidative stress and neuropathology. Other laboratory studies have demonstrated that pre-traumatic alpha-tocopherol supplementation reduces TBI-induced increases in lipid peroxidation and oxidative injury and impairments in spatial memory. (139)

As discussed above, phosphatidylcholine is an important constituent of the mammalian neuronal cell membrane. Under the right neuropermissive environment, repair of a neuron begins with neuritic extension of either axon or dendrite. It was found that alpha-tocopherol reduced Nogo-A expression in brain tissue after traumatic brain injury, and helped to promote nerve regeneration. (140)

Finally, gamma-tocopherol has been found to be the main anti-inflammatory component and has been found to be more effective in scavenging free radicals and nitrogen oxygen species that cause inflammation. Interestingly, the use of alpha-tocopherol supplements also significantly reduces serum gamma-tocopherol, and therefore, any potential health benefits of alpha-tocopherol supplements may be offset by deleterious changes in the bioavailability of other forms of potent tocopherols and tocotrienols. (141*)

Recommendation: Use of a mixed product containing vitamin E in the forms of gamma tocopherol 500mg and alpha tocopherol 400mg, two to three times a day.

Eicosanoids (Omega 3 and 6)

Omega-3 fatty acids (FA) are polyunsaturated fatty acids (PUFAs) having a double bond at the third position from the end of the FA chain. Omega-3 FAs are the major constituents of the cell membrane phospholipids, which suggest that supplementation of PUFAs, could help in reducing the irregular phospholipid metabolism that occurs during neuronal damage. They are highly essential for maintaining the cell membrane's fluidity and are present in all tissues, but are rich particularly in brain, retina, and spermatozoa. There are three important physiological omega-3 FAs available, including alpha linolenic acid (ALA), eicosapentaenoic acid (EPA), and docosahexaenoic acid (DHA). (142)

Epidemiological studies suggest that the ideal ratio of omega-6 to omega-3 essential fatty acids (EFA) is approximately 1/1 (whereas in a Western diet, the ratio is 15/1 or higher). This high omega-6/omega-3 ratio has been found to promulgate the pathogenesis of many diseases, including cardiovascular disease, cancer, osteoporosis, and inflammatory and autoimmune diseases; whereas, increased levels of omega-3 PUFA (a lower omega-6/omega-3 ratio) exert suppressive effects. (143)

In the initial stages of phase II injury after TBI, a characteristic progression herald by tissue damage, an imbalance in cerebral blood flow causing anoxia, ischemia, and hypoglycemia influences cellular metabolism. These conditional states can lead to an increased accumulation of lactic acid due to anaerobic glycolysis, with increased membrane permeability causing fluid retention and heightened risk for cerebral edema. As cerebral edema increases, intracranial pressure augments vascular stasis with further reduction in energy production (144). As a result of these events, there is depletion of ATP reserves as the cellular energy requirements become inadequate with anaerobic glycolysis. (145)

This ATP depletion, in turn, disrupts the membrane ion pumps. Therefore, the secondary stage of the TBI is initiated, which is characterized by the depolarization of terminal membrane leading to the release of excitatory neurotransmitters such as glutamate. The Ca^{2+} and Na^{+} influx becomes high due to the impaired ion pumps. The excess Ca^{2+} causes activation of lipases, proteases, and lipid peroxidases, and produces free FA and free radicals. Moreover, the activated caspases and endonucleases initiate the degradation of biomembranes and the nucleosomal DNA. This eventually leads to apoptosis, autophagy, and parthanatos of neuronal cells. The oxidative stress formed in response to TBI generates superoxides, NO, H_2O_2, and peroxynitrite. These reactive oxygen species lead to the peroxidation of cellular structures, phospholipid membranes, vascular endothelium in the brain, cleavage of DNA, and inhibition of the chemical actions within the mitochondria's electron transport chain. (146)

Okay, this is the punchline: It has been found that — as a consequence of TBI initiated cellular depletion of ATP reserves — there is reduced ubiquitous mitochondrial creatine kinase (uMtCK), an enzyme implicated in the energetic regulation of Ca^{2+}-pumps and in the maintenance of Ca^{2+}-homeostasis. Once Omega-3 supplements normalized the levels of uMtCK the pumps regulating Ca^{2+}-homeostasis can turn back on. (147)

Recommendation: Two to three grams (DHA/EPA) three times a day, and add 400 to 600mg of Alpha lipoic acid.

Zinc Citrate

After more than twelve years of monitoring the influence of zinc on the rate of conversion of testosterone to estradiol, in males, it is clear that if the patient is deficient in zinc they will produce more estradiol (E2). The Millennium treatment protocol uses only physiologic dosing of testosterone — based upon a number of studies looking at the diurnal production of testosterone in both genders. The addition of zinc will assure us of low conversion, as well as provide a long list of other biological benefits inherent to zinc.

In 1963, only three enzymes were identified that required zinc for their activities; however, in 2012, more than 300 enzymes, and more than 1000 transcription factors were identified as requiring zinc for their activities. (148) Two of my favorites are P53, the most important intranuclear anti-cancer factor, and Alpha Secretase, the enzyme that could alter the development of Alzheimer's disease — if there was adequate availability of zinc.

A recent article in the Journal of Affective Disorders found low dietary or supplemental zinc is associated with depression symptoms among women. (149) Therefore, we check levels in both genders.

Recommendation: If a male patient is on any form of testosterone (injectable or sublingual) we will place them on from 50 to 100mg of zinc citrate a day, and adjust upwards based upon intracellular testing (royal blue tube). Women can benefit from some conversion of testosterone to estradiol, but the added benefits to health based upon good levels of zinc cannot be underscored.

Mucuna Pruriens

Mucuna pruriens, also known as the velvet bean, contains L-DOPA, a precursor to the neurotransmitter dopamine. (150) Dopamine seems to be an important neurotransmitter for prefrontal functioning, which is expressed by the term "executive functions" that is meant to represent a wide range of cognitive abilities. Patients with damage to the prefrontal cortex show impaired judgment, organization, planning, and decision-making — as well as behavioral disinhibition and impaired intellectual abilities. (151)

Aside from compromise of executive functions, a patient with prefrontal injury can also exhibit daytime fatigue (not due to medications) or a degree of apathy. Mucuna, as a naturopathic agent, can help to improve upon these symptoms with increased levels of dopamine. A common allopathic agent is amantadine (listed next) which has an array of dopaminergic benefits in frontal lobe impacts, which are statically the most common in TBI cases.

Finally, we have had patients experiencing a noticeable improvement when they used the growth hormone Secretropin® because of its content of Mucuna in a nanoliposomal delivery vehicle, which enhances absorption through the oral and gastric mucosa.

Recommendation: A dose of 120mg a day is recommended for both TBI and Parkinson's disease.

Prescription Medications

Amantadine

Amantadine is a tricyclic water-soluble amine salt that affects the synthesis, accumulation, release, and reuptake of catecholamines in the central nervous system. It is rapidly absorbed, but it is not metabolized. Amantadine is 90 percent excreted unchanged in the urine, and the elimination half-life is 9.7 to 14.5 hours. Distribution is through all the tissues of the body, including the central nervous system, while peak plasma concentrations occur one to four hours after ingestion. Amantadine causes release of dopamine from central neurons, facilitates dopamine release by nerve impulses, and delays the reuptake of dopamine by neural cells. Amantadine appears to act through several pharmacological mechanisms, but no dominant mechanism of action has been identified. It is a dopaminergic, noradrenergic and serotonergic substance. It blocks monoamine oxidase A and NMDA receptors, and seems to raise beta-endorphin/beta-lipotropin levels. (152, 153)

Amantadine was approved by the U.S. Food and Drug Administration in October 1966 as a prophylactic agent against Asian influenza, and eventually received approval for the treatment of influenza virus A in adults. In 1969, the drug was also discovered by accident to help reduce symptoms of Parkinson's disease, drug-induced extrapyramidal syndromes, and akathisia.

Recommendations: We start with 100mg a day for about a month, and then increase to 100mg twice a day (200mg total). We have found that patients with apathy improve, as well as overall mental "energy," focus, determination, and quality of life.

Statins

Those of you who know me, and have seen my lecture, "Cholesterol: The Father of All Hormones," are probably thinking that I have gone crazy promoting the use of statins — nonetheless in TBI. While I might not fully agree with their traditional use to lower cholesterol, I have read enough logic relative to their use in the acute phase of TBI to present it here. I was convinced by one cardinal article: *Statins as Potential Therapeutic Agents in Neuroinflammatory Disorders and Statins in Traumatic Brain Injury.* (154) This review article addressed the roles of inflammation produced IL-6 and its generation of C-reactive protein (CRP) in the liver. Once IL-6 gets into the brain, it alters neuronal conduction causing a reduction in cognition. The increasing level of CRP can cause a decrease of nitric oxide, which leads to elevation in blood pressure and reduced blood flow in capillary networks throughout the body. (155)

The therapeutic effects of statins in traumatic brain injury may be divided according to mechanisms: acute lesional effects, anti-inflammatory and anti-excitotoxic effects, vascular and endothelial effects, anti-apoptotic effects, and positive effects on neurogenesis and angiogenesis.

Table 8.1: Statin Effects in Traumatic Brain Injury			
ACUTE		SUBACUTE	CHRONIC
Cerebral Blood Flow	Neuroinflammation	Apoptosis	Angiogenesis
▼Microthrombosis	▼Inflammatory cytokines	▼Bax/Bcl-2	▲VEGF, VEGFR2
▼Platelet Activity	▲BBB Integrity	▼Caspase 3	▲Akt/eNOS
▼Von Willebrand Factor	▼Cerebral Edema	Neuronal Injury	Neurogenesis & Plasticity
▲Endothelial Integrity	▼Microglial Activation	▼Excitotoxicity Death	▲BDNF, VEGF
▲eNOS	▼Oxidative Stress		▲PI3K/Akt

Recommendations: In an acute situation, within 24 hours of the TBI, use atorvastatin 10mg daily. In a chronic case you can use the C-reactive protein (CRP) level to direct treatment dosing and duration.

Selegiline

Selegiline, also known as L-deprenyl, is an irreversible and (relatively) selective MAO-B inhibitor. Meta-analysis of published clinical trials confirms it offers a cheap, safe and effective symptomatic treatment of early Parkinson's disease, and now, apathy in traumatic brain injury. (156)

Furthermore, selegiline may also be neuroprotective and act as an antidepressant. (157) Selegiline has immune-system-boosting and anti-neurodegenerative effects. (158) Its use increases the level of tyrosine hydroxylase, growth hormone, cerebral nitric oxide, and the production of key interleukins. Selegiline offers protection against DNA damage and oxidative stress by hydroxyl and peroxyl radical trapping, and protects against excitotoxic damage from glutamate. In addition, selegiline stimulates the release of superoxide dismutase (SOD). SOD is a key enzyme which helps to quench the production of damaging free-radicals. Potentially, selegiline may prevent or reverse iron-induced memory impairment. The deposition of excess iron in the brain is implicated in several neurodegenerative diseases.

Recommendation: A regimen of 2 x 5 mg daily of selegiline irreversibly inhibits over 90 percent of MAO-B in the basal ganglia, the location of over 80 percent of dopamine in the human brain. This level of MAO-B inhibition leads to a 40 to 70 percent increase in synaptic dopamine. The risk of a true serotonin syndrome with SSRIs and selegiline is quite low, and the combination can be taken together without event if caution is used. (159)

Bromocriptine

Bromocriptine is a prescription medication that has been around since the 60s, having been used in women who decide not to breastfeed their newborns. (160) This medication works by down-regulation of prolactin production from the pituitary by way of increasing dopamine, the prolactin inhibiting factor (PIF). A secondary benefit of bromocriptine is its dopaminergic, agonistic effect on the dopamine receptors — specifically, D2. This means that it can help individuals with Parkinson's symptoms associated with TBI, as well as improve upon the apathy that is common in mild to severe TBI. (161)

In individuals with post-TBI hyperprolactinemia, luteinizing hormone (LH) is proportionately suppressed, causing the loss of testosterone production in the male, and testosterone and estradiol production in the female. Menstrual irregularities (amenorrhea) with impotency in the female and diminished male characteristics with the rare occurrence of galactorrhea are risks if the level of prolactin is not returned to an optimal normal level. (162)

Additionally, in an article published in Brain, patients with TBI found "a selective effect of bromocriptine on cognitive processes, which involve executive control, and provide a foundation for potential therapies for patients with prefrontal damage causing dysexecutive syndromes." (163)

Recommendation: Bromocriptine at 2.5mg two to three times a day.

New Product Line

The Perfect Protocol™ - Cognitive Enhancers (TBI-1 and TBI-2)

The Cognitive Enhancers can be a two-part product: TBI-1 is used initially for a period of four weeks, and continued if there are noted benefits. If there is less than optimal improvement with TBI-1 alone, then TBI-2 is added to the regimen for a total of four weeks. At the end of that period, a decision needs to be made if there was a gestalt improvement on both

Cognitive Enhancers together or not. If there was no benefit, then it is suggested that only the Cognitive Enhancer TBI-1 be continued.

Perfect Protocol - TBI 1	1 cap	2 caps	4 caps
Quercetin	75	150	300
Pregnenolone	25	50	100
DL-Phenylalanine*	100	200	400
Phosphatidylcholine*	150	300	600
CoQ-10	25	50	100
Mucuna Pruriens	30	60	120
Sig: Initially two capsules twice a day.			
Perfect Protocol – TBI 2	1 cap	2 caps	4 caps
PQQ	10	20	40
Niacinamide	100	200	400
Carnosine	250	500	1000
Alpha Lipoic Acid	100	200	400
Phosphatidylserine	50	100	200
Sig: Initially two capsules twice a day.			

Table 8.2: Composition of Cognitive Enhancer TBI-1 & TBI-2. ®

Where to start: The following protocols are used in conjunction with the hormonal replenishment programs described in Chapter 9. The compositions of these progressive therapeutic protocols are supportive to the hormones used, as well as to enhance and improve the presence of antioxidants delivered into the brain. Many of the products contained are also within the domain of being neuro-permissive, fostering improvement of brain functioning as has been discussed elsewhere.

These should not be considered the last word in terms of composition and approach, but these are what we have presently provided to our patients. It is anticipated that there will be other options that might be even better. Therefore, please use these as a point of reference, and always do the best for your patients as science dictates.

The general directions in which the Millennium will add these selected supplements to a patient's protocol: This is the starting point for patients with less than optimal hormonal levels. These supplements are both supportive and additive to the individual's hormonal milieu. We have found that this step-wise approach, concurrent to hormonal replenishment, helps to embellish the ultimate outcome. We have seen improvement in those patients with minimal residual mood and cognitive impairment, such that they have regained more of who they were prior to injury. Again, these are fundamental supplementation protocols and are not to be considered the final lines in treatment — rather, as just a place to start.

Phase I	Supplement	Morning	Noon	Evening
Brain anti-oxidants and support	The Perfect Protocol TBI-1	2 caps		2 caps
Mood and Myelin	DHEA (25mg)			1-2 cap
A High-Potency Vitamins and Mineral	Perfect Protocol UltraVits	2 caps		2 caps
Phase II	Supplement	Morning	Noon	Evening
Brain anti-oxidants and support	The Perfect Protocol TBI-1	2 caps		2 caps
More Brain Support.	The Perfect Protocol TBI-2	1-2caps		1-2 caps
Myelin support (DHEA-s)	DHEA (25mg)			1-2 cap
A High-Potency Vitamins and Minerals	Perfect Protocol UltraVits	2 caps		2 caps
Phase III	Supplement	Morning	Noon	Evening
Brain anti-oxidants and support	The Perfect Protocol TBI-1	1-2 caps		1-2 caps
More Brain Support.	The Perfect Protocol TBI-2	1-2 caps		1-2 caps
A High-Potency Vitamins and Minerals	Perfect Protocol UltraVits	2 caps		2 caps
For apathy	Amantadine (100mg)	As directed above.		
For apathy and cognition	Selegiline (5mg)	As directed above.		

Table 8.3: The 3 steps of supplementation.

Intravenous Solution

The IV Bar

A few years ago, the Millennium started a new division called The IV Bar, which has the tagline: "Addressing health one solution at a time." We developed a number of unique solutions that address conditions ranging from simple fatigue due to over-working, to detoxification from alcohol. In the process of researching articles on oxidative stress and traumatic brain injury, we developed a solution that comes in two parts, which consist of B-12, B-complex, vitamin C, phosphatidylcholine, trace minerals, and glutathione.

Solutions	Directions
Myer's Solution	Once or twice a week for 10-12 weeks and can be continued indefinitely.
Phosphatidylcholine	Weekly 800mg-1000mg for 10-12 weeks or longer. Monitor blood levels at 6 weeks and 12 weeks initially to see where levels are attained.
Vitamin C	Check for G6PD deficiency before starting Vitamin C weekly for 10-12 weeks. Check serum levels of Vitamin C initially and after 6 weeks to achieve an ideal level of >400mg/dL.
Glutathione	Adding Glutathione to another solution containing Vitamin C will reduce glutathione to an inactive product. Glutathione is best as a slow push over 10 minutes or you can drip it over 30 minutes; use 1000mg weekly for 10-12 weeks.
Millennium-TBI IV	A two part IV with multiple nutrients and natural anti-oxidants to be given 1-3 times a week initially (1-3 months) then weekly based upon results.

Table 8.6 These are the most common solution that we are using for treating Oxidative Stress. The IV Bar: "Addressing health with one solution at a time." Licensing for the IV Bar are available.

Conclusion

The feasible benefits achievable from hormonal replenishment are generally unpredictable and too varied. But the goal in treatment will always be to improve upon the patient's expectations, and the predictive outcome for improved quality of life. How do we know that raising a patient's testosterone level from within the normal 25th percentile to the 30th or 40th percentile of the normal range will have any benefits? How do we know that adding amantadine, or even modafinil, in a patient with apathy and inanition will help to improve upon these symptoms? Simple, you don't know unless you try.

It appears that we have really failed in our scientific creativity due to the lack of knowledge about what we can do — since we are frequently told what we can't do. The knowledge that is needed only comes from the continued reading of an array of scientific literature on the basic science of application. That is, reading about how DHEA decreases glial cells from producing IL-6, which increases CRP and diminishes regional blood flow in the brain, causing the appearance of diminished capacity and cognitive impairment. Anoxia and hypoglycemia are the underlying mechanisms precipitating a direct rise in the production of IL-6 by astrocytes, which modify the ionic gates driving neuronal function by way of the GABA, NDMA, Sigma-1, and AMPA receptors. (164)

Concurrent to correcting any underlying hormonal deficiency or insufficiency, we begin the process of addressing the issue of oxidative stress (OS). This major component of the secondary phase of TBI is an important process to aggressively address with the use of one or more of the products listed above. Failing to specifically address OS will allow for the continued deterioration of neurons, and the persistence of a non-neuropermissive environment. Specifically, glutathione (GSH) depletion enhances peroxynitrite toxicity and tissue injury during circulatory shock, and a relationship between GSH depletion and enhanced peroxynitrite toxicity has also been proposed as contributing to the development of some neurodegenerative diseases such as Parkinson's disease, amyotrophic lateral sclerosis, Alzheimer's disease, and dementia. (165)

The goal in treating the second phase of TBI will be to establish a more neuro-permissive environment that allows for regeneration and repair of neuro-connectivity. We have provided a number of set protocols for you to try on your patients, but these are not the final words, since not everyone will respond as we would like to anticipate. Therefore, acquiring a modicum of knowledge about the process of oxidative stress will allow you to select, use, and improve the technology for better and more efficient protocols.

Now go read!

Chapter 9: Treatment of TBI

"Insanity is doing the same thing over and over again but expecting different results."

— Albert Einstein

"The secret of being a bore is to tell everything."

— Voltaire

Introduction

Over the course of the past ten years, relatives of individuals with mild TBI (mTBI) have called our office stating, "We have exhausted all (traditional) medical treatments with little or no improvement in our son's, daughter's, husband's, or wife's condition. We are desperate and you are our last hope." I cringe and think of how much could have been done sooner if we were not looked at as the "last hope," and had instead been at least their second or third option. Many of the patients and their families were told that "alternative" approaches to traumatic brain injury were not scientific and were unfounded due to the lack of empirical results. (1) But what hope and results did their traditional medicine offer and then deliver? These individuals are grasping for any vestige of hope, which was lost after years of traditional approaches failed to provide benefits. Yet, we are considered to be on the fringe when we are the ones reading over 8,700 peer review articles addressing post-TBI hypopituitarism (2) and over 18,500 articles on TBI and neurobehavioral changes. (3)

Nonetheless, these individuals, for the most part, never had loss of consciousness, amnesia, or sensorial confusion lasting more than a few hours, if not minutes. These are individuals who classically had an uneventful post-TBI period, were initially highly functional, and are representative of more than 85 percent of TBI cases. (4) Then, over the course of time, insidiously they developed changes in their personality involving: depression, isolation, and frequently, attempts at suicide. Evaluation and subsequent treatment generally included the standard laboratory testing to rule out any "major" biochemical imbalances, while never pursuing a more robust evaluation. Then, most were placed on one or more mood elevators and put out to pasture along with the other ten million plus with the same underlying condition subsequent to mTBI. (5)

Just recently, I reviewed two new patient intake forms from individuals who were requesting to be seen as new patients (under Interventional Endocrinology). I reviewed the first form, which was from a 37-year-old male requesting to transfer from a Men's Low Testosterone clinic to our offices. He had heard that we train our patients in how to self-inject with testosterone, instead of mandating weekly visits. I was intrigued and wanted to learn about his present franchised "Low T" clinic, so I called him and we had a nice 30-minute chat. In closing I asked him to send his pretreatment laboratories to us for review before accepting him as a patient.

When I received his laboratory results they were very limited — including only total and free testosterone, estradiol, FSH (but no LH), and an anemic blood chemistry panel. But what jumped out to me was that his total testosterone was below 200ng/ml (median 700ng/ml) and his FSH was below 0.1mIU/ml. In a 37-year-old male, this shouted out central hypogonadism. I called him back and asked if he had ever experienced any injuries to his body or head, at which point he said, "At 18, I was T-boned on the driver's side by another passenger vehicle, and my head hit the driver's window, shattering it." At that point he became a TBI patient and we ran a comprehensive TBI-hormonal evaluation panel, which found two central hormone issues. Within the first 30 days of his TBI protocol, he was feeling much better than he ever did on testosterone alone.

Another person called our office and talked with my incredibly astute office manager, Erin. Subsequent to that contact, the patient had filled out a TBImedlegal Intake Form where they indicated, "I just called your office to become a new patient for my long-term low thyroid problem that is not getting better. When I talked to your office (Erin) I was asked if I had experienced any head trauma. I was in fact involved in a head-on accident and my car was totaled. I did not know the relationship between head trauma and hormones." Instead of becoming a basic endocrine patient, she became a TBI patient and was found to have both central hypothyroidism and gonadotropic hormone deficiencies.

This brings up the importance of a comprehensive history as the prelude to optimal treatment. I believe that the underlying — and major cause of maturity onset hormonal dysfunctioning — is neurotrauma, not aging. In some individuals, it might be one major insult or the accumulation of many little ones that will influence the extent and nature of their hormonal homeostasis. Only through a comprehensive series of questions will we be able to elicit the presence of the predisposing event(s) that can precipitate central hormonal dysfunctioning. In some patients, there is a paucity of history to help pinpoint the timing of the precipitating event; but the labs tell no lies, and the symptoms follow suit.

Up to this chapter, you have learned the importance of the two phases of injury (primary and secondary), hormonal assessment and interpretation (the median rule), and the neuropsychiatric impact of neuro-hormonal deficiencies. The two main issues that will regulate the ability for improvement are the performance and interpretation of TBI-panel 3426 (also called Panel 1) and how to aggressively deal with a non-neuropermissive environment of inflammation and oxidative stress precipitated by the secondary phase of trauma. Failure to keep on track with both of these issues will yield a less than optimal response and poor recovery.

This chapter will present case studies that are geared to assist in the integration of each of these elements into a context that can be applied to all of your patients. We will present four major cases, and a few ancillary cases, to test your acumen and show you the way.

Goals of Treatment

It is obvious that the single most important goal of treatment is to return the individual to the closest proximity of their pre-injury status. The general expectation of the medical community is that the patient will achieve some degree of improvement with the use of medication, neuropsychiatric therapy, and rehabilitation. The belief that the patient will return to a pre-injury quality of life is looked at as unrealistic, especially after many years of treatment. After all, those that seek a non-traditional approach are usually many years post-TBI; therefore, it is assumed that their maximal achievable benefit has long since passed that elusive window of medical opportunity. Or has it?

There is always some modicum of improvement that can be achieved beyond that which was predicted, but the greatest magnitude of response will still be seen in those that receive evaluation and treatment soon after the precipitating injury. Exactly what "soon" means is impossible to define, since we have worked with patients 32 years post-TBI and their response was impossible to have predicted and some, if not most, unexpected. Therefore, since it is impossible to tell the patient that they "can/will" or "cannot/will not" expect some level of improvement, we only say that anything is possible and we are doing exactly what needs to be done, based upon results of laboratory testing and the support of current literature.

What is most important for the patient to understand is that we are not working off a palliative model, but on a rehabilitative one. We are not looking to cover-up the symptoms with medication that may make us feel good and do nothing for the underlying injury, but to provide a means by which there is the potential for regeneration and repair. The literature offers hope and direction in how best to provide the right biochemical environment (neuro-permissive environment) to help the brain regenerate some amount of what had been lost, and to protect the brain from any further damage. (6)

The inability of adult neurons to regrow after injury cannot be entirely attributed to intrinsic differences between adult CNS and all other neurons. As reported by Santiago Ramón y Cajal in 1928, based upon the research of Tallo (1911), it was shown that adult CNS neurons could regrow if they were provided access to the permissive environment of a conditioned sciatic nerve. Seventy years passed before Aguayo, in 1980, replicated those studies with new methods that definitively confirmed that adult CNS neurons have regenerative capabilities. This finding revealed that the failure of CNS neurons to regenerate was not an intrinsic deficit of the neuron, but rather a characteristic feature of the damaged environment (NNPE) that either did not support regeneration or prevented it. (7)

As was explained in Chapter 6 on the laboratory of TBI, our goal is to bring all the hormones (neurosteroids and neuroactive steroids) up toward the 75th percentile of the range and wait. The need for scheduled periodic laboratory testing is mandatory in order to monitor the patient's response to their specific protocol(s). Modification of a patient's initial treatment regimen, as well as all those that follow, is based upon serum testing. Failure to adhere to this concept can delay the onset of benefits, or delay the discovery of an impending problem. Again, we see patients on a monthly (1-3 months) basis for drawing labs, adjusting treatment, and adapting to the patients' needs with the addition of other supportive modalities of treatment.

In the earlier days of treatment, we did not have the level of success that we are encountering presently, which is due to our adherence to the established dogma pertaining to the interpretation of laboratory results. The ranges were gospel and the patients were pagans and therefore, we were listening to the wrong disciples. We frequently ignored the patient's remarks about how they felt just to treat the numbers. As failures mounted, newer articles grabbed at us to listen to the simplicity of the human race: We are all different but the same. Not everyone needs 60mg of testosterone. Some need 100mg, and others only 40mgs. How do you know if you don't try, or even consider it?

Physiologic versus Superphysiologic

For over 19 years, the concept of a physiologic treatment protocol has been at the foundation of how the Millennium has provided hormonal replenishment to its patients. Under this concept, the correction of the deficiency (or insufficiency) is achieved by replenishment of the hormone or hormones in question — with physiological doses — with the end-point being an optimal, physiological, median-normal level as seen in a healthy 25 to 35 year-old individual.

In terms of testosterone, the current and customary intramuscular dose is 200 to 300mg of Testosterone Cypionate (TC) once a week, once every two weeks, or even once a month. The problem with this is twofold: One, the dosing is beyond the physiological level and is more akin to that used by bodybuilders. Firstly, patients are not bodybuilders and there is no rationale to give such high does as described by the 1963 study, *Testosterone Production Rates in Normal Adults* (8) and the 1997 study, *Determination of Testosterone Production Rates in Men and Women Using Stable Isotope/Dilution and Mass Spectrometry.* (9) Testosterone, is produced in the human body at a rate of between 4mg to 11.8 mg daily in males (60mg/week) and 0.9 mg to 2.8 mg daily in females (20mg/week). These are the healthy physiologic amounts that need to be replenished.

Secondly, the use of a long-acting testosterone linked to esters such as Cypionate (36 to 48 hours), Enanthate (96 hours), or Undecanoate (200 hours) can cause them to circulate in the serum for days while they are needed in the brain — pronto. As a rule of thumb, seven times the average half-life of a compound is taken as the time it takes for that compound to be diminished into oblivion. Therefore, if you are dosing Testosterone Cypionate every two to four weeks, it drops into the background at 12.25 days. A more practical and beneficial approach would be to give a lower dose of a shorter acting testosterone more frequently, as we have done at the Millennium. Also, our monthly laboratory testing shows us objectively how efficiently low-dose testosterone therapy works.

With this said, there are reported benefits with the use of supraphysiological doses of testosterone, as in the article, *Testosterone Supplementation in Healthy Older Men Drives GH and IGF-I Secretion Without Potentiating Peptidyl Secretagogue Efficacy*. (10) Here, the high level of testosterone drives an increase in the production of growth hormone but, as a consequence of this high dose, there is an increase in the production of both estrogen (E2) and dihydrotestosterone (DHT). This occurs from the spike and induction of two enzymes: estradiol synthetase (ES) and 5-alpha-reductase (5AR). (11) This is the explanation accounting for the more rapid conversion of testosterone into E2 and DHT in those who have used or are using supraphysiological doses of testosterone. We do not get this response with physiological doses of testosterone in the range of 40 to 60mg/injection.

Under these conditions, an elevation in estrogen production in a male is usually met with a prescription for an aromatase inhibitor (anastrozole) and sometimes also an estrogen blocking agent (tamoxifen citrate). According to a number of well-written articles; Estrogen receptor alpha selectively modulates the waveform of GH secretory bursts in healthy women (12), they identified the presence of estradiol receptors (ERα) centrally, in both the hypothalamus and pituitary, that upregulates the production of growth hormone, as well as in the periphery. (13[1]) Also, in another article, *Tamoxifen Reduces Serum IGF-I* (14): the researchers found that Tamoxifen had a direct, dose-related, inhibitory effect on GH release from pituitary Somatotropes. It was cited that as small as a ten mumol/l dose consistently decreased both basal and growth hormone, releasing factor stimulated GH release — an inhibitory process of the hypothalamus (Somatostatin).

Therefore, when testosterone is used in supraphysiological doses, estradiol increases, an aromatase inhibitor is prescribed, and estradiol is reduced, thereby pulling down the normal production of growth hormone from the pituitary and suppressing IGF-1 from the liver. Additionally, the increase in estradiol can raise the risk of prostate cancer as documented in *Growth of LNCaP Human Prostate Cancer Cells Is Stimulated by Estradiol via Its*

Own Receptor (15) and can cause gynecomastia. So, how about just decreasing the amount of testosterone used?

In addition to the increase in estradiol from testosterone, there is also an increase in dihydrotestosterone (DHT) production, which is associated with oily skin, acne, hair loss, thinning of hair, enlargement of the prostate with concomitant increase in PSA, and shrinkage of the testes. (16) A response to this increase might be a prescription of finasteride or durastride. Unfortunately, both of these drugs pass through the blood-brain barrier down-regulating the enzyme 5-Alpha Reductase (5-AR), thereby inhibiting the conversion of Testosterone to DHT and progesterone to pregnanolone. The importance of DHT in the brain is its metabolites and their ability to modulate neuroreceptors, neurotransmission, and neurotransmitters like NMDA, Adenyl Cyclase, and the neuronal protection from pregnanolone and allopregnanolone. (17)

A comprehensive review of 73 papers on medical therapies for BPH was published on the site Indian Dermatology Online, with a focus on the effects of different pharmacological agents on sexual function. The review revealed that finasteride (Proscar) was associated with problems of ejaculation (2.1 to 7.7 percent), erection (4.9 to 15.8 percent), and libido (3.1 to 5.4 percent). (18) Yearly, we see two to three young men who were placed on a 5-AR blocker (5ARb) for protection of their hair, who subsequently developed erectile dysfunction and mild depression. These symptoms persisted for months after stopping the offending medication due to the long-term effect on neurosteroid production, which contributed to their symptoms. (19)

In The Prostate Cancer Prevention Trial (PCPT) reported in 2004, it conclusively stated that finasteride prevents or delays the detection of prostate cancer. They also identified one perplexing finding of more high-grade tumors in the finasteride treated group then in the controls. (20) These findings were subsequently challenged in 2009, stating that the results failed to take into account the alcohol consumption of those that developed prostatic cancer. (S20) How convenient!

Finally, in addition to catalyzing the rate-limiting step in the conversion of testosterone to DHT, both forms of the 5AR enzyme ($5AR^1$ and $5AR^2$) are responsible for the reduction of progesterone and deoxycorticosterone to dihydroprogesterone (DHP) and dihydrodeoxycorticosterone (DHDOC), respectively. (21) Recent data indicate that the subsequent 3-alpha-reduction of DHT, DHP and DHDOC produces steroid metabolites with rapid non-genomic effects on brain function and behavior (Gated-Ion Channels), primarily via an enhancement of γ-aminobutyric acid (GABA)-nergic inhibitory neurotransmission. (22)

Consistent with their ability to enhance the action of GABA at $GABA_A$ receptors, these neuroactive steroids possess anticonvulsant, antidepressant, and anxiolytic effects in addition to altering aspects of sexual- and alcohol-related behaviors. (23) Therefore, in a patient with TBI (or not) it is to their detriment to be placed on any of these products that pass through the blood brain barrier (BBB). The ideal way to avoid using these potentially counter-productive medications is to respect the body's needs for physiological dosing of not only testosterone but all hormones used in treatment of TBI and non-TBI patients.

Your success in treating TBI with testosterone can only be accomplished with attention to basic details involving feedback mechanisms of homeostasis throughout the body. This applies to both physiological and supraphysiological use of testosterone and its impact, and down-regulation of both DHEA-s and pregnenolone.

The ultimate loss of optimal levels of pregnenolone will not only decrease the production of DHEA-s, but will diminish the production of all downstream hormones that protect the brain from oxidative damage (allopregnanolone, progesterone, alloprogesterone, and their sulfated esters), induction of neuroregeneration (DHEA-s, GH, IGF-I,IGF-II, Estradiol), emotional stability (DHEA-s, DHEA, DHT, testosterone, GH, IGF-1), improve cognitive ability (DHT, testosterone, GH, IGF-1), augment immune protection (testosterone, DHEA-s, Estradiol,), extend cardiac protection (DHEA-s, DHT, Testosterone, Estradiol), and the adaptogenic benefits of cortisol and cortisone. (24)

Testosterone is regulated by luteinizing hormone (LH) through the conversion of cholesterol to 22-OH-Cholesterol (precursor to pregnenolone). High-normal and supraphysiological levels of testosterone will shut off LH production with a drop in both pregnenolone and DHEA in about four to six months. Concomitantly, there will be an increase (transient) in the level of cholesterol, since it will not be converted in the mitochondria (by P450scc) into pregnenolone. (25, 26)

While lecturing on Andropause (27[1]) to a group of physicians in Southeast Asia, one physician presented a case of a 47-year-old male with hypogonadism. The patient was started on low dose testosterone replenishment (60mg by weekly injections) and initially did very well until five months into his protocol. He felt as though the testosterone stopped working, so the doctor increased the dose to 80mg once a week without improvement. When I asked him if the patient was taking DHEA (25mg) and pregnenolone (30mg), he responded, "NO." Within two months of starting both of those omitted supplements, and dropping the testosterone back to 60mg a week, the patient's fatigue, depression, sense of well-being, physical stamina, and cognition all improved. Testosterone supplementation caused a negative feedback to shut down LH release, thereby decreasing all subsequently made hormones (neurosteroids).

Rational Treatment Based Upon Science

In the past twenty years, dozens of clinical trials for moderate to severe TBI have failed to produce beneficial responses in humans, in spite of the fact that over 130 drugs tested showed some efficacy in animal models of TBI. One major reason cited for these disappointing outcomes is that the complex and varied mechanisms associated with TBI are not being addressed by a single drug since the pathophysiology of TBI in humans is often much more heterogeneous and systemic, affecting many tissue systems and not just the brain itself. (28)

It is becoming more apparent, in the wake of these failures that an approach using multi-targeted pharmacotherapies holds more promise than drugs targeting specific pathobiological pathways (29), and that treatment may be optimized by combinations of agents acting on different mechanisms, or the same mechanisms, differently. (30, 31)

The natural tendency for expansion of the primary areas of damage (cavitation) can be tempered by the simultaneous use of neuroactive steroids and neurosteroids, and select supplements working synergistically to minimize oxidative damage and to promote neuroregeneration. (32) The success of Millennium's TBI protocols has been derived from applying these tenets using a multi-therapeutic approach with replenishment of all hormones to optimal physiological levels. Under the biological stress of injury, the brain is being attacked by a diversity of chemicals that, if unchallenged, will lead to further oxidative stress, cavitation, excitotoxicity, neurostimulation, and worsening of social functioning. (33[1])

No discussion of treatment in TBI would be complete without something being said about hypothermia, the process of chilling the body in an attempt to slow or stop damaging biochemical processes. The history of hypothermia predates modern medicine by thousands of years when Hippocrates (460 to 375 BC) advised "to surround badly wounded patients with ice and snow to reduce blood loss." Chinese physicians, Hua To (110 to 207 AD) submerged febrile patients in a stone trough filled with cold water as treatment. Robert Boyle (1672) James Currie (1798) and William Osler (1849 to 1919) all tried hypothermia as a treatment of typhoid fever. William Osler claimed a 17 percent absolute decrease in mortality, as published in the Johns Hopkins Medical News in 1892. (34)

The article, *Outcome Measures for Clinical Trials in Neuro-trauma* (2002), reviewed 40 years of research looking at different treatment modalities and the responses to medication and hypothermia in neurotrauma. Each study ended in what is referred to as "futility failure," where the studies were terminated prematurely due to the failure of the specific treatment to achieve at least a ten percent benefit to the patient, or the status of the patient worsened. (35) Dozens of medications were randomly tried — atropine, barbiturates, PEG-SOD, Nimodipine, tromethamine, to name a few — some with improvement in animal models, but none with significant benefit in human trials. (36)

In an NIH program called the American Hypothermia Trial, 390 patients were enrolled to test out Dr. Guy Clifton's theory on the benefits of hypothermia in TBI. Unfortunately, the trial reported a combined 27 percent overall mortality rate for the control and hypothermia-treated groups, and the pattern of complications and the causes of death have been similar to those reported in other severe head injury trials. No beneficial effect for prophylactic hypothermia was seen, but intracranial pressure (ICP) was lower in the cooled patients. (37)

A prior multicenter randomized study of surface induced moderate hypothermia in 392 patients with acute TBI showed no benefit (Clifton, 2001). In that study, hypothermia was induced at 4.3 to 1.1 hours after injury, and patients reached 33°C by 8.4 hours to three hours after injury. Hypothermia was maintained for 48 hours, and then patients were slowly rewarmed. Patients randomized to the hypothermia arm experienced an increased number of days with critical complications as compared to normothermia patients. (38)

Over 2,920 articles on hypothermia and traumatic brain injury have been added to the medical literature archives since 2008 (through January 2013). A recent review of these studies addressed the findings that treatment with hypothermia, with the body temperature reaching 33°C within eight hours after injury, is not effective in improving outcomes in patients with severe brain injury. (39)

Core Hormone Replacement

The approach taken in this chapter is based upon a number of case presentations with analyses. Information that has been presented throughout this text will be reasserted in relation to each case. In this manner, case scenarios, corresponding laboratory interpretation, and treatment protocols will be synchronized into a digestible and therefore, usable approach. Many of these case presentations come directly from our patient population and others are contrived to provide provocative approaches to both interpretation and treatment. (T9.1)

Hormone	Median M	Median F	Hormone	Median M	Median F
DHEA-s	200 ug/dL	277 ug/dL	Growth Hormone	5.0 ng/ml	5.0 ng/ml
T-Testosterone	690 ng/ml	44 ng/ml	IGF-1	200 ng/ml	200 ng/ml
F-Testosterone	14 pg/ml	2-4 pg/ml	IGFBP-3	4000 ng/ml	4000 ng/ml
DHT	52 ng/dl	<30 ng/ml	TSH	2.5 mcu/ml	2.5 mcu/ml
SHBG	45 pg/ml	75 ng/dl	fT4	1.5 ng/ml	1.5 ng/ml
Estrone	<60 pg/ml	<200 pg/ml	fT3	250 ng/dL	250ng/dL
Estradiol	25 pg/ml	90 pg/ml	rT3	165 ng/dL	165 ng/dL
Progesterone	0.8 ng/ml	5-7 ng/ml	fT3/rT3 Ratio	>1.06	>1.06
Pregnenolone	210 ng/dl	210 ng/dl	TPO	< 35 IU/ml	< 35 IU/ml
Vitamin D3	60 ng/dl	60 ng/dl	ACTH (am)	< 35 pg/ml	< 35 pg/ml
LH	5.1 mIU/ml	22 mIU/ml	Cortisol (am)	< 15 ug/dl	< 15 ug/dl
FSH	7.0 mIU/ml	8.6 mIU/ml	Cortisol (pm)	7.3 Ug/dl	7.3 Ug/dl
Prolactin	11.25 ng/ml	13.75 ng/ml	Insulin	< 25 miu/L	< 25 miu/L

Table 9.1: These are the median "normal" blood result from Access Medical Laboratories of Florida that we use to guide our interpretations. Please note that female hormone results need to be correlated to the on-set of their menses if still cycling. Otherwise, the numbers used here are for peri- and post-menopausal women.

Although we have organizationally presented the major hormones in four groups (growth factors, gonadotropins, thyroid, and adrenal), it is absolutely impossible (for me) to discuss any one group or member of a group in isolation without having a discussion on the multiple links that exists amongst them. To avoid the potential of confusion, we will start at a core approach and then spiral out into a more comprehensive understanding of how multifaceted and interactive each hormone's roll is in our well-being and resolve of TBI symptomatology. Remember, in reference to laboratory levels (Table 9.1, above), we are looking to accomplish an above the median result for each of the major hormones that are measured. Notwithstanding, there are a few results that we want below the median — like estrogens in males, and DHT in females. These issues will be discussed where appropriate, based upon the merits and gender of the case.

The lecture seminar associated with this publication is intended to provide an educational forum to solidify and accelerate your understanding and application of the information contained within. It is our goal and the demand of those suffering with the sequelae from TBI to help you approach their needs with the greatest of impact on their recovery and therefore, quality of life. It might appear to be complex or convoluted at first look, and you would be right, but there is a simplified means of grabbing the horns without being gored. Read on....

Growth Hormone Axis

Growth hormone, in my estimation, is the most unifying hormone in our body. It is pervasive or ubiquitous in not only being found in every cell and tissue in our body, but has influence over every other hormone and process therein. It exhibits both genetic and epigenetic capabilities just like we are finding with all the hormones. With that being said, growth hormone (GH) is not a hormone to be taken lightly — in that its presence is not of a secondary nature, but it is the captain of our preservation, perseverance, and regeneration. (40[1])

In a patient with compromised growth hormone homeostasis, the levels of GH will be below the median, which will also translate into low ranges of both IGFs and BPs (below the median). In patients with selective damage to the hypothalamus, you might find just the opposite with high levels of GH, IGFs, and BPs. This can be due to specific damage to the periventricular nucleus (41) where somatostatin (SS or SRIF) is produced. The loss of SS production will disable the negative feedback regulation of GH allowing for its unregulated production and release. (42)

Knowing that the half-life of GH is 20 minutes, IGF-1 about eight to ten minutes, and IGFBP-3 between 20 and 24 hours, gives us a better understanding of what to anticipate in terms of measured levels over time. We know that the majority of GH is produced between 8:00 p.m. and 4:00 a.m. and is carried by Growth hormone binding protein which is postulated to be derived from the extracellular portion of the GH receptor (S1). So, by the morning, we will anticipate that the level will be low or low-normal. In fact, the majority of our patients' results are between 0.5ng/ml and 0.05ng/ml, making a low morning reading a normal occurrence. On the other hand, IGF-1 has the carrier IGFBP-3, which can extend the half-life from ten minutes up to 20 to 24 hours. So, in the morning, it is not unusual to find levels of IGF-1 of 200ng/ml and above, even with an apparently low measured level of GH. Therefore, the long half-life of BP-3 makes it (IGFBP-3) the most reliable marker for assessing the adequacy of GH production. (43)

The importance of understanding the roll of IGFBP-3 in the GH/IGF-1 axis was illustrated in the paper by Baxter (44) where BP-3 was responsible for binding 95 percent of the IGF-I and IGF-II, making it the major carrier of IGFs in plasma. The principal function of IGFBP-3 therefore, is to extend the half-life of free IGFs and to regulate their availability for cellular use. Additionally, the serum level of IGFBP-3 appeared to be a constant over 24 hours, and was found to be GH dependent, which makes the detection of IGFBP-3 very useful in the evaluation of GH secretion. Furthermore, a single BP-3 measurement correlates significantly with the logarithm of the integrated spontaneous GH secretion. (45) This means that when GH is secreted, there is a corresponding production of IGFBP-3 by the liver, making its measurement mandatory when using a growth hormone secretagogue like Secretropin® (SRx).

Growth Hormone — General Recommendations

As indicated in Table 9.1 above, the ideal goal of treatment will be to bring GH to about 5ng/ml, IGF-1 to greater than 200ng/ml, and the IGFBP-3 level to greater than 4000 ng/ml. In reality, if the IGF-1 level is above 200ng/ml with an IGFBP-3 above 4000ng/ml then the morning GH level can be at any level. This is because whatever amount of GH was secreted during its peak production period has induced ideal levels of IGF-1 and IGFBP-3 production by the liver. However, this concept can be a "bitter pill" that is difficult to swallow. We normally look at lab results without considering any relevance to circadian rhythm; thereby, expecting everything to be at a constant and steady state. Not the case with growth hormone or other hormones with diurnal variations (cortisol, for one).

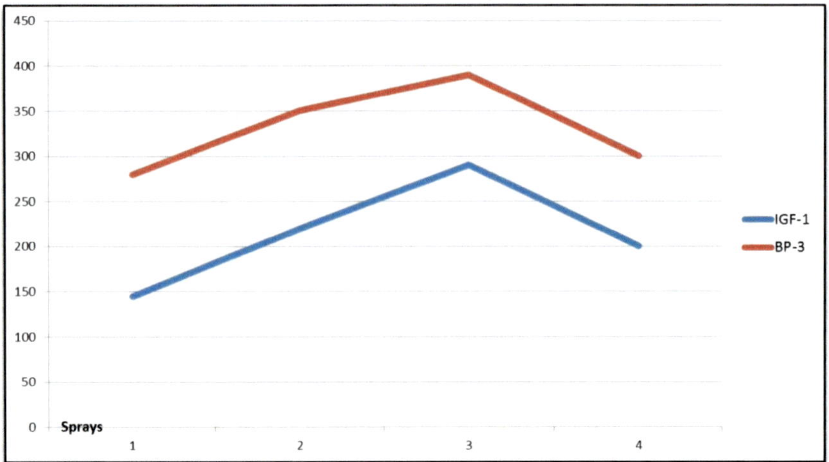

Graph 9.1: Response curve to progressive increases in Secretropin dosing over 3 months.

In our conservative approach to the initial treatment of patients with GH deficiency, or partial deficiency (insufficiency), we tend to start with a secretagogue for a period of three months. The rationale behind this is threefold: (1) legal hurdles to prescribing GH, (2) high cost per month, and (3) impact of recombinant human growth hormone (rhGH) use on the endogenous production of growth hormone.

Legally, in order to prescribe growth hormone, the physician must perform one of the growth hormone challenge tests (46) to be in compliance with the "standards of care." Failure to perform a challenge test can have grave consequences on the longevity of a physician's license to practice. Cost-wise, growth hormone continues to increase in price beyond most patients' reach. Finally, as shown by Muller and Locatelli (47), within 48 hours of using growth hormone there is 40 percent suppression of endogenous GH production and by 30 days, a 100 percent reduction. This means that eventually 100 percent of the circulating GH is derived from an exogenous source (the injections), leaving the individual's natural production suppressed. This is why so many individuals using growth hormone have a difficult time when they want to stop.

Secretropin® is our product of choice for these reasons: (1) I helped develop it in 2001, (2) it uses a number of neuroendocrine pathways to stimulate GH production, not just one, (3) it has a 100 percent natural composition, (4) it became a physician-only dispensed product in 2006, (5) two clinical studies show its effectiveness in 90 percent of patients, and (6) it is cost effective. National distribution is by University Compounding

Specialty of San Diego, California, USA (attention: Ms. Susan Dolinger 866-444-9475) and internationally by Millennium Health Centers, Inc. of Encino, California USA; (Secretropin@gmail.com).

We initially start treatment with Secretropin® at two sprays under the tongue (2015 protocol), which is held for one minute before swallowing. This is done for 30 days and then a blood test is drawn to look at the response levels of GH, IGF-1 and BP-3. When compared to the initial levels, if there is an increase in IGFBP-3, it is an indication that GH production was increased; therefore, deferring the need to use injectable GH. Remember that: IGFBP-3 has the longest half-life, it is logarithmically related to the GH pulses, and it carries IGF-1. Therefore, the ideal pattern to find will be one that has an elevation of both IGFBP-3 and IGF-1.

It is important that you also understand the other potential patterns of a Secretropin® induced response so that you do not jump to any conclusion about it not working. Secretropin® works within the regulatory system of the hypothalamic-pituitary GH/IGF-1 axis; therefore, if GH goes up above the set point (threshold) it triggers the production and release of Somatostatin, causing a drop in GH, IGF-1, and BP-3. Lowering the nighttime dose of Secretropin® is all that is required.

Other reasons why Secretropin® has failed to increase IGF and BP-3 production are: (1) pituitary trauma, (2) failure to hold the sprays under the tongue for one minute, (3) acute liver disease, and (4) certain medication or supplements (such as melatonin, DHEA, dopamine, and testosterone) can increase GH production so that the set-point limit is breached more readily (S2).

In regard to acute liver disease, we have a GE VScan™ unit in the office to perform bedside ultrasounds to look for issues of hepatic cysts, fatty degeneration, and any other hepatic pathology. More times than not, it comes up negative; however, it has found Peliosis hepatis associated with abusive levels of testosterone, as well as many with fatty liver degeneration.

In our lecture on the use of Secretropin® we discuss how to increase and decrease the number of sprays based upon the patient's response as reflected in production of GH, IGF-1, and BP-3. If the levels go down when the patient is using three sprays a night, it means that we have caused a negative feedback, thereby increasing somatostatin (SS) production. Increased SS will cause a drop in GH production and release.

To correct this, we decrease from three sprays a night to two sprays a night, following the hold for 60 seconds before swallowing. We keep decreasing the number of sprays from three to one, as directed by the patient's response to its use.

On the other hand, if there is an increase of IGF-1 and IGFBP-3 on three sprays a night, we increase to four sprays opting to reach the highest production of GH as possible. We know that we have exceeded the regulatory mechanism (threshold tolerance) when increasing the number of sprays causes a sudden drop in the amount of GH factors made.

We have also developed a combination protocol that uses low-dose rhGH in the morning and Secretropin® at bed time. If the patient has had benefit from the use of Secretropin® (SRx), it can be combined with rhGH in the following manner: ½ IU of GH in the morning and two to three sprays of SRx at bedtime. The rationale behind this is that the composition of SRx® not only decreases the production of SS, but also stimulates other pathways to maintain the tonus of the anterior pituitary and the production of GH. This is important when rhGH is discontinued and the natural production of GH has been suppressed so long that it might take up to if not more than a year for GH production to restart.

Glucagon Stimulation Test (GST)

In the event that the secretagogue (Secretropin®) does not give an optimal response, we will offer the patient a glucagon stimulation test (GST). The GST was initially described as a four-hour test, but recent studies have suggested that the test could be shortened to a three-hour test, and that serum GH levels can be evaluated at five time points (zero, 90, 120, 150, and 180 minutes) as the majority of GH peaks occurred between 120 and 180 minutes (85 percent) after the glucagon injection. (48)

The procedure involves the patient coming into the office on a twelve-hour fast (or so) at which time a baseline serum GH level is drawn (Time Zero). You can place an indwelling catheter, a butterfly, or single needle sticks with a Vacutainer® system to get blood. Subsequent to the baseline blood draw, a subcutaneous injection of 1mg of glucagon is given for a patient weighing less than 90kg and 1.5mg for over 90kg. Blood is drawn according to the simplified protocol, with results according to a study by Berg, which revealed an optimal peak GH cutoff value of 2.5 ng/mL with 95 percent sensitivity and 79 percent specificity (this has been rounded up to 3.0 ng/ml). (49) The most common side effects experienced during the

GST included: nausea, vomiting, and headaches and have been reported to range from less than ten percent to 34 percent. In our offices we rarely see any reactions other than caffeine withdrawal for those who have missed their morning coffee.

As an aside, the GST can also function as an adrenal challenge test to evaluate the patient for adrenal insufficiency (adrenal fatigue). Cortisol levels are drawn along with GH and the cutoff is 3ug/dl (100 nmol/liter), which provides high reliability for the diagnosis of adrenal insufficiency. (50)

Once the results are in, a report is written addressing the patient's history (TBI), symptomatology, results of the test, and your decision to place them on a trial of growth hormone for three to six months. Many times, the report is submitted to the insurance company who rejects it because you failed to use the "gold standard" test called the ITT — insulin tolerance test. (51) If you indicate in your report that the ITT was not chosen because the patient has had a TBI and that there is a chance of seizure, or that they have coronary artery disease with prior cardiac event(s), they might accept it. (See the supplement to this book entitled, *Office Documentation for TBI.*)

If Secretropin® has failed completely (an issue somewhere in the HP axis), then use a low-dose regimen of rhGH starting with 1/2IU (.334mg) of recombinant human growth hormone (rhGH) for either male or female, and adjust up in 1/4IU steps at one month intervals until optimal levels are achieved.

Monitoring: We tend to monitor our patients closely during the first three months of treatment with labs once a month (1-3 months). Many of the patients have their blood drawn remotely, and then a report is written and sent to them. Their follow-up visits can be in the office, by Skype, or phone call.

Laboratory Testing: (1) GH, (2) IGF-1, (3) IGFBP-3, (4) DHEA-s, and (5) free testosterone.

Side Effects: Due to GH's involvement in all the major processes throughout the body, there are a number of potential side effects that can be transient and therefore, avoidable. Hence, the need to move up, and not down, with the dosing of growth hormone:

(A) A potential early occurrence of fluid retention (high-dose and high-salt intake).

(B) Fatigue secondary to an increase in IGF-1, which has a ten percent crossover to insulin receptors (hypoglycemia). This can manifest in patients with complaints of fatigue, headaches or change in sleep pattern. This is why an insulin level is important in the pretreatment laboratory testing.

(C) Additionally, GH is associated with lipolysis, thereby increasing blood lipid levels, which can also exacerbate insulin levels in a patient with known metabolic syndrome. Since this is all individualized, dose-dependent responses will need you to be vigilance in order to respond appropriately.

(D) Elevation in blood glucose, secondary to lipolysis, with blocking of insulin receptors may lead to a diagnosis of metabolic syndrome. Check the chromium levels.

Gonadotropins:

We have decided to group the reproductive hormones (testosterone, estrogen, and progesterone) under this heading since in terms of TBI treatment protocols; they have highly synergistic roles to play. Additionally, we have found that the term "reproductive hormones" might be a misnomer (56), as is the case with vitamin D, now a Seco-hormone (57), since these hormones have been found to regulate many neurocognitive, neuroregenerative, neurosynaptic, neo-neurogenic, and neuroprotective functions within the CNS, as well as structural and protective functions outside the CNS. In the twenty-three years that I have focused on the non-reproductive aspects of hormones (TBI related), I would venture a guess that they function 40 to 60 percent of the time on other important bodily functions, and not just sex.

Furthermore, these same hormones produced in the periphery have been found to also be produced by glial cells of the CNS. The expanding recognition of the significant roles that these neuroactive (NAS) and neurosteroids (NS) have on neuropsychology and neurophysiology make them an important consideration in both laboratory assessment, and in all treatment protocols. (58)

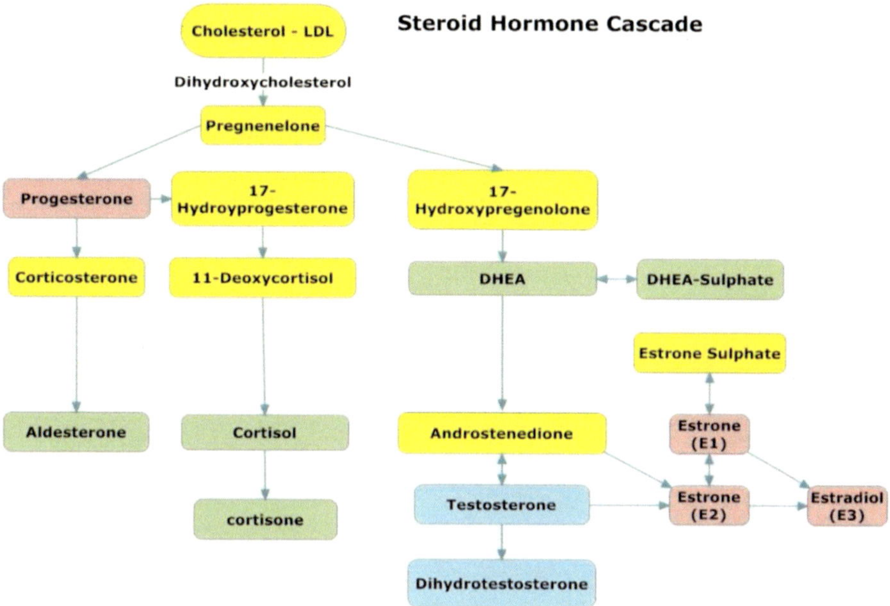

Chart 9.1: The Steroid Hormone Cascade shows the relationship and metabolism of cholesterol to all the important neuroactive steroids produced in the peripheral glands and also those produced as neurosteroids in the brain.

Testosterone

The optimal goal with replenishment of testosterone is to get the highest level of free testosterone into the patient's brain, which is determined by the type of testosterone and the route of its delivery. In the brain, testosterone becomes a significant neuroactive steroid, promoting improvement in the limbic system (amygdala) (59), and hippocampus (memory, both recent and remote) to name a few, while its major metabolites [dihydrotestosterone and estradiol (60)] influence neuronal survival, regeneration, synaptogenesis, and decrease oxidative stress related damage. (61) Testosterone has also been found to stimulate CD+4 cells, thereby inducing increase in IL-10 and the reduction of inflammatory cytokines and interleukins. (62)

Aside from its overt importance in human sexuality, testosterone has a range of benefits influencing cognitive functioning and memory, neurobehavior (63), immunity and inflammation, cardiovascular protection, wound healing, and muscle strength and maintenance that overshadow its sexual functions. What is apparent now is that our "sex hormones" have a greater responsibility in all aspects of our bodily functions and well-being.

Testosterone Treatment

The Millennium has divided the treatment of males with hypogonadism into two classifications: the below forty and the above forty classifications. Our general assumption is that those below forty have not finished having a family, while those above have. Nevertheless, we always verify and have them sign a "Testosterone Disclosure and Waiver" form, which acknowledges all the possible side effects from the chronic use of testosterone. I am happy to say that since we use physiological doses of testosterone and perform scheduled laboratory testing, we rarely run into any of the listed issues. But we monitor consistently.

In the case of a male under 40 years of age, we will use one of the following protocols: (1) HCG 500IU a day, (2) Clomid® 50mg a day, or (3) HCG 500IU five days a week with Clomid® 50mg five days a week. The decision as to which one to use will be based upon cost and patient compliance issues. Sometimes, an oral medication is selected over the injectable. I personally have not been able to decide which protocol is better than the other since results are unpredictable. If either the HCG or the Clomid® fails to perform in a single agent approach, I will combine them as stated. Recently, we have had very good results using a lower dose regimen of 50mg Clomid® on a Monday-Wednesday-Friday schedule.

In those males over 40 who have an established family, vasectomy, homosexuals, or just plain lazy, we will discuss the different forms of testosterone that are available. Based upon their lifestyle, and perception of ease of life issues, we choose a manner in which to pursue a physiologic level of testosterone.

In women, the same issues apply, as do the many options for treatment. Generally speaking, we frequently add testosterone to their intra-vaginal hormone creams, as will be discussed in Case 2 and also under the section labeled: Estradiol (E2): Estrone (E1) and Progesterone Treatment.

Regardless of the patient's age, we will offer them a provocative testosterone test (PTT). This consists of giving a male 60mg, or a female

20mg, of our proprietary blend of testosterone (Cypionate and propionate) as an intramuscular or subcutaneous injection. These dosages represent the average weekly testosterone production in a healthy male and female, respectively. We use the PTT as a means of teaching the patient, in the office, how to perform a hygienic self-injection of testosterone and, just as important, to see how they respond to a physiological dose of testosterone.

Once the patient has injected themselves, they are given a *PTT-Questionnaire* to fill out in five to seven days, at which time they email the form back to our office and we arrange a brief phone or Skype conversation to review their response. We also decide on a treatment protocol based upon their results.

In the event that the patient does not have significant benefits from the initial injection, we will invite them back for a second injection. This occurs in about five percent of the patients, and almost 100 percent of them experience a benefit when given a second shot. It is important that you do not give up if the first shot does not work. Not everyone responds to what we call a "physiological dose" of medication; but, for the most, they do. Also, do not assume that supraphysiological dosing of testosterone is the only way to get a response. You will get a response along with the potential of side effect like acne, gynecomastia, clitoromegaly, excessive estrogen, and mood swings.

How to Inject

We use a 5/8", 25gauge, 1cc, zero-waste needle from BD. Our proprietary testosterone is compounded privately by UCP of San Diego for our patients. Our associate physicians that want to use our Tc/Tp 200mg/cc product must receive authorization from our office. Otherwise, we do not share the product with non-participating physicians. Since this is a compounded product, we use a depo-testosterone (Cypionate) in the office to teach the patient how to self-inject in their thigh. Many patients are initially hesitant to stick a needle into their own body due to the anxiety of pain. With support and clear directions, and rarely shouting, "Do it now," the patient will inject themselves and frequently respond with, "I didn't even feel it."

When we do have that follow-up phone/Skype call, we are looking for noticeable responses that include improvement in each of the three sections that they are being assessed; psychological, physiological and physical. There is also one question that addresses the duration of their responses in days. This will help us to establish if they will do well on a one shot a week regimen or if a shot "every-third-day" regimen will be better. Based upon the summation of this interaction, we decide if the benefits outweigh the risks, then we place them on the agreed weekly dose regimen. After one month, and every month thereafter, the patient fills out a *Monthly Program Questionnaire (MPQ)*. Labs are drawn based upon the program, and any changes that have occurred in the interim.

In the past three years, we have been moving patients from a weekly 60mg of testosterone to the 40mg every third day protocol — with much better quality of life responses. This has recently influenced our prescribing pattern to preference the every-third-day protocol. There is less drop-off (sudden loss of testosterone effects) and further control of estradiol and DHT because we lowered the spike-effect (sudden rise in testosterone induces 5-Alpha reductase and estradiol synthetase).

Soon you will hear about Testosome® 2 percent, a compounded form of oral testosterone gel (emulsion). Using nanoliposomal technology, the Millennium Health Centers, Inc. has developed a carrier that takes a highly lipophilic material (testosterone) and delivers it into an ultra-nanoliposomal emulsion that is carried rapidly into the blood from the oral, esophageal, and gastric mucosa. Clinical testing shows a 200 percent increase in base line blood levels for total testosterone and a 237 percent increase in free testosterone levels in just one hour. The majority of patients have also noted a remarkable increase in mental and physical energy, a sense of well-being, confidence, improved focus, cognitive enhancement, and some with increased libido. All these taking place within 60 minutes of a ten to 20mg dose.

Unfortunately, the rapid clearance of nanoliposomal-testosterone from the blood means that it needs to be taken on a daily regimen. This also means that it can be easily titrated to the needs of the patient without the risk of long-term effects since the half-life is so short. At present, the recommended dosing is one pump (10mg) for women over 40 years and two pumps (20mg) for men over 40 year of age.

This will be available in mid-2016 from a number of major compounding laboratories.

Topical Testosterone

Topical testosterone, as a cream or gel, when placed on the skin is converted at a rate from 20 to 40 percent to dihydrotestosterone (DHT) by the 5-alpha reductase (5-α Reductase) present in the hair follicles. This greatly reduces the amount of free testosterone delivered to the blood that can be available to pass through the blood brain barrier to convert to the neuroactive steroid DHT. Patients who use topical testosterone usually have elevated levels of DHT, which accounts for thinning of the hair, oily skin and acne, enlargement of the prostate with increased PSA, and testicular atrophy. (64) Additionally, DHT acts as a hematopoietic agent causing an increase in the red cell mass, which can cause thickening of the blood due to polycythemia. (65)

Testosterone Product	Application	Serum Level	Comments
AndroGel 1%	1-4 Pumps/day	T(T) 500-800 ng/dl	**Apply to shoulder or upper arms only.**
AndroGel 1.62%	1 pump/day	T(T) 350-800 ng/dl	**High DHT and Estradiol levels.**
Testim 1% Gel	5-10 grams/day	T(T) 500-800 ng/dl	**High DHT and Estradiol levels.**
TestoCream 10%	½- 1 gram a day	F(T) 12-14 ng/dl	**Apply to flank if not in contact with others.**
Testosterone Cypionate	M: 40-80mg/wk F: 10-30mg/wk	T(T) 500-800 ng/dl F(T) 12-14 ng/dl	**Weekly subcutaneous or IM injection.**
Testosterone Cypionate Testosterone Propionate		T(T) 500-800 ng/dl F(T) 12-14 ng/dl	**Most physiologic and consistent level of Free (T) with quick on-set of actions. Low aromatization. 40-80mg a week in single or divided dose every 3rd day. (40mg Q3rd day)**
Testosterone Pellets	Based upon weight	T(T) 500-000 ng/dl F(T) 12-14 ng/dl	**Initial high levels dropping over 4-6 months. Can't remove once implanted.**
Testosterone Troches	M: 25-50mg BID 3/wk F: 12.5-25mg BID 3/wk	T(T) 500-800 ng/dl F(T) 12-14 ng/dl	**Short half-life. Frequent dosing needed.**
Testosome 2%	M: 10-20mg Qday F: 5-10mg Qday	M: F(T) 12-14 ng/dl F: F(T) 2-4 ng/dl	**Excellent absorption. CNS benefits dominate with improved focus, concentration, decreased depression, rise in libido, and increased mental energy.**

Table 9.3: Testosterone products Learn all of these options to offer to the patient based upon their comfort and life style. Encourage the patient to experience a number of these options.

The recommended daily dose of topically applied testosterone can vary between five to ten grams of a ten percent gel. Adequacy of treatment has commonly been based upon the amount of total testosterone, although for treatment in TBI cases it is the free testosterone that provides us with the level of responses that have made our protocols successful — this finding, thanks in part to one of my mentors, and a hell of a nice man, Dr. Ronald Swerdloff, Professor of Medicine, David Geffen School of Medicine at UCLA, Chief Division of Endocrinology, Harbor-UCLA Medical Center, Senior Investigator Los Angeles Biomedical Research Institute. (66)

Sublingual Testosterone (Lozenges)

Sublingual testosterone (lozenges) is another approach to replenishment through the oral cavity with testosterone suspended in sesame oil as drops or in paraffin lozenges or troches. These work well at delivering free testosterone rapidly into the blood, but have a short half-life of about four hours. Therefore, these must be dosed once or twice a day and between three to five days a week, if not daily. They are associated with spiking levels of free testosterone and elevation in estradiol (E2). Dosing must be individualized since absorption is erratic. Once the ideal dosing is established, the benefits are quite impressive.

We start males on 25 to 50mg(¼ to ½ of a 100mg lozenge) once or twice a day, three days a week to start, and then increase the number of days based upon the patient's response — and not blood levels of free testosterone. Blood levels of testosterone [f(T), t(T), DHT, and E2] are done on the morning of the off day (if taking on Monday-Wednesday-Friday, draw blood on Tuesday or Thursday).

We start females on 12.5 to 25mg(¼ to ½ of a 50mg lozenge) once or twice a day, three days a week to start, and then increase the number of days based upon the patient's response — and not blood levels of free testosterone. Blood levels of testosterone [f(T), t(T), DHT, and E2] are done on the morning of the off day (if taking on Monday-Wednesday-Friday, draw blood on Tuesday or Thursday).

Testosterone by Injection

Testosterone by injection is my most common approach to the solution of insufficiency or deficiency associated with TBI. It allows for weekly adjustment in the dosing based upon the patient's subjective response and their serum level. Most important here is that the dose of testosterone given is physiologic. In the subsection, *Physiologic versus Supraphysiologic*, we learned that 60mg is an ideal dose to start in 70 percent of our patient population. That is to start! Within one week of the patient's initial dose of testosterone, they fill out a *Provocative Testosterone Testing (PTT) Questionnaire.* Based upon the response, the dose is either optimal and needs no change, thereby continuing on a once a week injection, or the patient goes to step two testosterone replenishment. This consists of placing the patient on 40mg of our blended testosterone every third day. This protocol actually turns out to be the best in terms of low dose and optimal physiological levels.

Testosterone Implants (Pellets)

The insertion of testosterone pellets is a simple office procedure that can be an ideal solution for some individuals with testosterone insufficiency. The number of pellets and the total milligrams of testosterone placed into the subcutaneous tissue vary based upon the patient's weight, age, liver functions, and lifestyle. Many times, this calculation works to the patient's benefit, but sometimes it is inaccurate leading to either hyper- or hypo-testosterone states. Therefore, it is wise to initially start the patient on intramuscular or subcutaneous injections of Testosterone Cypionate weekly for a few months to see how the patient responds, then to use the dosage as the means of selecting the pellets.

General Testosterone Recommendations

Females: Start with a 20 to 30mg IM injection of blended testosterone (Propionate and Cypionate) when the patient is in the office. This is the provocative testing we use to see if the patient has a beneficial or adverse response to the hormone, and that the normal physiologic dose is adequate for the patient. Give them the *PTT Questionnaire* (as discussed above), and follow-up by phone in five to seven days.

Males: Start with a 60 to 80mg IM injection of blended testosterone (Propionate and Cypionate) when the patient is in the office. This is the provocative testing we use to see if the patient has a beneficial or adverse response to the hormone and that the normal physiologic dose is adequate for the patient. Give them the *PTT Questionnaire* (as discussed above), and follow-up by phone in five to seven days.

Side Effects: Due to the low-dose protocol, we infrequently encounter: oily skin, acne, testicular atrophy, or elevation in PSA with prostatic enlargement. Also, the reason why we try not to use testosterone in males less than 40, or those without a family, is to avoid azoospermia and infertility.

Monitoring: We tend to monitor our patients closely during the first three months of treatment with labs once a month. Many of the patients have their blood drawn and a report on their chart before follow-up. When in the office, we can immediately adjust their protocol, based upon the results as opposed to a one to two week delay in any adjustments.

Laboratory Testing: (1) free testosterone, (2) total testosterone, (3) DHEA-s, (4) DHT, and (5) estradiol (E2).

In the years that the Millennium has existed, we have never used Arimidex® (anastrozole) because our effective low dose regimen of testosterone supplemented with zinc citrate (50mg twice a day) controls estrogen production. (67, 68)

Finasteride

Finasteride is the first 5α-reductase inhibitor that received clinical approval for the treatment of human benign prostatic hyperplasia (BPH) and androgenetic alopecia (male pattern hair loss). These clinical applications are based on the ability of finasteride to inhibit the Type II isoform of the 5α-reductase enzyme, which is the predominant form in human prostate and hair follicles, and the concomitant reduction of testosterone to dihydrotestosterone. (71)

In addition to catalyzing the rate-limiting step in the reduction of testosterone, both isoforms of the 5α-reductase enzyme are responsible for the reduction of progesterone and deoxycorticosterone to dihydroprogesterone (DHP) and dihydrodeoxycorticosterone (DHDOC), respectively. Recent preclinical data indicate that the subsequent 3α-reduction of DHT, DHP, and DHDOC produces steroid metabolites with rapid non-genomic effects on brain function and behavior, primarily via an enhancement of ɣ-aminobutyric acid (GABA)nergic inhibitory neurotransmission. Consistent with their ability to enhance the action of GABA at $GABA_A$ receptors, these steroid derivatives (termed neuroactive steroids) possess anticonvulsant, antidepressant and anxiolytic effects in addition to altering aspects of sexual- and alcohol-related behaviors. (72)

Therefore, the use of either finasteride or durastride will lead to potential clinical changes in the neurosteroids produced centrally, as well as those neuroactive steroids produced peripherally. In our practice, we have seen cases of central impotency, depression, cognitive impairment, as well as clinical studies addressing cases of cardiovascular disease associated with their use. (73)

Therefore, the option here is to use natural products such as saw palmetto (74), Pygeum Africanum (75) and pumpkin seed extracts, which have all been found to regulate the 5-alpha-reductase gene.

Estradiol (E2), Estrone (E1), Pregnenolone, and Progesterone

General Estrogen/ Regulatory crosstalk between estrogens and progesterone are too interwoven to allow for a separate discussion on each merit. Nonetheless, the presence of a condition referred to by Dr. John Lee as estrogen dominance is an important subject to broach at this time. (76)

Estrogen dominance is an increasingly problematic issue being experienced by young menstruating women, as well as poorly treated and monitored peri- and menopausal women.

Gamma-aminobutyric acid (GABA) is an inhibitory neuro-transmitter. Estradiol inhibits GABA activity in the cerebellum, hippocampus, and hypothalamus. (77) Progesterone on the other hand modulates anxiety, and these effects are probably mediated by its metabolite allopregnanolone. This neurosteroid potentiates the inhibitory actions of GABA by modulation of the $GABA_A$ receptor. (78) The net affect when progesterone and its metabolites dominate is calm, while the reverse is true when estradiol dominates.

Progesterone and allopregnanolone administration usually produce an anxiolytic effect by the action on the amygdala and basal ganglia, which is lost in ED and can account for the development of the symptoms such as: agitation, insomnia with sleep deprivation, emotional lability, and cognitive impairment. (79)

Estrogen dominance will also tend to cause copper toxicity. Progesterone will tend to reduce copper in the body. But in estrogen-dominant women, copper levels remain elevated because progesterone is not available to counter copper's effects. As copper and estrogen build, they will give way to many symptoms including: PMS, irregular menstruation, fibroids, migraines, ovarian cysts, insomnia ,and many other symptoms. (80)

Progesterone Treatment Recommendations

This patient's treatment would begin with the PTT using 20mg of blended testosterone, followed by a *PTT Questionnaire* and a short phone conversation in one week.

The Millennium has preferred the use of vaginally applied BHRT over topical because the absorption is better, and you can add testosterone to the formulations. If testosterone is applied to the skin of a woman, it can cause hair growth and darkening of hair that already exists.

The Millennium's Female BHRT Products					
	Estradiol	Estriol	Prog	Test	Apply
Basic V	0.2mg	2.0mg	100mg	1mg	Vaginal
Breast	0.1mg	2.0mg	100mg	1mg	Vaginal
Fatigue	0.2mg	2.0mg	50mg	1mg	Vaginal
Libido	0.2mg	2.0mg	100mg	2mg	Vaginal
Basic T	0.2mg	2.0mg	100mg	NO	Topical
Breast	0.1mg	2.0mg	100mg	NO	Topical
S/P Cancer	None	2.0mg	100mg	1-2mg	Vaginal

Table 9.4: Estrogen Replenishment. These compounded hormonal creams are balanced for optimal benefits in both BHRT and TBI patients.

We therefore start with ½ gram of the "standard" preparation, which has been found to fit for the majority of patients with either TBI, or in need of a comprehensive BHRT.

Side effects: If we start the "standard" BHRT and the patient complains of breast tenderness, we move to the "breast" formula. If the patient is sensitive to 100mg of progesterone, as in the "standard" preparation, and develops morning tiredness or fatigue, we use the 'fatigue" formulation. If the patient needs more of a libido boost, we use the "libido" formulation. As shown, up to this point all are vaginal products.

When testosterone converts to DHT it can cause oily skin that can predispose the female patient to acne. If this occurs, add saw palmetto 160mg once a day for four weeks, and increase to twice a day if there is a need for a stronger response. Topical ten percent benzoyl peroxide soap or lotion can help too.

Monitoring: We tend to monitor our patients closely during the first three months of treatment, with labs once a month. Many of the patients have their blood drawn and a report on their chart before follow-up. When in the office, we can immediately adjust their protocol based upon the results, as opposed to a one to two week delay in any adjustments. When using ½ gram of the vaginal preparation, the patient has used it the night before and labs are drawn in the morning. Adjustments up or down are made based upon these results.

Laboratory: (1) estradiol, (2) estrone, (3) DHEAs, (4) free testosterone, (5) DHT

Comments: When we treat women with estrogens (E2 and/or E3), we add Diindolylmethane (DIM) 75 to 100mg twice a day to preferentially convert all estrogens to the non-genotoxic 4(OH) forms. In the past, indole-3-carbinol (I3C) was primarily used for the same purpose, being the unpredictable precursor to DIM. Now that DIM is readily available and inexpensive, we no longer exclusively use I3C, but may use a combination of the two with more weight on DIM.

Pregnenolone

Pregnenolone is the first pro-hormone derived from cholesterol and is both a neurosteroid and neuroactive steroid. Pregnenolone (86) and its sulfated derivative, pregnenolone sulfate enhance learning and memory in animal models at concentrations that are physiologically relevant. In clinical application, pregnenolone was very well tolerated with minimal side effects, and did not affect weight, heart rate, blood pressure, menstrual cycle, or glucose levels. (87, 88)

Neurosteroids hold great promise for the treatment of diseases of the central nervous system (CNS). In an interesting study led by Ducharme, participants were given either intranasal or an IV labeled pregnenolone and progesterone. Uptake and distribution was followed with the identification of eleven regions in the brain of preferential concentration. Both neurosteroids appeared in blood and brain after either method of administration, but with important differences in uptake. Bioavailability based on appearance in arterial serum showed that about 23 percent and 14 percent of the intranasal administered doses of pregnenolone and progesterone, respectively, entered the blood. Brain levels were about twofold lower after intranasal administration for the two neurosteroids. With intranasal administration, brain levels of the two steroids did not vary over time (two to 120 minutes), whereas brain levels were higher early (ten minutes or less) after IV administration. With IV administration, uptake by brain regions did not vary, whereas the olfactory bulb, hippocampus, and hypothalamus had high uptake rates after intranasal administration. Intranasal administration of pregnenolone improved memory, whereas progesterone decreased anxiety, thus demonstrating that therapeutic levels of neurosteroids can be delivered to the brain by intranasal administration. These results show that either the IV or intranasal routes of administration can deliver neurosteroids to blood and brain, but that the two routes have significant differences with intranasal administration favoring some brain regions. (89[1])

Recommendations for Pregnenolone

Females: Start with 50mg of oral, natural pregnenolone at bedtime. Although a rare occurrence, if the patient complains of morning fatigue, we reduce the dose in half until there are no further symptoms.

Males: Start with 30mg of oral, natural pregnenolone at bedtime. Although a rare occurrence, if the patient complains of morning fatigue we reduce the dose in half until there are no further symptoms.

Nanoliposomal Pregnenolone: A number of nanoliposomal products for TBI and BHRT are in the dietary and compounding pipeline. The convenience of the delivery system allows for a significant reduction in overall dosage of a product, as well as enhanced delivery to the circulatory system and therefore, brain.

Side Effects: In 18 years we have maybe seen one or two patients who developed morning fatigue on 60mg of pregnenolone. Since pregnenolone is the direct precursor to progesterone, there is the infinitesimal possibility that similar side effects can occur but, to date, we have not seen them. (See the next section on progesterone.)

Monitoring: We tend to monitor our patients closely during the first three months of treatment with labs once a month. Many of the patients have their blood drawn and a report on their chart before follow-up. When in the office, we can immediately adjust their protocol based upon the results as opposed to a one to two week delay in any adjustments.

Laboratory Testing: (1) pregnenolone, (2) progesterone, (3) DHEA-s, (4) estradiol, and (5) DHT.

Comment: Pregnenolone Steal Syndrome

Progesterone

Clinical data accumulating over the last several years indicates that progesterone may be highly effective in the treatment of TBI. (90[1]) A neuroactive steroid, progesterone has been shown to improve behavioral and functional recovery and to reduce inflammation, oxidative damage, cerebral edema, and neuronal cell death. (91) The specific manner in which progesterone provides these actions has not been clearly illustrated, but it appears to function across a number of biochemical and molecular mechanisms. (92) Progesterone is therefore a hormone with multiple mechanisms of action and can even be considered a "combination therapy" in itself. Given its demonstrated effectiveness and safety in human patients, it is reasonable to consider progesterone as a basis for combinations with other potential therapies.

In both males and females, the presence of an optimal level of progesterone can have significant benefits since it is a neuroactive steroid, shown to improve behavioral and functional recovery, and to reduce: inflammation, oxidative damage, cerebral edema, and neuronal cell death. (93)

Progesterone — General Treatment Recommendations

Females: Start with 100mg of oral, natural progesterone at bedtime. If the patient develops sleepiness in the morning, reduce the dosing to 50mg a night. If the patient continues with sleepiness, reduce it further to 25mg a night. If the sleepiness is tolerable and the patient does not drive a car or operate machinery, have them continue and reassess in seven days. Many patients develop a tolerance to this potential side effect.

Males: Start with 10mg of oral, natural progesterone at bedtime. If the patient develops sleepiness in the morning, reduce the dosing to 5mg a night. If the sleepiness is tolerable and the patient does not drive a car or operate machinery, have them continue and reassess in seven days. Many patients develop a tolerance to this potential side effect. Additionally, there is a risk in males of suppression to LH leading to a reduction of testosterone and DHT production, which will affect libido.

Nanoliposomal Progesterone: A number of nanoliposomal products for TBI and BHRT are in the dietary and compounding pipeline. The convenience of the delivery system allows for a significant reduction in overall dosage of a product, as well as enhanced delivery to the circulatory system and therefore, brain.

The compounded P-Somal (progesterone liposomal) 5mg is taken at bedtime and titrated up until one of the following occurs: (1) side effects, (2) supraphysiological levels of progesterone, or (3) significant reduction in dihydrotestosterone (DHT).

Side Effects: Sleepiness is the most common side effect of excessive progesterone, but also:

> Down-regulation of estrogen receptors causing a decrease in serotonin production (depression), and also central growth hormone production(ER-Alpha).
>
> Lowered libido due to blocking LH release and the conversion of testosterone to DHT.
>
> Edema (water retention).
>
> An increase in androgen production by blocking conversion of testosterone to DHT.

Laboratory Testing: (1) pregnenolone, (2) progesterone, (3) DHEA-s, (4) estradiol, and (5) DHT.

Comment: Progesterone is a precursor to cortisol and cortisone, and may help in individuals with adrenal insufficiency or fatigue. In the past 18 years, the Millennium has always tried to provide the natural pre-cursors to adrenal hormones before giving a synthetic medication that can (does) further shut down the normal hypothalamic-anterior pituitary-adrenal axis.

Dehydroepiandrosterone (DHEA and DHEA-s)

Dehydroepiandrosterone sulphate (DHEA-s) is one of the most important neurosteroids in the brain that is synthesized from dehydroepiandrosterone (DHEA). The concentration of DHEA-s in the brain is sometimes higher than in the peripheral system. DHEA-s has been shown to target $GABA_A$, NMDA, sigma-1 receptors and metabotrophic glutamate receptor (mGluR), and also modulates a variety of neurotransmitter systems, including the cholinergic, GABAergic, dopaminergic and glutamatergic systems. DHEA-s has been found to have multiple effects on important brain functions, such as: memory enhancing, emotional behavior modulating effects, neurodevelopment-modulating effects, and anxiolytic effects, and it has a beneficial relationship to Alzheimer's disease (AD) and addiction. (94)

In a double-blind, crossover study of 30 subjects, age 40 to 70 years, supplementing 50 mg/day DHEA or placebo for three months, 67 percent of men and 84 percent of women in the DHEA group reported a remarkable increase in physical and psychological well-being, with no response in the control group. (95)

According to a study led by Ioannis Charalampopoulos, DHEA and allopregnanolone can protect the sympathoadrenal medulla cells against apoptosis by increasing the presence of anti-apoptotic Bcl-2 proteins. This would diminish the loss of volume of the adrenal medullary cells that are responsible for the production and secretion of epinephrine (adrenaline), norepinephrine (noradrenaline), and a small amount of dopamine in response to stimulation by sympathetic preganglionic neurons. (96)

DHEA Recommendation

Contrary to the unofficial dictum on dosing of DHEA in the morning, there is more literature support for giving DHEA at bedtime. Women given DHEA at bedtime had an increase in GH production by 20 percent. (97)

Females: Start with a 25mg at bedtime.

Males: Start with a 60 to 80mg IM injection of blended testosterone (Propionate and Cypionate) when the patient is in the office. This is the provocative testing we use to see if the patient has a beneficial or adverse response to the hormone, and that the normal physiologic dose is adequate for the patient. Give them the *PTT Questionnaire* (as discussed earlier), and follow-up by phone in five to seven days.

Nanoliposomal DHEA: A number of nanoliposomal products for TBI and BHRT are in the dietary and compounding pipeline. The convenience of the delivery system allows for a significant reduction in overall dosage of a product, as well as enhanced delivery to the circulatory system and therefore, brain.

Side Effects: DHEA in some females (more than males) can cause oily skin and acne. If this occurs, we decrease the frequency of dosing from seven days a week to five days a week, and even to three days a week. We have also added 7-Keto DHEA to the regimen which seems to influence the conversion of DHEA to DHT, which is causing the sebum problem.

Monitoring: We tend to monitor our patients closely during the first three months of treatment with labs once a month. Many of the patients have their blood drawn and a report on their chart before follow-up.

Laboratory Testing: (1) cortisol, (2) ACTH, (3) DHEA-s, (4) pregnenolone, and (5) progesterone.

Thyroid Hormones

The range of TSH is presently accepted as from 0.5 to 4.5mcu/ml, making the median at 2.5mcu/ml. Therefore, when TSH is above the median it would indicate that the body is attempting to increase the production of thyroid hormone from the gland, and when below the median there is a sufficient amount of circulating T4 — the main regulator of the HPT (hypothalamic-pituitary-thyroid) axis. When there is post-traumatic dysfunction of the HPT, the peripheral levels of T4 and T3 diminish without the corresponding increase in TSH. Over time, the TSH level falls or is maintained at a fixed low level that is inconsistent with the peripheral hormone levels. This is one of the most common reasons why central hypothyroidism is missed: Because assessment is frequently based only upon this one test — TSH.

In adult hypopituitary patients, GH replenishment has been reported to unmask central hypothyroidism in 36 to 47 percent of apparently euthyroid patients. Alterations in the hypothalamo-pituitary-thyroid axis have been reported following GH administration in both adults and children, with and without growth hormone deficiency [somatostatin (SS) decreases TSH release from the pituitary]. (S1) Reductions in serum fT4 increased T3 with or without a reduction in serum TSH secretion have been reported following GH use. This appears to occur because GH participates in the peripheral conversion of T4 to T3. When GH is replenished, the conversion of T4 to T3 returns to its normal rate, decreasing the amount of T4 and raising the amount of T3. The dysfunctional HPT axis does not respond to the low and continually dropping level of T4; therefore, eventually, T4 and T3 become pathologically low, exposing the central dysfunction. (98)

A debate that has been heating up over the past five to seven years is the issue of monotherapy (T4) versus combination therapy (T4 and T3) in the treatment of hypothyroidism. The standard of care has always been a monotherapy regimen with L-thyroxin (T4), which is being challenged due to reports of there being an improvement in cognition and a sense of well-being with combination therapy — both T4 and T3. (99)

Also, be aware that medications such as dopamine agonists (100) and glucocorticoids can suppress the central production of TSH (101), which now includes Metformin in patients with a history of diabetes and hypothyroidism. (102) Avoiding these pitfalls can lead to added improvement in a TBI patient.

Thyroid — General Treatment Recommendation

Common Interpretation Error

When one sees an rT3 level that is above 250 pg/ml, this should make you stop and think about all the reasons why rT3 might be elevated. Yes, there have been many articles written in the past five years that acknowledge the influence of cortisol on the conversion of T4 to rT3. We know that cortisol goes up in those with stress: physiologic, nutritional, emotional, and chemical. We are also seeing the literature speaking of low B-12, ferritin and iron levels associated with elevated production of rT3. Look at your CBC results and if the MCV is elevated, it can tell you deficiency in B-12 of folic acid, and if low the iron and ferritin levels need to be assessed.

If the T3/rT3 ratio is less than 1.06, I will add 5mcg of T3 to the patient's regimen in the morning. I will initially separate the dosing of the AT30 and 5mcg T3 by one to two hours. If there is no adverse reaction over an initial week of testing, I will have the patient combine the two in the morning on an empty stomach. Based upon the patient's response, but subjectively and biochemically (laboratory testing), we might add another 5mcg of T3 in the afternoon.

As has been presented elsewhere, the benefit of optimal T4 and T3 are relative to a sense of well-being, reduced depression, and a happier life.

Side Effects: On a rare occasion, even natural thyroid (i.e., Armour® Thyroid) can cause racing of the heart (tachycardia), sweating (hyperhidrosis), anxiety, and diarrhea. These symptoms can occur more frequently with the use of triiodothyronine (T3) if not started at a low level and slowly built up.

Monitoring: Following our standard protocol of laboratory testing once a month during the first three months of initiating treatment, under certain situations we might delay re-testing or perform it sooner.

Laboratory Testing: (1) TSH, (2) fT4, (3) fT3, (4) rT3, and (5) TPO only if there is suspicion of Hashimoto's Thyroiditis or an iodine deficiency.

Comment: Elevation in estradiol can cause hepatic production of thyroglobulin ,which will bind to T4, decreasing its availability to provide

T3. A relative hypothyroidism can develop with the symptoms associated with a real hypothyroidism.

ACTH/Cortisol

The two major peripheral limbs of the stress system are the hypothalamic-pituitary-adrenal (HPA) axis and the sympathetic nervous system. (106) Stress-induced activation of the HPA axis is associated with the release of hypothalamic CRH and vasopressin (AVP), the principal regulators of anterior pituitary corticotropin (ACTH) secretion. Central activation of the sympathetic neurons leads to activation of both the systemic sympathetic nervous system and, through the splanchnic nerves, the adrenal medullae. (107)

Subacute or chronic stress, like major surgery, traumatic brain injury, physical trauma, chronic infections, and chronic autoimmune diseases are associated with the health of the adrenals. Only recently has it become evident that in these states, a condition of dissociation between central activation of the HPA axis and the adrenal cortex may occur. (108) This is why we can measure normal or low-normal levels of ACTH with concurrent elevation in cortisol. The sympathetic nervous system, working through the splanchnic nerve, can directly control the adrenal medullary cells production of cortisol.

Neuroendocrine regulation of the adrenal zona fasciculata may depend on neurotransmitters released from nerve endings that originate from two different sources but terminate in the adrenal cortex. Neurons originate in cell bodies from within the adrenal medulla, and may be regulated by splanchnic nerve activity. (109) These adrenal nerves are mainly catecholaminergic and peptidergic, storing the catecholamines dopamine, epinephrine, and norepinephrine and a wide variety of neuropeptides, including: opioid peptides, neuropeptide, and others. (110*) These neurotransmitters and neuropeptides have been shown to modulate adrenocortical function.

Adrenal insufficiency is a common finding in TBI survivors. Commonly, the practice is to supplement the patient with doses of Cortef, Solu-medrol, Medrol, and so forth. The Millennium chose to take a different approach and since we began treating patients with compromised adrenal function, we have never used these products. What we have done instead is to use pregnenolone and DHEA together to provide the body with the precursors to cortisol (progesterone, cortisone, and aldosterone too) hoping that this would force the production of cortisol, or to replenish the diminished substrates in a patient who has been on corticoids in the past, or suffers from adrenal fatigue or adrenal shut-down.

Don't be impatient. As long as the patient is able to walk and talk, the presence of an Addison-like condition is unlikely and therefore, not an emergency. Obviously, when looking at the patient's complete laboratory panel, this will help to fine tune the final approach to treatment.

In 1998, Dr. Genazzani identified the effects of corticotropin-releasing hormone (CRH) and ACTH produced under stress on the neurosteroids progesterone, allopregnanolone, and DHEA — noting that these were initially increased, while suppression occurred with the use of dexamethasone (a common medication given in the acute phase of neurotrauma). (111[1]) As discussed above, the presence of these neurosteroids (and NAS) are important to the protection and promotion of recovery in cases of TBI.

Prolactin

Pituitary prolactin secretion is regulated by endocrine neurons in the hypothalamus. Dopamine (aka Prolactin Inhibitory Hormone, or PIH) is secreted by the hypothalamus to act on the D_2 receptors of lactotrophs cells located in the anterior pituitary, causing inhibition of prolactin secretion, while gamma-aminobutyric acid (GABA) is secreted to act as the prolactin-releasing factor (PRF). Additionally, thyrotropin-releasing hormone (TrH) has a stimulatory effect on prolactin release acting as a PRF. (113)

Prolactinemia (hyper-) associated with traumatic brain injury is indicative of a significant trauma to the hypothalamus. Unlike the other anterior pituitary hormones, the hypothalamic control of prolactin release is predominantly of tonic inhibition. Therefore, patients usually present with galactorrhea (114) or hypogonadism (sexual dysfunction) due to suppression of LH by elevated levels of prolactin.

Prolactin as a growth factor binding to cytokine-like receptors also influences hematopoiesis and angiogenesis, and is involved in the regulation of blood clotting through several pathways. In summary, "More than 300 separate actions of PRL have been reported, including effects on water and salt balance, growth and development, brain and behavior, reproduction, and immune regulation and protection." Prolactin acts in endocrine, autocrine, and paracrine manner through the prolactin receptor and a large number of cytokine receptors. (115)

Medications and Herbs Associated with Galactorrhea					
Psychotropic	SSRI	Antihypertensive	H_2-receptor blockers	Other	Herbs
Buspirone	Citalopram (Celexa)	Atenolol (Tenormin)	Cimetidine (Tagamet)	Amphetamines	Cannabis
MAO Inhibitors	Fluoxetine (Prozac)	Methyldopa	Famotidine (Pepcid)	Opiate	Anise
Moclobemide	Paroxetine (Paxil)	Reserpine (Serpasil)	Ranitidine (Zantac)	Cyclobenzaprine	Fennel
Anxiolytics	Sertraline (Zoloft)	Verapamil (Calan)	PPI	Anesthetics	Nettle
Antipsychotics			Cisapride (Propulsid)	Arginine	Red raspberry
Phenothiazines	Tricyclic Meds		Rimantadine	Sumatriptan (Imitrex)	Red clover
Chlorpromazine				Danazol (Danocrine)	Blessed thistle
Prochlorperazine				Valproic acid	Fenugreek seed

Table 9.5: A diversity of commonly used medicines and natural products can contribute to the cause of Galactorrhea. A complete investigation of the patients use of medication and alternative products is important to elucidate any non-TBI causes.

In patients with galactorrhea, Table 9.5 lists many common medications and herbs that function as either a PIH or directly as a PRF.

General Treatment Recommendations

Medication: Dopamine agonists are the first-line treatment for the majority of patients with hyperprolactinemic disorders. Cabergoline is a long-acting dopamine agonist that is very effective and well tolerated in patients with pathological hyperprolactinemia. Treatment with cabergoline normalized serum PRL levels in: 86 percent of all 292 patients; 92 percent of the 244 patients with idiopathic hyperprolactinemia (TBI?) or a microprolactinoma; and 77 percent of the 181 patients with macroadenomas. (116)

Dosing: The median dose of cabergoline at the start of therapy was 1.0mg/week, but could be reduced to 0.5mg/week once control is achieved.

Medication: Amantadine was originally an anti-influenza medication (1966) until it was found to function as a dopamine agonist in the treatment of neurological diseases such as Parkinson's syndrome, and in the treatment of neuroleptic side effects such as dystonia, akinthesia, and neuroleptic malignant syndrome. Unfortunately, nothing lasts forever, and amantadine has come under attack since newer and more expensive medications (which are protected by patents) have been developed and released. Nonetheless, amantadine increases dopamine release and receptor sensitivity, thereby acting as a PIF. Additionally, a number of recent studies have shown efficacy of amantadine in TBI patients with apathy. (117)

Dosing: We start with 100mg a day for about 30 days, and then increase by 100mg every two to four weeks, up to 300mg a day.

Side Effects: Euphoria, hallucinations, causing or worsening psychosis, orthostatic hypotension, increased orgasmic intensity, weight loss, anorexia (symptom), nausea, insomnia, unusual tiredness or weakness, dizziness, drowsiness, lightheadedness, syncope, twitching, twisting or other unusual body movements, pericardial effusion, fibrous thickening of lining that covers some of the internal organs [including the heart or the lungs (fibrotic reaction)], and pathological addiction (gambling, shopping, internet pornography, hyper-sexuality).

Monitoring: We tend to monitor prolactin in conjunction with calcium levels — initially, every three months for six months, then every six months with regular follow-up visits.

Laboratory Testing: (1) prolactin. (2) Luteinizing hormone

Comment: In the past ten years we have had no issues with amantadine toxicity (our primary dopamine agonist) since we titrate the dosing up from 100mg to 300mg a day. We use amantadine for the apathy and to increase motivation, sex drive, and sense of well-being. We have not had the opportunity to treat hyperprolactinemia as of yet.

Four Case Presentations

The following four case presentations were taken from a challenging group of patients that each offer a slight twist on the interpretation and diagnosis of hormonal dysfunction. Not all are due to overt trauma but all have a significant effect on the neurohormonal status of the patient.

Case 1, Section a: Male (57 y/o) — no specific TBI history

Symptoms: Over the past two years, this patient has experienced a subtle progression of fatigue, mood swings, irritability, weak erections, diminished libido, easy exercise fatigue, and increasing musculoskeletal complaints.

Medication: Rosuvastatin 20mg for ten years.

Chart 1: GH 0.62ng/ml, IGF-1, 168ng/ml, IGFBP-3, 3,750 ng/ml, drawn at 9:00 a.m.

Chart 1: Male (57) Unknown TBI		
Marker	**Result**	**Median**
Growth Hormone	**0.62**	**5.0 ng/ml**
IGF-1	**168**	**200 ng/ml**
IGFBP-3	**3750**	**4000 ng/ml**

In Case 1, a morning GH of 0.62ng/ml with a corresponding low-normal IGF-1 and borderline IGFBP-3 is not indicative of a central GH insult, but more representative of just suboptimal production. The cause for this low production could be secondary to TBI, but it could also be due to compromise of GH, IGF-1 and BP-3 production in the liver (main organ) by alcohol, obesity, a high carbohydrate and/or fat diet, low estradiol, low ghrelin, low DHEA-s, low melatonin, or in someone that has had been injecting recombinant human growth hormone (rhGH) in the recent past.

Chart 2: DHEA-s 79.6ug/dL, total testosterone 234ng/ml, free testosterone 4.35ng/ml, DHT 14ng/dl, SHBG 9.0pg/ml, estrone 3.0pg/ml, estradiol 34pg/ml, progesterone 0.34 ng/ml, pregnenolone: 97ng/dl, LH 16.7miul/L, FSH 9.2mIU/L, Zinc 31.3 mcg/dL, and vitamin D3 23.0 ng/dL.

Chart 2: Male (57) Unknown TBI		
Marker	**Result**	**Median**
DHEA-s	79.6 L	200 ug/dL
Total Testosterone	234 L	690 pg/ml
Free Testosterone	4.35 L	14 ng/ml
DHT	14 N	< 52ng/dL
SHBG	9.0 N	<45 pg/ml
Estrone	3.0 N	60 pg/ml
Estradiol	34.0 HN	25 pg/ml
Pregnenolone	97 LN	210 ng/dl
Progesterone	0.34 LN	0.8 ng/ml
FSH	9.2 HN	7.0 mIU/ml
LH	16.7 H	5.1 mIU/ml
Zinc	31.3 L	95 mcg/dL
Vitamin D3	23 L	60 ng/dL

What you are seeing here is more than just testosterone results, but also laboratory tests that are related to the production and metabolism of testosterone. DHEA-s is the sulfated ester of DHEA and a metabolite of pregnenolone, which comes from cholesterol. Therefore, patients taking statin drugs can (will) have a diminished amount of cholesterol to be used in making pregnenolone and all the hormones that follow in this important cascade. (S68) Additionally, cholesterol is the precursor of vitamin D (another hormone), Co-Q10, and RAS (a cell regenerating compound). No doubt this is why pregnenolone was given the name "Mother of all hormones," and in my testosterone lecture, I refer to cholesterol as the "Father of all hormones." No children without mom and dad.

In this patient who has been on a substantial dose of statins for many years, it is clear that DHEA-s, testosterone, estrogens, pregnenolone, progesterone, and vitamin D have all been negatively affected. Since his testosterone and estrogen levels are sub-optimal, the liver is not being stimulated to make SHBG; thereby minimizing binding to what little free-testosterone is available. Elevated release of both FSH and LH tells us that the HPG axis is still intact and functioning in regard to the gonads. Finally, there is a red herring here in the elevation of estradiol, which can be perceived as strange, but can be explained by the low level of zinc, a natural aromatase inhibitor. In a normal individual, a low zinc level can increase the conversion of testosterone to estradiol, so look for it. (69)

One final note, the recent proliferation of papers on the expanding functionality of vitamin D, now identified as a hormone with both genomic and non-genomic roles, has advanced the finding that a low level of vitamin D is associated with hypogonadism — specifically, an inability of the body to make testosterone. (70) Hence, the rational for its inclusion in this section on androgens becomes clear.

Chart 3: TSH 3.86mcu/ml, fT4 1.04ng/ml, fT3:2.7pg/dl, rT3 210 ng/dl, T3/rT3 ratio 1.28

Chart 3: Male (57) Unknown TBI		
Marker	**Result**	**Median**
TSH	**3.86 HN**	**2.5 mcu/ml**
Free T4	**1.04 LN**	**1.5 ng/ml**
Free T3	**2.7 N**	**2.5 pg/dl**
Reverse T3	**210 HN**	**165 ng/dl**
T3/rT3 ratio	**1.28 N**	**Above 1.06**

This patient's TSH is elevated above the median, with a corresponding low level of fT4. The fT3 is normal, with an elevated rT3, but the T3/rT3 ratio is normal. This pattern should start you thinking about why the TSH is above the median and that would be because of the low T4 which brings up the question of why? Could it be because of Hashimoto's thyroiditis (103), a frequently missed cause of hypothyroidism that is easily diagnosed with a TPO (thyroid peroxidase) test? The question is: Could it be due to the conversion of T4 to rT3 because of low B-12, low ferritin, low iron, and elevated cortisol? (104, 105) These are all issues that will need to be evaluated for the optimal recovery of the patient. A low dose regimen of a natural thyroid of 15mg to 30mg a day might help with his overall improvement.

Chart 4: ACTH 27pg/ml, cortisol 18, DHEA-s 79.6 ug/dl, pregnenolone 97ng/dl

Chart 4: Male (57) Unknown TBI		
Marker	**Result**	**Median**
ACTH	**27 N**	**35 pg/ml**
Cortisol	**18 HN**	**15ug/dl_am /7.3ug/dl_pm**

The result of ACTH is normal, while there is an elevation in the level of cortisol.

In some patients with a history of long-term high-dose statins, we also find cortisol insufficiency, which might be looked at as adrenal fatigue since cholesterol to pregnenolone to progesterone to 11-hydroxycorticosterone is reduced and therefore, so is Cortisol. This is not the situation in this patient, since his elevation in cortisol might be a compensatory response due to stimulation of the adrenals to produce DHEA.

Case 1 — Summary

This is not an overt traumatic brain injury case although, I believe everyone has some degree of neurotrauma (mTBI) influencing their hormones, cognition, and behavior. Nonetheless, the true nature of this case and the major point being made is that statins have a wide-reaching deleterious effect on all organ systems throughout our body's — the brain being the most important. In this patient, we would refer them back to their primary physician to decease or stop the statin immediately. (118, 119, 120)

The GH/IGF-1 axis in this patient is low-normal, which can reflect his age and accumulation of mTBI insults throughout his lifetime. Many traumas are ignored and forgotten since they did not draw blood or send them to the ER. Also, a significant TBI might have induced a retrograde amnesia, causing them to forget the incident. This is the reason we take a thorough inventory of all physical activities using the *TBI History Form*, and ask specific questions about injuries. Many times when this form is reviewed with the patient, they remember forgotten injuries that are sometimes major.

In terms of a protocol, we would offer this patient a three month trial of Secretropin®, starting out with 2-3 sprays at bedtime. Re-evaluation to assess a response would be performed in one to three months, based upon their complete treatment protocol (see the end of this case review).

This patient's combined hormone results are a classic picture of deficiency, possibly induced by his statin use. In patients that stopped their statin drug, it can take six to nine months before they start regenerating these hormones. Pregnenolone being the first hormone off of cholesterol is the substrate for the two main pathways (with one pathway going to progesterone and cortisol, and the other going to DHEA to feed production of testosterones and estrogens). A deficiency in vitamin D increases the risk for diminished testosterone production (121) — as does the lack of adequate zinc increases the conversion of what little free testosterone is available to estradiol. The protocol at this point is testosterone replenishment, zinc citrate, and vitamin D.

Thyroid functions are not directly affected by the statins, but the lack of cortisol production peripherally can cause an increase in corticotropin-releasing hormone (CRH). The elevation in TSH with a low T4 is consistent with an impending hypothyroidism; or, based upon his symptoms, he already has a pre-clinical form of it. The rT3 is in the high-normal range with a T3/rT3 ratio that is normal. As part of his complete treatment protocol, a low dose of natural thyroid might be considered to increase his fT3 and add T4 to his thyroid hormone pool.

Cortisol is high-normal, with a normal level of ACTH, which could imply that at some point in time, the ACTH was higher and now has decreased due to the negative feedback loop. This might be a cause for the high-normal level of rT3. Perform a laboratory follow-up in six to twelve weeks to evaluate.

Case 1, Diagnoses: (1) GH — partial growth hormone deficiency, (2) androgens — primary hypogonadism versus statin-induced hypogonadism (3) subclinical hypothyroidism, (4) elevated cortisol, and (5) hypovitaminosis D.

Case 1, Treatment:

Case 1: Products	What we did	Options
Secretropin	3 sprays at bedtime to start	
Testosterone	Injection 40mg every 3rd day	60mg Provocative Testing
DHEA	25mg – 50mg at bedtime	
Pregnenolone	50mg at bedtime.	100mg at bedtime.
Zinc Citrate	30mg BID	
Armour Thyroid 30mg	Upon arising, AT30mg	T4:0.125 plus T3:5ug-25ug
Vitamin D3	10,000IU daily	

Case 2, Section a: Female (44 y/o) — motor vehicle accident (MVA) at age 41 w/o LOC, GCS 15

Symptoms: Although this individual did not have loss of consciousness (LOC), she suffered with post-TBI headaches accompanied with nausea for the first nine months. This was also associated with progression of daytime fatigue, irritability, photophobia, craving sweets, and an interrupted sleep pattern. About a year after the MVA, she developed mood swings, anxiety, loss of tolerance/patience, depression, and loss of libido. She states that she has gained weight around the mid-section, chest and face with sensitivity of her nipples. Her menstrual cycles went from being regular to heavy with variation from 28 to 32 days (whereas normally, "It was 28 days like clockwork").

Medication: Gabapentin.

Chart 5: GH 0.05ng/ml, IGF-1, 101ng/ml, IGFBP-3, 2100 ng/ml, drawn at 9:00 a.m.

Chart 5: Female (44) MVA		
Marker	**Result**	**Median**
Growth Hormone	**0.05 L**	**5.0 ng/ml**
IGF-1	**101 L**	**>200 ng/ml**
IGFBP-3	**2100 L**	**>4000 ng/ml**

In Case 2, the patient's level of GH at 0.05ng/ml with concurrent low levels of both IGF-1 and BP-3 are suggestive of damage to the pituitary somatotropes. Considering the mechanism of her TBI injury (MVA) and the delay of three years before she exhausted her primary care physician, it is reasonable to consider that she has sustained an injury to the HP axis. Note: In female patients with a regular menstrual cycle, we draw blood on or about day 21. As you read thousands of hormone levels in women you will eventually be able to guestimate where they are in their cycle (Estrogens, Progesterone, Testosterone, FSH, and LH).

Chart 6: DHEA-s 147ug/dL, total testosterone 17.4ng/ml, free testosterone 0.57ng/ml, DHT 11.7ng/dl, SHBG 88pg/ml, estrone: 212pg/ml, estradiol:

127pg/ml, progesterone 0.13/ng/ml, pregnenolone 380/ng/dl, EP ratio 2607, LH 3.7mIU/L, FSH 5.3 mIU/L, zinc 59, and Vitamin D3 55ng/dl.

Chart 6: Female (44) MVA		
Marker	**Result**	**Median**
DHEA-s	**147 LN**	**277 ug/dL**
Total Testosterone	**17.4 N**	**44 pg/ml**
Free Testosterone	**0.57 L**	**2-4 ng/ml**
DHT	**11.7 N**	**<30 ng/dL**
SHBG	**88 HN**	**75 pg/ml**
Estrone	**212 H**	**60 pg/ml**
Estradiol	**127 HN**	**90 pg/ml**
Pregnenolone	**380 HN**	**210 ng/dl**
Progesterone	**0.13 L**	**6 ng/ml**
EP Ratio	**2607 H**	**<250**
FSH	**5.3 LN**	**7.0 mIU/ml**
LH	**3.7 LN**	**5.1 mIU/ml**
Zinc	**59 L**	**95 mcg/dL**
Prolactin	**9.15 N**	**13.75 ng/ml**
Insulin	**8.0 N**	**12.5 miu/L**
Vitamin D3	**55 N**	**>60 ng/dL**

The National Institute on Aging reports that the average age of menopause for an American female is 51 years. (81) Nonetheless, they also state that it can also happen in a woman's forties or fifties. That's another example of well spent tax dollars. In this case, what stands out the most are the high-normal levels of estrone (E1) and estradiol (E2) with low progesterone. Whether this is a sign of the body trying to squeeze out the last vestige of hormones from the ovaries, or the peripheral conversion of DHEA by the adrenals, it has been a difficult question to answer. Nonetheless, the estrogen-progesterone ratio (EP ratio) is significantly elevated, making this an issue of estrogen dominance.

The high levels of E1 and E2 stimulate the liver to produce SHBG in a proportional manner, which can bind free testosterone, as well as free estrogen, thereby lowering their circulating amounts. Since estrogens regulate LH and FSH, we do not know for certain if their levels reflect the TBI, or just the levels of estrogens. Furthermore, the patient's androgens are on the low to low-normal side, requiring correction. Zinc is low and vitamin D3 is acceptable at this present level.

Chart 7: TSH 2.1mcu/ml, fT4 1.4ng/ml, fT3 2.9pg/dl, rT3 123ng/dl, T3/rT3 ratio 2.35

Chart 7: Female (44) MVA		
Marker	**Result**	**Median**
TSH	**2.1N**	**<2.5 mcu/ml**
Free T4	**1.4 N**	**>1.5 ng/ml**
Free T3	**2.9 N**	**>2.5 pg/dl**
Reverse T3	**123 N**	**<165 ng/dl**
T3/rT3 ratio	**2.35 N**	**> 1.06**

Overall, these parameters for thyroid are normal, based upon a TSH less than 2.5mcu/ml, a low rT3, and a good T3/rT3 ratio. As you will see, the T3/rT3 ratio becomes a very important meter of thyroid health.

Chart 8: ACTH 37.45pg/ml, cortisol: 3.12ug/dL.

Chart 8: Female (44) MVA		
Marker	**Result**	**Median**
ACTH	**37.45**	**35 pg/ml**
Cortisol	**3.12**	**15ug/dl_am /7.3ug/dl_pm**

The morning level of ACTH is above the median, with the cortisol level low-normal. Taking a second look at the DHEA-s and pregnenolone levels, we see that DHEA-s is below the median, with the pregnenolone in the high-normal range.

What appears to be happening here is the "Pregnenolone Steal" syndrome. This seems to occur under stressful conditions when the necessity for cortisol increases. In order to supply substrate for cortisol's production demands, DHEA's production is down-regulated to boost pregnenolone availability. This can be harmful to the body when the stressor is long-term, causing a down-stream deficiency DHEA, an important substrate for testosterone, DHT, 5-Androstenediol, estradiol, estrone, and estriol.

In this case, it appears that pregnenolone is taking a significant amount of DHEA from testosterone production and is not producing cortisol or significant amounts of testosterone, but is generating estrogens. Why this is occurring is not clear, but is most likely relative to the elevated levels of pregnenolone.

Case 2 — Summary

Quite frequently, the progression of symptoms associated with TBI after an MVA can be insidious and diverse. In this case of a 44-year-old female, three years post-TBI, without loss of consciousness, she has developed a litany of symptoms, both psychological and physical. A rhetorical question that needs no response is, "What amount of her symptoms is relative to her peri-menopausal hormones, and those that were impacted by the MVA?"

The GH/IGF-1 axis in this patient is low, and a glucagon stimulation test (GST) will help to see her GH reserves, and clarify any damage to the pituitary. It will also fulfill the requirement for dispensing recombinant human growth hormone (rhGH). Due to the expense associated with the GST, we offer a three month trial of Secretropin®, starting out with 2-3 sprays at bedtime. Re-evaluation to assess a response would be performed in one to three months, based upon her complete treatment protocol (see the end of this case review).

The complexity in this case is to recognize the sequelae of the MVA on her HP axis in terms of hormonal dysfunctioning, with the loss of hormonal homeostasis. Unfortunately, the pattern here is not that clear; high-normal pregnenolone in association with decreases of DHEA-s (DHEA), free and total testosterone, cortisol, and progesterone suggests the Pregnenolone Steal Syndrome. Elevated estrone (E1) plus a normal estradiol (E2) with a low progesterone is creating an estrogen dominance environment, as noted by the elevated EP ratio [(E1+E2)/Progesterone]. Elevated estradiol with a low free testosterone is not going to create the hormonal environment to trigger positive feedback with increases to LH and/or FSH. Issues relative to Zinc and vitamin D are moot at this point.

Thyroid functions are normal. The rT3 is normal at this time, but should be watched since an increase in cortisol could cause the rT3 to rise.

This section is a little convoluted. Due to the Pregnenolone Steal Syndrome, DHEA is being taken away from producing testosterones and estrogens; therefore, the diminished levels. Pregnenolone is being preferred so that it can be metabolized to progesterone and then cortisol. Progesterone is low due to the contributing effects of elevated estrogen and therefore, what progesterone is presented to the adrenals is not being converted to cortisol. This is highly suggestive of adrenal fatigue. (122)

Case 2, Diagnoses: (1) GH – r/o Central GH deficiency, (2) estrogen dominance (3) low testosterone, and (4) adrenal fatigue.

Case 2, Treatment:

The key for this patient will be to prioritize the Pregnenolone Steal Syndrome and the Estrogen Dominance issues. The patient's amount of E2 is not the problem, as is the E1. We have used 7-Keto-DHEA to suppress the production of E1(estrone) since it does not aromatize and appears to down-regulate DHEA's conversion to E1. At the same time, we give the DHEA orally and testosterone by injection or intra-vaginally. We perform a follow-up monitoring panel in six-twelve weeks.

Case 2: Products	What we did	Options
Secretropin	4 sprays at bedtime to start	Or perform a GST (rhGH)
Testosterone	Intra-vaginal 1mg a night.	Injection 20mg once a week
DHEA	25mg at bedtime	
Pregnenolone	50mg at bedtime	
Progesterone	100mg at bedtime	
Adrenal Support	One capsule BID	
7-Keto-DHEA	25mg BID	

Case 3, Section a: Female (51y/o) — pedestrian hit and run at age 49 with LOC, GCS 9

Symptoms: Chronic pain in traumatic fractures to her right femur, hip/pelvis, and right ulna/radius. She has chronic fatigue upon arising, anosmia, and hypogeusia with some visual cortex disturbance. Her symptoms of depression with anxiety are poorly controlled on a poly-pharma regimen.

Medication(12): Lamotrigine 10mg, Venlafaxine 37.5mg, Paroxetine 20mg, Hydrocodone 10mg Lorazepam 5mg, Adderall 10mg BID, Carisoprodol 500mg, Ibuprofen 800mg, Pantoprazole 20mg, apixaban 2.5mg, Trazodone 150mg, Aripiprazole dosage pending.

Chart 9: GH 0.07ng/ml, IGF-1, 76 ng/ml, IGFBP-3, 1600 ng/ml, drawn at 9:00 a.m.

Chart 9: Female (44) P vs MV w/LOC		
Marker	**Result**	**Median**
Growth Hormone	**0.07 L**	**5.0 ng/ml**
IGF-1	**76 L**	**>200 ng/ml**
IGFBP-3	**1600 L**	**>4000 ng/ml**

This is a case of moderate TBI with significant features, aside from the musculoskeletal trauma, presenting with hyposmia and hypogeusia, which is a tell-tale sign of hypothalamic and pituitary damage. The resulting GH/IGF-1 pattern of deficiency is a common pattern we are seeing in patients with a central disruption of hypothalamic-pituitary axis (HP) homeostasis.

Chart 10: DHEA-s 119ug/dL, total testosterone 3.7ng/ml, free testosterone 0.04ng/ml, DHT 4.8ng/dl, SHBG 37pg/ml, estrone 7pg/ml, estradiol 23pg/ml, progesterone 0.09ng/ml, pregnenolone 234ng/dl, EP ratio 333, LH 2.1mIU/L, FSH 3.3 mIU/L, zinc 41, prolactin 18.9 ng/ml, insulin 11.25mIU/L, and vitamin D3 35ng/dl.

Chart 10: Female (44) P vs MV w/LOC		
Marker	**Result**	**Median**
DHEA-s	**119 L**	**277 ug/dL**
Total Testosterone	**3.7 L**	**44 pg/ml**
Free Testosterone	**0.04L**	**2-4 ng/ml**
DHT	**4.8 L**	**<30 ng/dL**
SHBG	**37 N**	**75 pg/ml**
Estrone	**7 N**	**60 pg/ml**
Estradiol	**23 LN**	**90 pg/ml**
Pregnenolone	**204 N**	**210 ng/dl**
Progesterone	**0.09 L**	**5-7 ng/ml**
EP Ratio	**333 H**	**<250**
FSH	**3.3 LN**	**7.0 mIU/ml**
LH	**2.1 LN**	**5.1 mIU/ml**
Zinc	**41 LN**	**95 mcg/dL**
Prolactin	**18.9 HN**	**13.75 ng/ml**
Insulin	**11.25 N**	**12.5 mIu/L**
Vitamin D3	**35 LN**	**60 ng/dL**

Clearly, this case has a number of central issues aside from the significant growth hormone disruption. Following the cascade from DHEA-s through to estrogens, all the hormones are low. Low testosterone and low estrogens with low LH and FSH are highly suggestive of a central hypogonadism.

Prolactin is high-normal, which is most likely due to loss of the negative regulation from the hypothalamus by prolactin inhibiting factor (dopamine). Therefore, this is further corroboration of hypothalamic injury causing interruption of potentially all hormones — in addition to hypocretin (82), leptin (83), and ghrelin. (84) One might want to repeat the Prolactin level with the next group of lab tests.

Over the past 15 years we have seen elevation in many of the hormones which I believe is associated with some of the psychotropic medication that these patients are taking. Sifting through the literature you will come across a number of articles support this perception. (S3)

If this was a younger female, I would be concerned about her having hypothalamic amenorrhea (85), a condition that will need leptin to help regulate her menstrual cycle.

Chart 11: TSH 0.79mcu/ml, fT4 1.08ng/ml, fT3 1.62pg/dl, rT3 232ng/dL ,T3/rT3 ratio 0.69

Chart 11: Female (44) P vs MV w/LOC		
Marker	**Result**	**Median**
TSH	**0.79 LN**	**<2.5 mcu/ml**
Free T4	**1.08 LN**	**>1.5 ng/ml**
Free T3	**1.62 LN**	**>2.5 pg/dl**
Reverse T3	**232 HN**	**165 ng/dl**
T3/rT3 ratio	**0.69 L**	**> 1.06**

TSH is not responding to the circulating low-normal levels of T4. Additionally, rT3 is elevated, creating a T3/rT3 ratio below the 1.06 cutoff, the **Low T3 Syndrome**. This is a case of central hypothyroidism with elevated rT3, both commonly missed due to limited thyroid function testing. This is a very deep problem which was compounded recently when a colleague in New Zealand asked me to write a letter of support for her having ordered fT3 and fT4. In New Zealand these tests are considered outside the standard of care since TSH is considered the only necessary test to determine thyroid functioning. What about central hypothyroidism? I sent a four-page dissertation supported by some 17 articles in defense of the doctor and condemnation of their shoddy testing parameters. The cumulative effect of a group of our letters helped to avert punitive medical board actions against her.

Chart 12: ACTH 4.00pg/ml, Cortisol 19.2ug/dL.

Chart 12: Female (44) P vs MV w/LOC		
Marker	**Result**	**Median**
ACTH	**4 LN**	**35 pg/ml**
Cortisol	**19.2 HN**	**15ug/dl_am /7.3ug/dl_pm**

ACTH is low in relation to the high-normal morning level of cortisol, which suggests damage to the HPA axis. Only recently has it become evident that in cases of TBI there can be dissociation between the central regulatory activation of the HPA axis and the adrenal cortex. Normally, the pituitary produces ACTH to stimulate adrenal production of cortisol, but under central damage and overwhelming stressors, the sympathetic nervous system steps in and directly stimulates production of cortisol from the adrenal cortex without using ACTH. This dissociation cannot be explained by the different half-lives of the pituitary and adrenal hormones, and suggests a reset of the HPA axis and/or the presence of extra-pituitary mechanisms of adrenal regulation. (112*)

Case 3 — Summary

This case represents a significant interruption of function between the HP (hypopituitary-pituitary) axis, with the patient experiencing: anosmia, hypogeusia, weight gain, prolactin elevation, low GH, disruption of the HPG and HPT axes, and dissociation of the HP axis.

If it is truly the case that the deficiency of GH is from the hypothalamus' inability to produce GHRH, performance of an ITT or the glucagon stimulation test (GST) will give a normal response if the pituitary is intact. Additionally, if damage had occurred to the region of the hypothalamus where somatostatin is produced (ventromedial nucleus), the patient's level of GH might have been elevated. Considering the severely low levels of GH, IGF-1, and BP-3, it would be appropriate to have this patient placed on rhGH.

The presence of central hypogonadism is unequivocal here, and therefore requires an approach of treatment that provides the replenishment of testosterone, estrogens, progesterone, and DHEA. Looking at the EP ratio, even though the levels of estrogen and progesterone appear to be low, it is above the 250 cutoff. This is an indication to give the patient additional progesterone not only to treat the deficiency, but also to have the benefits of central progesterone working for us (improved sleep, mood, reduced panic and anxiety, and increased GABA). (123) Additionally, vitamin D and zinc need to be supplemented.

The diagnosis of central or tertiary hypothyroidism has been made based upon low TSH and low fT4 and fT3. This patient will need replenishment with a combination thyroid product adding some selenium and iodide too.

The cortisol that is being produced is not coming from pituitary ACTH stimulation of the adrenals, but from a peripheral sympathetic signal that, at this time, is not clearly understood. The Millennium has never used synthetic supplements of cortisol (hydrocortisone, methylprednisolone), but a combination of DHEA and pregnenolone, and a desiccated adrenal extract.

Case 3, Diagnoses: (1) central growth hormone deficiency, (2) hypothalamic amenorrhea or central hypogonadism, (3) estrogen dominance, (4) low free testosterone (5) elevated prolactin, (6) subclinical hypothyroidism, (7) hypovitaminosis D, and (8) elevated cortisol.

Case 3, Treatment:

After performing a GST for the records, we started 0.5IU of rhGH with the intent of increasing the levels of IGF-1 and IGFBP-3 to the median levels. Using our standard estrogen-progesterone cream with 2mg/gram of testosterone, the patient applies 0.5gram intravaginally every night. Additionally, we gave the patient 100mg of progesterone orally each night to boost nocturnal levels to help with sleep and provide an improved neuro-permissive environment to optimize neuroregeneration, stabilize receptors, and reduce oxidative stressors. Schedule a laboratory follow-up in four to twelve weeks (P1521).

Case 3: Products	What we did	Options
rhGH 0.5IU a day	Glucagon Stim Test (GST)	Secretropin*
EstroCream 2%	Basic EstroCream with 2mg Testosterone **E2:0.2mg, E3:2mg, Prog:100mg, T:2mg**	20mg injectable testosterone once a week.
DHEA	25mg at bedtime	
Pregnenolone	50-100mg at bedtime	
Progesterone	100mg at bedtime for a month.	
Desiccated Adrenal	One capsule twice a day (AD1).	
Armour Thyroid	30mg on empty stomach, AM	T4:0.125 plus T3:5ug-25ug

<u>Case 4, Section a: Male (38 y/o), Afghanistan Green Beret — IED and artillery blast traumas</u>

Symptoms: Late afternoon fatigue, apathy, lack of interest in activities, poor concentration and focus, sudden onset of anger, irritable, memory faltering, mad for no reason, occasional isolation, lack of libido, drinking more. He has noted increased pain in both knees and right shoulder (traumatized in blast-related fall).

Medication: bupropion, amantadine, ibuprofen.

Chart 13: GH 2.78ng/ml, IGF-1, 224 ng/ml, IGFBP-3, 4200 ng/ml, drawn at 9:00 a.m.

Chart 13: Male (38) IDE, Blast Trauma		
Marker	**Result**	**Median**
Growth Hormone	**2.78 LN**	**5.0 ng/ml**
IGF-1	**224 N**	**>200 ng/ml**
IGFBP-3	**4200 N**	**>4000 ng/ml**

These results for growth hormone parameters are basically normal with appropriate levels of GH for the morning, IGF-1, and BP-3. In fact, the GH level might be a little suspicious since it is above 1.0ng/ml. Looking at hundreds of GH levels in the past three years, we infrequently see levels above one let alone two. Taking a close look at the medication this patient is on might answer the question. Amantadine (52) and bupropion (53) both interact with dopamine and the dopamine 2 receptors, having the side effect of increasing the production of growth hormone. (54) In this case, their anticipated benefits are to improve upon the patient's levels of apathy and general inanition. (55)

Chart 14: DHEA-s 189ug/dL, total T 323ng/ml, free T 7.53ng/ml, DHT 31.5ng/dl, SHBG 48pg/ml, Estrone 11pg/ml, Estradiol 17.3pg/ml, progesterone 0.78ng/ml, pregnenolone 317ng/dl, LH 2.04mIU/L, FSH 3.56mIU/L, zinc 48.9mcg/dL, prolactin 5.55ng/ml, insulin 4.3mIU/L, Vit D 29ng/dl.

Chart 14: Male (38) IDE, Blast Trauma

Marker	Result	Median
DHEA-s	189 LN	200 ug/dL
Total Testosterone	323 LN	690 pg/ml
Free Testosterone	7.53 LN	14 ng/ml
DHT	31.5 N	52ng/dL
SHBG	48 HN	45 pg/ml
Estrone	11 N	60 pg/ml
Estradiol	17.3 N	25 pg/ml
Pregnenolone	317 HN	210 ng/dl
Progesterone	0.78 N	0.8 ng/ml
FSH	3.56 LN	7.0 mIU/ml
LH	2.04 LN	5.1 mIU/ml
Zinc	48.9 LN	95 mcg/dL
Prolactin	5.55 N	11.25 ng/ml
Insulin	4.31 N	12.5 miu/L
Vitamin D3	29 L	60 ng/dL

DHEA-s is low-normal, as are both free and total testosterones. DHT and SHBG are normal, as are estrone and estradiol. Progesterone is normal with a high-normal pregnenolone. Luteinizing hormone (LH) is low at a time that it should be elevated to compensate for a low free testosterone. FSH is low too. Zinc is low-normal. Prolactin is normal. Insulin is normal. Vitamin D is Low.

Chart 15: TSH 1.85mcu/ml, fT4 1.44ng/ml, fT3 2.8pg/dl, rT3 137ng/dL, T3/rT3 ratio 2.04

Chart 15: Male (38) IDE, Blast Trauma

Marker	Result	Median
TSH	1.85 N	< 2.5 mcu/ml
Free T4	1.44 N	> 1.5 ng/ml
Free T3	2.8 N	> 2.5 pg/dl
Reverse T3	137 N	165 ng/dl
T3/rT3 ratio	2.04 N	> 1.06

Overall, the results of this thyroid panel are normal, based upon the TSH and T3/rT3 results.

Chart 16: ACTH 25.50pg/ml, cortisol 14.5ug/dL

Chart 16: Male (38) IDE, Blast Trauma		
Marker	**Result**	**Median**
ACTH	**25.5 N**	**35 pg/ml**
Cortisol	**14.5 N**	**15ug/dl_am** **7.3ug/dl_pm**

In this patient, the results of the HPA axis testing is normal.

Case 4 — Summary

These results for the GH/IGF-1 axis are important as a learning point. Without looking at the medication this veteran is being prescribed, I would think that he was supplementing with growth hormone (rhGH). As it turns out, he is on a number of medications that stimulate the Dr2 receptors, thereby increasing production of GH. The question then becomes, what is his natural level of GH? Once he is off his psychotropic medication we will learn.

Beginning with DHEA-s down the cascade to testosterone, these are all low-normal with a non-reactive LH suggesting HP axis disruption. The healthy normal levels of estrogens that one would expect to be proportionately (to testosterone) lower could be the effect of low-normal zinc levels.

Pregnenolone is high-normal with a normal cortisol and low-normal DHEA-s, and subsequent androgens suggesting the presence of a pregnenolone steal state. Insulin is normal. Vitamin D3 was low, which can account for a number of this patient's symptom. (124)

Prolactin is produced by the anterior pituitary, but is under constant hypothalamic suppression by the constant release of PIF (dopamine and GABA). When there is interruption of PIF production by the hypothalamus, the levels of prolactin surge, causing a depression in the level of prolactin release. This patient is on a number of medications that are listed as dopaminergic; therefore, there would be a suppression of prolactin secretion. The importance of this is to acknowledge that as dopamine levels rise, there can be an increased occurrence of anxiety, agitation, and insomnia. (125)

As dopamine levels rise, there is an increase in GH, which increases SS, which leads to a decrease in TSH levels, as well as prolactin — as we just learned. This patient's TSH level appears to be normal in that it is below 1.5mcu/ml; but, is this a normal level, or is it artificially reduced? His T3/rT3 ratio is good and therefore, we will answer that question when he is off the potentially offensive medications.

ACTH is normal with a cortisol that is just about high-normal. Whether this is due to the Pregnenolone Steal Syndrome or from direct stress is not clear, but it will be taken into consideration.

Case 4, Diagnoses: (1) central hypogonadism, (2) Pregnenolone Steal Syndrome (3) hypovitaminosis D.

Case 4, Treatment:

Because of the age of the patient being less than 40 years of age we usually do not use injectable or even topical testosterone in order to protect their sperm production. In those with completed families or in a few early vasectomies we will discuss the options of Clomid, HCG and injectable testosterone.

In 2014, we started a three year Clomid Experience Project (CEP) where we looked at a few regimens of dosing Clomid 50mg. During the first year we saw that a Monday-Wednesday-Friday vs a Monday-Friday regiment was able to double or even triple the baseline testosterone levels. In the second year we went to an every third day regimen and found that over 95% of those on the protocol were able to mount a significant elevation in testosterone levels associated with cognitive and psychological improvement.

When the patient is in the office having a review of their lab results and is found to be hypogonadal we will offer them a Provocative Testosterone Challenge Test (PTT). We give a male a one-time 60mg injection of testosterone and have them fill out a *Provocative Testing Questionnaire in 5 to 7 days*. On the most part, we have found the results of this process to be predictive in anticipated responses when on their final treatment protocol (injectable testosterone or Clomid). Rarely, do we have failures to respond, but when they do occur, we invite the patient back for a second injection of 60mg. That usually does it!

Case 4: Products	What we did	Options
A. Clomid 50mg	Every 3rd day in the AM.	60mg Provocative Testing
B. Testosterone and Clomid	60mg Provocative Testing	40mg every 3rd day with 50mg Clomid three days a week.
DHEA	25mg – 50mg at bedtime	
Pregnenolone	50mg at bedtime.	100mg at bedtime.
Zinc Citrate	50mg BID	
Vitamin D3	10,000IU daily	
N-AcetylCysteine (NAC)	500mg BID	2 grams twice a day
Quercetin	2 capsules twice a day	
B-Complex with PQQ	2 capsule twice a day	

Conclusion

Historically, medical advancements have been made by hardworking scientists who committed themselves to the ideas of change, based upon the need to improve diagnostic and treatment paradigms. In past epochs, many of these forward-thinking individuals were thwarted and held back by religious, political, and collegiate jealousy. Presently, it seems like it is more a cookie-cutter format, where everyone gets a symptomatic approach to treatment instead of a diagnostic one.

One of those mythological stories that I was told some years back about one of the last interviews that Thomas Edison had with a cub-reporter serves me to inspire others that think. The reporter asked Mr. Edison, "When you were developing the light bulb, how did you feel about the 1080 failures that you had before finding the right filament?" To that, Edison supposedly responded, "Sonny, I did not think of them as failures, but as what just did not work." That story, true or not, has inspired me and many like-minded individuals to push forward from one "what just did not work" to the next — hoping to find a working solution.

In the 20 years since starting on the path that led me to write *A Clinical Approach to Interventional Endocrinology* (2007), I noticed that many of the hormonally deficient and partially deficient patients I was treating had experienced significant improvement in their psychological well-being. It was not until 2004, while reading about growth hormone deficiencies in Turkish pugilists, did my epiphany appear. (126) I myself sought medical evaluation in 1997 for mounting depression, anxiety, and cognitive decline. I was not a happy camper. I had had a number of head traumas starting at four years of age, as well as sports-related concussions. My depression was medicated, without full improvement, suggesting treatment resistant depression. (127, 128, 129)

In August 1997, I was started on hormonal replenishment, and by November 1997, I returned to a living life. At that time, I did not have the knowledge to understand what happened, but I sought the information. I fortunately was a volunteer clinical professor for USC, which gave me unlimited access to the Norris Medical Library. My focus, comprehension, and speed reading abilities returned upon treatment, and I read 20-30 articles a week, leading up to that epiphany article of 2004.

Throughout this workbook, I have laid out the information as best I can, realizing that there are many blank spaces or holes that could have been filled with more information. As compensation, I have loaded this digital format with about 1,500 references to the literature I consumed (these are context-sensitive). Many of the reference points are to full articles or locations on the internet, which are filled with information on neuroendocrinology and more.

It is my hope that you will read this workbook and accept my positions on laboratory interpretation and treatment. Thereafter, you can meld, warp, and enhance what I have started looking for into something even more effective. But at this time, I can only say that things seem to be working well for our patients, as made evident by Petty Officer Matthew Gosney's response on the Joe Rogan Experience #574.

The ball and the knowledge have now been passed to you.